NATIONAL ACADEMIES *Sciences Engineering Medicine*

NATIONAL ACADEMIES PRESS
Washington, DC

Leveraging Advances in Modern Science to Revitalize Low-Dose Radiation Research in the United States

Committee on Developing a Long-Term Strategy for Low-Dose Radiation Research in the United States

Nuclear and Radiation Studies Board

Division on Earth and Life Studies

Consensus Study Report

THE NATIONAL ACADEMIES PRESS 500 Fifth Street, NW Washington, DC 20001

This activity was supported by a contract between the National Academy of Sciences and the Department of Energy. Any opinions, findings, conclusions, or recommendations expressed in this publication do not necessarily reflect the views of any organization or agency that provided support for the project.

International Standard Book Number-13: 978-0-309-27577-4
International Standard Book Number-10: 0-309-27577-6
Digital Object Identifier: https://doi.org/10.17226/26434

This publication is available from the National Academies Press, 500 Fifth Street, NW, Keck 360, Washington, DC 20001; (800) 624-6242 or (202) 334-3313; http://www.nap.edu.

Copyright 2022 by the National Academy of Sciences. National Academies of Sciences, Engineering, and Medicine and National Academies Press and the graphical logos for each are all trademarks of the National Academy of Sciences. All rights reserved.

Printed in the United States of America.

Suggested citation: National Academies of Sciences, Engineering, and Medicine. 2022. *Leveraging Advances in Modern Science to Revitalize Low-Dose Radiation Research in the United States.* Washington, DC: The National Academies Press. https://doi.org/10.17226/26434.

The **National Academy of Sciences** was established in 1863 by an Act of Congress, signed by President Lincoln, as a private, nongovernmental institution to advise the nation on issues related to science and technology. Members are elected by their peers for outstanding contributions to research. Dr. Marcia McNutt is president.

The **National Academy of Engineering** was established in 1964 under the charter of the National Academy of Sciences to bring the practices of engineering to advising the nation. Members are elected by their peers for extraordinary contributions to engineering. Dr. John L. Anderson is president.

The **National Academy of Medicine** (formerly the Institute of Medicine) was established in 1970 under the charter of the National Academy of Sciences to advise the nation on medical and health issues. Members are elected by their peers for distinguished contributions to medicine and health. Dr. Victor J. Dzau is president.

The three Academies work together as the **National Academies of Sciences, Engineering, and Medicine** to provide independent, objective analysis and advice to the nation and conduct other activities to solve complex problems and inform public policy decisions. The National Academies also encourage education and research, recognize outstanding contributions to knowledge, and increase public understanding in matters of science, engineering, and medicine.

Learn more about the National Academies of Sciences, Engineering, and Medicine at **www.nationalacademies.org**.

Consensus Study Reports published by the National Academies of Sciences, Engineering, and Medicine document the evidence-based consensus on the study's statement of task by an authoring committee of experts. Reports typically include findings, conclusions, and recommendations based on information gathered by the committee and the committee's deliberations. Each report has been subjected to a rigorous and independent peer-review process and it represents the position of the National Academies on the statement of task.

Proceedings published by the National Academies of Sciences, Engineering, and Medicine chronicle the presentations and discussions at a workshop, symposium, or other event convened by the National Academies. The statements and opinions contained in proceedings are those of the participants and are not endorsed by other participants, the planning committee, or the National Academies.

Rapid Expert Consultations published by the National Academies of Sciences, Engineering, and Medicine are authored by subject-matter experts on narrowly focused topics that can be supported by a body of evidence. The discussions contained in rapid expert consultations are considered those of the authors and do not contain policy recommendations. Rapid expert consultations are reviewed by the institution before release.

For information about other products and activities of the National Academies, please visit www.nationalacademies.org/about/whatwedo.

COMMITTEE ON DEVELOPING A LONG-TERM STRATEGY FOR LOW-DOSE RADIATION RESEARCH IN THE UNITED STATES

JOE W. GRAY (NAM) (*Chair*), Oregon Health & Science University (emeritus), Portland
SIMON D. BOUFFLER, UK Health Security Agency, Chilton, United Kingdom
SHAHEEN A. DEWJI, Georgia Institute of Technology, Atlanta
ANDREW P. FEINBERG (NAM), Johns Hopkins University School of Medicine, Baltimore, Maryland
BENJAMIN FRENCH, Vanderbilt University, Nashville, Tennessee
BERNARD D. GOLDSTEIN (NAM), University of Pittsburgh (retired), Pennsylvania
JOHN D. GRAHAM, Indiana University, Bloomington
ELIZABETH M. JAFFEE (NAM), Johns Hopkins University, Baltimore, Maryland
EVAGELIA C. LAIAKIS, Georgetown University, Washington, District of Columbia
LINDSAY M. MORTON, National Cancer Institute, Bethesda, Maryland
DAVID B. RICHARDSON, University of California, Irvine
DÖRTHE SCHAUE, University of California, Los Angeles
RASHID A. SHAIKH, Health Effects Institute (retired), Cambridge, Massachusetts
RICHARD L. WAHL (NAM),[1] Washington University School of Medicine in St. Louis, Missouri
GAYLE E. WOLOSCHAK, Northwestern University, Evanston, Illinois

Staff

OURANIA KOSTI, Study Director
LAURA D. LLANOS, Finance Business Partner
DARLENE GROS, Senior Program Assistant

---

[1] Resigned from the committee effective September 2, 2021.

NUCLEAR AND RADIATION STUDIES BOARD

WILLIAM H. TOBEY (*Chair*), Los Alamos National Laboratory, Los Alamos, New Mexico
JAMES A. BRINK (*Vice Chair*), Massachusetts General Hospital, Boston
SALLY A. AMUNDSON, Columbia University, New York, New York
STEVEN M. BECKER, Old Dominion University, Norfolk, Virginia
AMY BERRINGTON DE GONZÁLEZ, National Cancer Institute, Bethesda, Maryland
MADELYN R. CREEDON, The George Washington University, Washington, District of Columbia
SHAHEEN A. DEWJI, Georgia Institute of Technology, Atlanta
PAUL T. DICKMAN, Argonne National Laboratory, Washington, District of Columbia
ALLISON M. MacFARLANE, The University of British Columbia, Canada
ELEANOR MELAMED, National Nuclear Security Administration (retired)
PER F. PETERSON (**NAE**), University of California, Berkeley
R. JULIAN PRESTON, Environmental Protection Agency, Chapel Hill, North Carolina
MONICA C. REGALBUTO, Idaho National Laboratory, Idaho Falls
HENRY D. ROYAL, Washington University School of Medicine in St. Louis, Missouri

Staff

CHARLES D. FERGUSON, Senior Board Director
JENNIFER HEIMBERG, Senior Program Officer
MICHAEL T. JANICKE, Senior Program Officer
OURANIA KOSTI, Senior Program Officer
LAURA D. LLANOS, Finance Business Partner
DARLENE GROS, Senior Program Assistant
LESLIE BEAUCHAMP, Program Assistant

Acknowledgments

A number of people and organizations contributed to the successful completion of this report. The committee wishes to thank the following individuals:

Dr. Todd Anderson (Office of Biological and Environmental Research, Biological Systems Science Division, Department of Energy [DOE]) sponsored the study and provided information on activities related to low-dose radiation research. Dr. Anderson also served ably as the sponsor liaison to the committee and was effective in coordinating several information requests for the committee including on funding of DOE's national laboratories to carry out low-dose radiation research and their capabilities. **Dr. Steve Binkley** (Office of Science, DOE) provided views on DOE's potential role in the government-wide effort to coordinate low-dose radiation research in the United States.

The speakers are too numerous to name here; all gave high-quality presentations during the public meetings listed in Appendix C, and many of them responded to follow-up questions from the committee.

Dr. Guy Garty (Columbia University), **Colonel (Dr.) Mohammad Naeem** (Armed Forces Radiobiology Research Institute), **Dr. Guy Savard** (Argonne National Laboratory), **Dr. Marcelo Vazquez** (Loma Linda University Medical Center), **Dr. Jason Weeks** (National Aeronautics and Space Administration's Johnson Space Center), and **Dr. Michael Weil** (Colorado State University) responded to the committee's request for information on the characteristics and capabilities of the radiation facilities in their institutions. The committee found the responses comprehensive and a valuable asset to the radiation community and has included these responses in Appendix E.

Ms. Lilly Adams (Union of Concerned Scientists) assisted National Academies' staff with identifying individuals from the communities impacted by nuclear weapons production and testing and moderated the presentations and discussion during the committee's October 28, 2021, meeting. Ms. Adams also coordinated follow-on communications with the impacted communities and advocacy groups.

Ms. Lisa Meissner (Hobbs Straus Dean & Walker, LLP) coordinated with the Navajo Nation Office of the President and the Department of Health for presentations to the committee by Navajo President Jonathan Nez and Health Administrator Dr. Jill Jim.

Ms. Lisa Robinson (Harvard T.H. Chan School of Public Health) assisted the committee with retrieving information on current and historic government processes for cost-benefit analyses and rulemaking.

Mr. Armond Cohen (Clean Air Task Force) proposed several speakers for the committee's meeting focused on risk communication and public engagement and provided comments in writing.

Ms. Virgini Donaldson (CANDU Owners Group [COG]) facilitated the presentation on the COG-supported low-dose radiation program and access to its report.

Dr. Kimberly Applegate (University of Kentucky, retired), **Professor Perry Charley** (Diné College), **Ms. Barbara Hamrick** (University of California, Irvine, Medical Center), **Dr. Kathy Held** (National Council on Radiation Protection and Measurements), **Dr. Arjun Makhijani** (Institute for Energy and Environmental Research), **Dr. Noelle Metting** (DOE, retired), **Mr. John Tappert** (U.S. Nuclear Regulatory Commission), and **Colonel (Dr.) Alvin Young** (U.S. Air Force, retired) provided comments in writing.

Several members of impacted communities and advocacy groups provided detailed commentaries with recommendations for the committee's consideration. Those members are as follows (in the order they signed the commentaries): **Dr. Bemnet Alemayehu** (Natural Resources Defense Council), **Terrie Barrie** (Alliance of Nuclear Worker Advocacy Groups), **Mary Dickson** (Utah Downwinders), **Daniel Hirsch** (Committee to Bridge the Gap), **Keith Kiefer** (National Association of Atomic Veterans), **Trisha Pritikin** (Author, *The Hanford Plaintiffs*), **Benetick Kabua Maddison** (Youth, Climate, and Nuclear Issues), **Dr. April L. Brown** (Marshallese Educational Initiative), **Beata Tsosie** and **Belin Marcus** (Breath of My Heart Birthplace), **Robert Alvarez** (Consequences of Radiation Exposure), **Jeff Carter** (Physicians for Social Responsibility), **Tina Cordova** (Tularosa Basin Downwinders Consortium), **Diane D'Arrigo** (Nuclear Information and Resource Service), **Dr. Thomas De Pree** (Rensselaer Polytechnic Institute), **Denise Duffield** (Physicians for Social Responsibility–Los Angeles), **Cindy Folkers** (Beyond Nuclear), **Susan Gordon** (Multicultural Alliance for a Safe Environment), **Dr. Robert M. Gould** (San Francisco Bay Physicians for

Social Responsibility), **Wenonah Hauter** (Food & Water Watch and Food & Water Action), **Dennis Nelson** (Support and Education for Radiation Victims), **Mary Olson** (Gender and Radiation Impact Project), **Dr. Linda Marie Richards** (Corvallis, Oregon), **Anna Marie Rondon** (New Mexico Social Justice and Equity Institute, Indigenous Lifeway, Inc.), **Lukas Ross** (Friends of the Earth), **Adrian Shelley** (Public Citizen, Texas), **Chris Shuey** (Southwest Research and Information Center), **Tyson Slocum** (Public Citizen), and **Dr. Sasha Stiles** (Atomic Workers Advocacy).

The committee also thanks other individuals who provided comments in writing or during the committee's public meetings.

The committee is grateful to the staff of the Nuclear and Radiation Studies Board of the National Academies of Sciences, Engineering, and Medicine (the National Academies) for organizing and facilitating this study. Study director **Dr. Ourania Kosti** organized the committee meetings and assisted the committee with collecting the information it needed to write its report. **Ms. Darlene Gros** managed the logistics of the meetings, report review, and publication. Additional National Academies' staff assisted with report production: **Eric Edkin,** Division on Earth and Life Studies, assisted with figure design, and **Christopher Lao-Scott**, National Academies' Research Library, assisted with report production.

Reviewers

This Consensus Study Report was reviewed in draft form by individuals chosen for their diverse perspectives and technical expertise. The purpose of this independent review is to provide candid and critical comments that will assist the National Academies of Sciences, Engineering, and Medicine in making each published report as sound as possible and to ensure that it meets the institutional standards for quality, objectivity, evidence, and responsiveness to the study charge. The review comments and draft manuscript remain confidential to protect the integrity of the deliberative process.

We thank the following individuals for their review of this report:

BEMNET ALEMAYEHU, Natural Resources Defense Council
SALLY AMUNDSON, Columbia University
KIMBERLY APPLEGATE, University of Kentucky (retired)
AMIR BAHADORI, Kansas State University
JAN BEYEA, Consulting in the Public Interest
PAUL DICKMAN, Argonne National Laboratory
AMY KRONENBERG, Lawrence Berkeley National Laboratory
KERSTIN LINDBLAD-TOH (NAS), Broad Institute
TIMOTHY MOUSSEAU, University of South Carolina
SHEILA OLMSTEAD, The University of Texas at Austin
ARISTIDES PATRINOS, New York University (retired)
TRISHA PRITIKIN, Author, *The Hanford Plaintiffs: Voices from the Fight for Atomic Justice* (University Press of Kansas, 2020)
STEVEN SIMON, National Cancer Institute (retired)
JEFFREY ULLMAN (NAS/NAE), Stanford University

RICHARD WAKEFORD, University of Manchester
LANCE WALLER, Emory University
LYDIA ZABLOTSKA, University of California, San Francisco

Although the reviewers listed above provided many constructive comments and suggestions, they were not asked to endorse the conclusions or recommendations of this report, nor did they see the final draft before its release. The review of this report was overseen by **MARYELLEN GIGER,** University of Chicago, and **BARBARA HAMRICK,** University of California, Irvine, Medical Center. They were responsible for making certain that an independent examination of this report was carried out in accordance with the standards of the National Academies and that all review comments were carefully considered. Responsibility for the final content rests entirely with the authoring committee and the National Academies.

Preface

It has been an honor and privilege to chair the committee tasked with developing a strategy for low-dose radiation research in the United States. Throughout my career as a biomedical scientist, I have led large biomedical programs that have been at the forefront of scientific innovation in translational research with the goal of improving human health. Chairing this committee allowed me an opportunity to gain an appreciation of how scientific research can influence and guide policy decisions that impact the lives of the U.S. population.

Ionizing radiation occurs in a wide range of medical, industrial, military, and commercial settings and the number of individuals exposed or potentially exposed to radiation in these settings is increasing. While these exposures may yield individual or societal benefit, they may also adversely affect human health. Past and present environmental exposures are especially concerning to some communities which are typically exposed involuntarily and may not receive or even agree with the presumed societal benefit. These include Indigenous communities; atomic veterans; nuclear workers; uranium miners, millers, transporters, and their families; and those individuals or communities impacted by radioactive contamination or nuclear fallout due to nuclear weapons testing, offsite radiation releases from nuclear weapons production sites, and nuclear waste cleanup activities. Disparities in infrastructure, social and behavioral risk factors for disease, and complex environmental stressors exacerbate risks for disease to some community members and raise important health questions as to whether these communities are also at higher risk of developing disease from low-dose radiation exposures. These disparities also raise social questions regarding environmental injustice. It is imperative that risks to all exposed populations be known as well as is scientifically possible and that risk mitigation efforts be guided by that knowledge.

Much of what we know about risk from low doses of radiation comes from epidemiological studies of exposed populations including the Japanese atomic bombing survivors, and occupationally and medically exposed individuals. These studies give most attention to cancer as the adverse health effect, but there is increasing evidence that low-dose radiation exposure may be associated with non-cancer health outcomes such as cardiovascular disease, neurological disorders, immune dysfunction, and cataracts. The present study focuses on developing a low-dose and low-dose-rate research strategy for the United States and is built on the concept that recent advances in epidemiology, biological understanding of disease occurrence, and computational and analytical technologies can be leveraged by a revitalized low-dose radiation research program to improve assessment and understanding of the risks of adverse health effects that result from the radiation exposures received by the U.S. population. Other fields embrace these advancements. Radiation research must do the same.

During its seven public meetings, the committee received more than 80 presentations including from representatives of government and Congress, nongovernmental agencies, the national and international radiation research community, managers of the previous low-dose radiation program and collaborators, the U.S. biomedical research community, and, importantly, from impacted communities. The committee also received solicited and unsolicited information in writing. The presentations and recordings of the public meetings are posted on the National Academies' study webpage[1] and the written comments are available to the public upon request through the study's public access file.[2]

The committee and I clearly heard the concerns raised by some of the presenters about possible bias on the part of some of the committee members including myself as a result of my past work in the Department of Energy (DOE)-supported national laboratories and publications on aspects of low-dose radiation effects. We discussed these concerns at length and were mindful of them during our deliberations. It was our intent to develop a strategic research plan that was neutral in terms of the impact of the proposed research on assessment of radiation health risk and consequently its potential impact on radiation protection policy and practice in the United

---

[1] See https://www.nationalacademies.org/our-work/developing-a-long-term-strategy-for-low-dose-radiation-research-in-the-united-states.

[2] Inquiries and requests for the list of the public access file materials can be made to the National Academies' Public Access Records Office (see https://www8.nationalacademies.org/pa/managerequest.aspx?key=DELS-NRSB-21-02).

States. I believe that we succeeded in defining a research program that will provide the best possible information on risk so that risk mitigation efforts can be as scientifically well-grounded as possible. The committee also gave special attention to discovery or better quantification of health effects other than cancer that might be caused by low-dose radiation exposures. The essence of the proposed plan is captured in a list of nine findings and two recommendations.

The committee recognized that, while DOE has been the historical research home for radiation research in the United States, other federal agencies in the United States and programs in other countries carry out or support low-dose radiation research. The committee identified eight essential elements of a low-dose radiation research program that should be considered during the development of a revitalized low-dose radiation research program in the United States. Coordination with other research efforts in low-dose radiation is an important one.

I hope the audience of this report finds that this is an unbiased and forward-looking document that builds a strong case that a revitalized, focused, and comprehensive multidisciplinary low-dose radiation program that leverages advances in biotechnology and research infrastructure can provide evidence on risks at low doses of radiation for different health outcomes, thereby alleviating the need to rely on risk estimates derived from higher doses.

Joe W. Gray, *Chair*
Committee on Developing a Long-Term Strategy
for Low-Dose Radiation Research in the United States

Contents

COMMON ACRONYMS AND ABBREVIATIONS   xxi

SUMMARY   1

1   INTRODUCTION   15
    1.1 Low-Dose Radiation Exposures to the U.S. Population, 19
    1.2 Low-Dose Radiation Research in the United States, 22
    1.3 Study Task and Approach, 28
    1.4 Report Roadmap, 30

2   LOW-DOSE RADIATION EXPOSURES AND
    HEALTH EFFECTS   31
    2.1 Low-Dose Radiation Sources and Exposures, 33
       2.1.1 Natural Sources, 38
       2.1.2 Medical Exposures, 43
       2.1.3 Occupational Exposures, 47
       2.1.4 Nuclear Power Operations, 49
       2.1.5 Nuclear or Radiological Incidents, 53
       2.1.6 Nuclear Weapons Program, 56
       2.1.7 Nuclear Waste Management, 61
    2.2 Current Epidemiological Evidence on Low-Dose
       Radiation Health Effects, 64
       2.2.1 Cancer, 64
       2.2.2 Cardiovascular Disease, 66
       2.2.3 Neurological Disorders, 67

2.2.4 Immune Dysfunction, 68
2.2.5 Cataracts, 70
2.2.6 Heritable Genetic Effects, 71
2.3 Chapter Summary and Finding, 73

3 SCIENTIFIC BASIS FOR RADIATION PROTECTION 75
3.1 The Radiation Protection Framework, 75
3.2 Agencies with Radiation Protection Responsibilities in the United States, 80
3.3 Science Behind Radiation Protection, 82
3.3.1 The Regulatory Development Process, 84
3.3.2 Decision-Making Frameworks for Radiation Protection, 85
3.3.3 Characterization of Risk in the Regulatory Development Process, 86
3.4 Potential Economic Impacts of the Low-Dose Radiation Research Program, 93
3.5 Chapter Summary and Findings, 95

4 STATUS OF LOW-DOSE RADIATION RESEARCH 97
4.1 Low-Dose Radiation Research in the U.S. Government, 97
4.1.1 Department of Energy, 98
4.1.2 National Aeronautics and Space Administration, 101
4.1.3 National Institutes of Health, 104
4.1.4 Centers for Disease Control and Prevention, 106
4.1.5 Department of Defense, 108
4.1.6 National Science and Technology Council, 109
4.1.7 Intelligence Advanced Research Projects Activity, 110
4.2 Low-Dose Radiation Research in National Laboratories, 110
4.3 Low-Dose Radiation Research in Universities, 113
4.4 Support for Low-Dose Radiation Research by Other U.S. Entities, 113
4.4.1 National Council on Radiation Protection and Measurements, 113
4.4.2 Electric Power Research Institute, 114
4.4.3 Health Physics Society, 114
4.4.4 American Nuclear Society, 115
4.5 Support for Low-Dose Radiation Research Internationally, 115
4.5.1 Multidisciplinary European Low-Dose Initiative, 116
4.5.2 International Commission on Radiological Protection, 117

CONTENTS   xix

        4.5.3 United Nations Scientific Committee on the Effects of Atomic Radiation, 117
        4.5.4 Nuclear Energy Agency/Organisation for Economic Co-operation and Development, 119
        4.5.5 Support for Low-Dose Radiation Research in Canada, 120
        4.5.6 Support for Low-Dose Radiation Research in Japan, 122
    4.6 Chapter Summary, 126

5   PRIORITIZED RESEARCH AGENDA   127
    5.1 Low-Dose Radiation Research Challenges and Overview of Research Priorities, 127
    5.2 Epidemiological Research Priorities, 134
        5.2.1 Develop and Deploy Analytical Tools for Radiation Epidemiology (Priority E1), 134
        5.2.2 Improve Estimation of Risks for Cancer and Non-Cancer Health Outcomes from Low-Dose External and Internal Radiation Exposures, Including Suitable Surrogate Biomarkers of Health Risk Where Appropriate (Priority E2), 139
        5.2.3 Determine Factors That Alter the Low-Dose and Low-Dose-Rate Radiation-Related Adverse Health Effects (Priority E3), 142
    5.3 Biological Research Priorities, 146
        5.3.1 Develop More Accurate Model Systems for Study of Low-Dose and Low-Dose-Rate Radiation-Induced Health Effects (Priority B1), 146
        5.3.2 Develop Biomarkers for Radiation-Induced Adverse Health Outcomes (Priority B2), 151
        5.3.3 Define Health-Effect Dose-Response Relationships Around 10 mGy or 5 mGy/h (Priority B3), 154
        5.3.4 Identify Factors That Modify or Confound Estimation of Risks for Radiation-Induced Adverse Health Outcomes (Priority B4), 157
    5.4 Research Infrastructure Priorities, 160
        5.4.1 Tools for Sensitive Detection and Precise Characterization of Aberrant Cell and Tissue States (Priority I1), 160
        5.4.2 Harmonized Databases to Support Biological and Epidemiological Studies (Priority I2), 168
        5.4.3 Dosimetry for Low-Dose and Low-Dose-Rate Exposures (Priority I3), 170

          5.4.4 Facilities for Low-Dose and Low-Dose-Rate
                Exposures (Priority I4), 174
    5.5 Estimated Timeline and Costs, 180
    5.6 Comparison of the Committee-Recommended
        Research Agenda to Those of Other Entities, 184
    5.7 Chapter Summary, Findings, and Recommendation, 185

6   ESSENTIAL COMPONENTS OF THE LOW-DOSE
    RADIATION PROGRAM   189
    6.1 Programmatic Commitment, 190
    6.2 Independent Advice and Evaluation, 191
    6.3 Transparency, 195
    6.4 A Prioritized Strategic Research Agenda, 196
    6.5 Research-Sponsorship Mechanisms, 196
          6.5.1 Development of Research Solicitation, 197
          6.5.2 Review of Applications, 197
          6.5.3 Funding Mechanisms, 197
          6.5.4 Research Oversight, 199
          6.5.5 Data Management and Sharing, 199
          6.5.6 Dissemination of Scientific Results, 200
    6.6 Training, 201
    6.7 Engagement and Communications with Stakeholders, 204
    6.8 Coordination, 209
          6.8.1 Mechanisms for Coordination, 209
          6.8.2 Leadership, 212
    6.9 Department of Energy and Management of the
        Low-Dose Program, 214
          6.9.1 Congress's Views, 215
          6.9.2 DOE's Views, 215
          6.9.3 Views of Members of the Scientific Community, 216
          6.9.4 Views of Members of the Impacted Communities, 216
          6.9.5 The Committee's Views, 216
    6.10 Chapter Summary, Findings, and Recommendation, 217

REFERENCES   221

APPENDIXES
A   Consolidated Appropriations Act, 2021   267
B   Committee and Staff Biographies   271
C   Information-Gathering Meetings   281
D   Projects Designated by the Department of Energy as
    "Low-Dose Radiation Projects" Carried Out at National
    Laboratories (2016–2021)   289
E   Unedited Responses from Radiation Facilities   295

Common Acronyms and Abbreviations

ABCC	Atomic Bomb Casualty Commission
ABM	agent-based model
ACERER	Advisory Committee for Energy-Related Epidemiologic Research
AEC	Atomic Energy Commission
AFRRI	Armed Forces Radiobiology Research Institute
AI	artificial intelligence
ALARA	as low as reasonably achievable
ALSDA	Ames Life Sciences Data Archive
ANL	Argonne National Laboratory
ANS	American Nuclear Society
AOP	adverse outcome pathway
ATLAS	Argonne (National Laboratory) Tandem Linac Accelerator System
BEIR	Biological Effects of Ionizing Radiation
BER	Biological and Environmental Research
BEST	Biomarkers, Endpoints and other Tools
BMI	body mass index
BNL	Brookhaven National Laboratory
CANDLE	CANcer Distributed Learning Environment
CANDU	CANada Deuterium Uranium
CDC	Centers for Disease Control and Prevention

CERCLA	Comprehensive Environmental Response, Compensation, and Liability Act
CIF	Community Involvement Fund
CIRRPC	Committee on Interagency Radiation Research and Policy Coordination
CNSC	Canadian Nuclear Safety Commission
COG	CANDU Owners Group
COHERE	Canadian Organization on Health Effects from Radiation Exposure
CRESP	Consortium for Risk Evaluation with Stakeholder Participation
CT	computed tomography
DoD	Department of Defense
DOE	Department of Energy
DOE-BER	Department of Energy's Biological and Environmental Research
DOE-EM	Department of Energy's Office of Environmental Management
DTRA	Defense Threat Reduction Agency
EMR	electronic medical record
EPA	Environmental Protection Agency
ERR	excess relative risk
FAIR	findable, accessible, interoperable, and reusable
GAO	Government Accountability Office
GPU	graphics processing unit
HHS	Department of Health and Human Services
HLG-LDR	high-level group in low-dose radiation
HPS	Health Physics Society
HRP	Human Research Program
HTAN	Human Tumor Atlas Network
HuBMAP	Human BioMolecular Atlas Program
ICGC	International Cancer Genome Consortium
ICRP	International Commission on Radiological Protection
IES	Institute for Environmental Sciences
IND	improvised nuclear device
INWORKS	International Nuclear Workers Study
IoMT	Internet of Medical Things

IoT	Internet of Things
ISCORS	Interagency Steering Committee on Radiation Standards
LANL	Los Alamos National Laboratory
LBNL	Lawrence Berkeley National Laboratory
LET	linear energy transfer
LLNL	Lawrence Livermore National Laboratory
LNT	linear no-threshold
LSS	Life Span Study
MD	molecular dynamic
MEI	maximally exposed individual
MELODI	Multidisciplinary European Low-Dose Initiative
ML	machine learning
MOU	memorandum of understanding
MRI	magnetic resonance imaging
MTA	Monitoring and Technical Assistance
NASA	National Aeronautics and Space Administration
NCI	National Cancer Institute
NCRP	National Council on Radiation Protection and Measurements
NEA/OECD	Nuclear Energy Agency/Organisation for Economic Co-operation and Development
NIAID	National Institute of Allergy and Infectious Diseases
NIEHS	National Institute of Environmental Health Sciences
NIH	National Institutes of Health
NIOSH	National Institute for Occupational Safety and Health
NORM	naturally occurring radioactive material
NSF	National Science Foundation
NSTC	National Science and Technology Council
OMB	Office of Management and Budget
ORNL	Oak Ridge National Laboratory
OSHA	Occupational Safety and Health Administration
PAG	Protective Action Guide
PDE	partial differential equation
PET	positron emission tomography
PNNL	Pacific Northwest National Laboratory
PSC	posterior subcapsular
PTM	post-translational modification
PUMA	Pooled Uranium Miner Analysis

QALY	quality-adjusted life year
QST	National Institutes for Quantum and Radiological Science and Technology
RadBio-AI	radiation biology research using artificial intelligence and machine learning
RDD	radiological dispersal device
REAC/TS	Radiation Emergency Assistance Center/Training Site
REB	Radiation Epidemiology Branch
RECA	Radiation Exposure Compensation Act
REE	rare earth element
RERF	Radiation Effects Research Foundation
REVCA	Radiation-Exposed Veterans Compensation Act
RNCP	Radiation and Nuclear Countermeasures Program
SPEERA	Secretarial Panel for the Evaluation of Epidemiological Research Activities
TCGA	The Cancer Genome Atlas
TCR	T-cell receptor
TEI-REX	Targeted Evaluation of Ionizing Radiation Exposure
TENORM	technologically enhanced naturally occurring radioactive material
UNSCEAR	United Nations Scientific Committee on the Effects of Atomic Radiation
U.S. NRC	United States Nuclear Regulatory Commission
USCG	United States Coast Guard
VSL	value of a statistical life
WMD	weapon of mass destruction

Summary

Ionizing radiation occurs in a wide range of medical, industrial, military, and commercial settings, and the number of individuals exposed or potentially exposed to radiation in these settings is increasing. There are longstanding concerns that exposures in these settings, even at low doses (defined as doses below 100 milligray [mGy]) or low dose rates (delivered at rates below 5 mGy/h), can adversely affect human health. Today, these concerns influence patient acceptance of medical diagnostic procedures, U.S. government decisions related to the future of nuclear power and clean energy policies, continuing efforts to assess the full range of radiogenic health outcomes of legacy exposures to fallout from nuclear weapons production, testing, and waste sites, management of nuclear waste, and plans for responding to radiological threats. These concerns also raise questions as to whether the public and workers are adequately protected from current environmental and occupational radiation exposures and from potential new sources of exposure such as rare earth element and lithium mining to support green energy and long-term energy policies in the United States.

Low-dose and low-dose-rate radiation effects on human health outcomes and the biological mechanisms of these effects are not fully understood. Cancer is the health outcome most commonly studied for its association with low doses of radiation, and heritable genetic effects are assumed to be associated with low-dose exposures, despite minimal evidence to date of such effects in humans. There is also increasing evidence that low-dose radiation exposure may be associated with non-cancer health outcomes such as cardiovascular disease, neurological disorders, immune dysfunction, and cataracts. For some of these health outcomes, experts rely on risk estimates from studies of individuals who were primarily exposed to higher doses. As a result, the uncertainties associated with current estimates of adverse health effects that result from low-dose and low-dose-rate exposures of relevance to the U.S. population are considerable. Advances in epidemiological study design and analysis, radiation biology research, and biotechnology and research infrastructure make it possible to obtain more direct information on health effects that result from exposures to low-dose and low-dose-rate radiation. The increasing low-dose radiation exposures and the improved capabilities to quantify health risks and study the underlying mechanisms make it both urgent and feasible to improve understanding of the adverse human health effects from exposures to doses and dose rates of relevance to the U.S. population.

Research in low-dose and low-dose-rate radiation in the United States is currently limited and fragmented, lacking leadership and an overarching prioritized strategic research agenda. The Consolidated Appropriations Act, 2021 (Public Law 116-260) directed the Secretary of Energy to enter into an agreement with the National Academies of Sciences, Engineering, and Medicine (the National Academies) to develop a long-term strategic and prioritized research agenda for low-dose radiation research within the Department of Energy. A separate congressional directive (American Innovation and Competitiveness Act of 2017, Public Law 114-329) aims to develop a strategy for coordination of low-dose radiation research conducted across federal agencies. This congressional directive tasks the National Science and Technology Council within the White House's Office of Science and Technology Policy with the coordination strategy.

The National Academies appointed an expert committee to define the essential components and to set priorities to guide research for a multidisciplinary coordinated low-dose radiation program that is developed neutrally in terms of the impact of the research on assessment of radiation health risk and consequently its potential impact on radiation protection policy and practice in the United States. The proposed program as outlined in this report involves the broad research enterprise and goes beyond the resources of any one federal agency. This summary contains the complete list of the committee's findings and recommendations in response to the seven charges of the Statement of Task (see Box S.1).

> **BOX S.1**
> **Statement of Task**
>
> The National Academies of Sciences, Engineering, and Medicine will perform a study and provide a report with findings and recommendations on the current status and development of a long-term strategy for low-dose radiation research in the United States. Specifically, the objectives of the study will be to:
>
> 1. Define the health and safety issues that need to be guided by an improved understanding of low-dose and low-dose-rate radiation health effects.
> 2. Identify current scientific challenges for understanding low-dose and low-dose-rate radiation health effects.
> 3. Assess the status of current low-dose radiation research in the United States and internationally.
> 4. Recommend a long-term strategic and prioritized research agenda to
>   a. address scientific research goals for overcoming the identified scientific challenges in coordination with other research efforts and
>   b. support education and outreach activities to disseminate information and promote public understanding of low-dose radiation.
> 5. Define the essential components of the research program that would address this research agenda within the universities and National Laboratories.
> 6. Address coordination between federal agencies (including the National Institutes of Health, the National Science Foundation, the National Aeronautics and Space Administration, and different Department of Energy offices) and with international efforts to achieve objectives.
> 7. Identify and, to the extent possible, quantify potential monetary and health-related impacts to federal agencies, the general public, industry, research communities, and other users of information produced by such research program.

IMPACT OF A MULTIDISCIPLINARY LOW-DOSE RADIATION PROGRAM

The following three findings address the goals and impact of a multidisciplinary low-dose radiation program in the United States (see Chapters 2 and 3).

Finding 1: A coordinated multidisciplinary low-dose radiation research program in the United States can improve understanding of adverse human health effects from exposures to radiation at doses and dose rates of relevance to the U.S. population. In addition, this program can identify mechanisms for induction of these health effects, develop improved risk models for doses and dose rates at which direct measurement of risks is not currently possible, and ultimately develop more individualized risk estimates.

Finding 2: Comprehensive understanding of adverse human health effects emerging from the multidisciplinary low-dose radiation program will enable better assessment of whether current risk estimates (primarily for cancer) at low doses and low dose rates are accurate, underestimated, or overestimated and provide improved risk estimates for other adverse health outcomes. This assessment may impact radiation protection by confirming that current regulations and guidance sufficiently protect human health or by supporting either more restrictive or less restrictive regulations and guidance.

Finding 3: The committee is unable to quantify the low-dose radiation program's economic impacts because comprehensive estimates of overall costs to comply with current radiation standards are unavailable. Additionally, any changes to the current estimates will depend on new information on adverse health effects that will be generated by the low-dose radiation research program. When adjustments in radiation protection standards and guidance are proposed based on new information, agencies can estimate the economic impacts of the changes and perform benefit-cost and cost-effectiveness analyses of alternative measures.

Costs for complying with radiation protection standards and guidelines, administering radiation compensation programs, or for using technologies that utilize radiation in medical and other applications are balanced with the health, societal, and other benefits based on current scientific understanding of low-dose radiation health effects. To the committee's knowledge, comprehensive estimates of overall costs to federal agencies and the society to comply with current radiation protection standards and guidelines are unavailable. Similarly, comprehensive estimates for the overall cost savings for protecting the U.S. population's health by implementing these standards and guidelines are also unavailable. Without these current estimates as a starting point, preparing comprehensive estimates of overall costs to comply with prospective radiation protection standards or guidelines is not possible.

PROPOSED RESEARCH AGENDA PRIORITIES

Epidemiological and biological research of low-dose and low-dose-rate radiation faces several challenges. These arise because the effects of low-dose and low-dose-rate radiation exposures are assumed to be subtle and difficult to distinguish from those caused by other stressors or "spontaneous" changes that adversely affect the normal functions of cells, tissues, and organs. Moreover, a full understanding of possible effects may be complicated by change in the magnitude of observed effect with dose, dose rate, type of radiation, and duration of exposure.

The following three findings and one recommendation address the proposed research agenda priorities (see Chapter 5).

Finding 4: Epidemiological studies have played a crucial role in identifying risks (primarily for cancer) from medical, occupational, and environmental radiation exposures at low doses. Existing epidemiological studies are unable to address a number of outstanding questions of low-dose and low-dose-rate exposures of concern to the U.S. population including the full range of potential adverse health effects, risks associated with doses around 10 milligray, and the potential impacts of genetic, lifestyle, environmental, and other factors that may also affect radiation-related risk estimates. Epidemiological studies designed to overcome these limitations can better elucidate adverse health effects of radiation exposure at low doses and low dose rates relevant to the U.S. population today.

Finding 5: Radiation biology studies have contributed to the mechanistic understanding of the effects of radiation on molecular pathways and intra- and extracellular processes. The application of novel and developing technologies will enable more precise definition of the cellular and molecular processes that are affected by low-dose and low-dose-rate exposures. Integration of this information with that from epidemiological studies will enable better quantification of the adverse health effects from low-dose and low-dose-rate exposures relevant to the U.S. population, increase understanding of the involved mechanisms, and inform on the most appropriate risk assessment models to be used.

Finding 6: Advances in biotechnology and research infrastructure have been driven by the vast research and development enterprise in the United States. These include new observational and experimental systems, tools for measurement and genetic manipulation, increased computational power, improved interpretative algorithms, and shared data access systems. These advances have enabled innovation and breakthroughs in many scientific areas including cancer research and treatment, environmental health effects research, and vaccine production. A revitalized low-dose radiation research program can likewise leverage and further develop these capabilities to enable scientific innovation and breakthroughs in radiation biology and epidemiology.

Recommendation A: Agencies responsible for the management of the multidisciplinary low-dose radiation program should fund low-dose and low-dose-rate radiation research in the 11 high-priority research topics identified by the committee and can address the scopes outlined in Finding 1. (See Table S.1 for listing and approach for addressing the recommended priorities.) These research priorities are broadly classified as epidemiological research, biological research, and research infrastructure and are of equal importance.

Criteria used to identify priorities for low-dose and low-dose-rate research included (1) existing human, laboratory model, and cellular evidence for adverse health effects resulting from radiation exposure; (2) limitations in the current radiation protection system in the United States; (3) feasibility of improving low-dose and low-dose-rate risk estimation models given newly available technologies and resources as well as increased understanding of human disease mechanisms; and (4) issues of concern for exposed populations.

The proposed research will address cancer and non-cancer health outcomes including cardiovascular disease, neurological disorders, immune dysfunction, cataracts, and heritable genetic effects for both internal and external exposures. The committee strongly emphasizes the need for integration across the research lines and anticipates that the most impactful research projects will include work in more than one research line and will be carried out by multidisciplinary teams. The specific tactics for addressing the recommended priorities and for integrating the research lines will be developed with input from the extended research community and other stakeholders. Importantly, the list of priorities will likely evolve as biological understanding and research tools advance and as the research community and other stakeholders are engaged with the program.

Finding 7: Significant investments over a sustained period spanning several decades are necessary to develop and maintain a multidisciplinary low-dose radiation research program in the United States that leverages existing and developing research infrastructure that will achieve the goals outlined in Finding 1. The committee's best estimate is that the investments required during the first 10–15 years of the program are at the level of $100 million annually and periodic reassessments are required as large epidemiological studies and necessary research infrastructures are established.

The committee's research agenda extends for 15 years, through 2037. By that time, several of the biological research priorities (e.g., development of model systems [Priority B1] and development of biomarkers for radiation-induced adverse health outcomes [Priority B2]) and research infrastructure priorities (e.g., tools for detection and precise characterization of aberrant cell and tissue states [Priority I1] and dosimetry for low-dose and low-dose-rate exposures [Priority I3]) are expected to be completed or to be approaching completion and providing critical information. However, it is likely that the epidemiological research priorities will extend further into the future, based on progress with improving dosimetry for epidemiological studies (Priority I3), further establishment of database infrastructure (Priority I2), and advances on the most biologically important components of low-dose and low-dose-rate radiation (e.g., through research on Priorities B2 and B4).

The committee estimates that funding needed for the program is on par with the congressionally authorized funds for 2023 and 2024, that is, at the level of $30 million and $40 million, respectively, but needs to rise to the level of $100 million annually thereafter and remain at that level through 2037. Although the committee recognizes that the exact form of the program will be determined by the funding agency after consultation with stakeholders, it provided a prototypical program that comprises interacting hubs focusing on basic and translational biology, analytical and computational technologies, and epidemiology, intended to justify the $100 million annual funding level. The committee also notes that appropriations at the level of $5 million per year are not adequate to even initiate a meaningful low-dose radiation research program—as seen in 2021 and 2022 when funds for the program were at that level and the program was not initiated. Inadequate funding for the program will lead to continued scientific and policy debates about risks of low doses of radiation to the possible detriment of adequate protection of patients, workers, and members of the public from the adverse effects of radiation.

ELEMENTS OF A SUCCESSFUL LOW-DOSE RADIATION RESEARCH PROGRAM

The following two findings and one recommendation address the essential elements of a successful low-dose radiation research program (see Chapter 6).

Finding 8: The Department of Energy's (DOE's) Office of Science has a long history leading and supporting radiation research at national laboratories and universities to advance knowledge of radiation health effects and mechanisms of these effects. However, since about 2016, the Office's focus has been directed away from radiation health effects research, resulting in a lack of leadership and scientific activity in this

TABLE S.1 Committee-Recommended Research Priorities for Low-Dose and Low-Dose-Rate Radiation Research

Priority Research Goal Epidemiological Research

E1 Develop and deploy analytical tools for radiation epidemiology.

E2 Improve estimation of risks for cancer and non-cancer health outcomes from low-dose and low-dose-rate external and internal radiation exposures.

E3 Determine factors that modify the low-dose and low-dose-rate radiation-related adverse health effects.

Biological Research

B1 Develop appropriate model systems for study of low-dose and low-dose-rate radiation-induced health effects.

B2 Develop biomarkers for radiation-induced adverse health outcomes.

B3 Define health-effect dose-response relationships below 10 mGy and below 5 mGy/h.

B4 Identify factors that modify or confound estimation of risks for radiation-induced adverse health outcomes.

Research Infrastructure

I1 Tools for sensitive detection and precise characterization of aberrant cell and tissue states.

I2 Harmonized databases to support biological and epidemiological studies.

I3 Dosimetry for low-dose and low-dose-rate exposures.

I4 Facilities for low-dose and low-dose-rate exposures.

[a]The broader field of "-omics" includes genomics, transcriptomics, proteomics, metabolomics, and radiomics.
NOTES: Examples of integration across the priorities are described in Chapter 5. mGy = milligray.

Approach	Integration Across Research Lines
Develop cohorts of sufficient size, with detailed health information and biosample collection and accurate dosimetry, to support epidemiological studies of radiation-induced health effects in medically, occupationally, and environmentally exposed U.S. populations.	B2–B4; I1–I3
More precisely define health outcomes to enable exclusion of diseases caused by other effects, identifying easily measured signatures that can serve as disease surrogates, by improving dosimetry and identifying and compensating for confounding and modifying factors.	B1–B4; I1–I3
Assess the impact of genetic makeup, epigenomic status, DNA repair efficacy, comorbidities, exposure history to radiation and other agents, lifestyle and psychosocial factors, and immune status on radiation-induced adverse health outcomes.	B1–B4; I1–I3
Identify laboratory model systems in which molecular, cellular, and pathological features of radiation-induced health effects are similar to humans.	E2–E3; I1–I4
Identify radiation-induced changes in cellular and molecular features that causally link to adverse health effects in appropriate model systems.	E1–E3; I1–I4
Establish radiation dose-response curves for molecular and cellular endpoints and for associated early- and late-stage diseases at doses below 10 mGy and dose rates below 5 mGy/h.	E1–E3; I1–I4
Assess the impact of genetic makeup, epigenomic status, DNA repair efficacy, comorbidities, exposure history to radiation and other agents, lifestyle factors, and immune status on low-dose and low-dose-rate radiation-induced adverse health effects and associated cellular and molecular response endpoints.	E1–E3; I1–I4
Identify, develop, and deploy bulk and single-cell -omics[a] and image measurement and computational analysis workflows to quantify disease-linked cellular and molecular signatures that are sufficiently sensitive, reliable, and low cost for wide-scale application.	E1–E3; B1–B4
Develop accessible databases that document exposure levels, rates, types, and durations as well as cell, molecular, and health outcomes for human populations and experimental models.	E1–E3; B1–B4
Elucidate biological localization of internalized radionuclides; directly measure radiation-induced damage and associated response mechanisms; develop high-fidelity anatomically and physiologically based dosimetry; develop and apply modern statistical and computational methods for dose reconstruction.	E1–E3; B1–B4
Ensure access to low-dose and low-dose-rate exposure facilities, including those allowing internal exposure in model systems by a variety of routes (e.g., inhalation, ingestion) or invest in new facilities.	B1–B4

area. Separate offices within DOE and within other federal agencies and national and international organizations have relevant expertise and have supported and continue to support research in radiation health effects. Except for the National Aeronautics and Space Administration, radiation research carried out by these other entities has not been coordinated with that supported by DOE's Office of Science.

DOE and its predecessor organizations have a long history of leading research on radiation effects in academia, national laboratories, and elsewhere, starting in the 1940s in support of the U.S. nuclear weapons program. From 1999 to 2016, DOE's Office of Science Biological and Environmental Research (BER) managed the low-dose radiation program. The program took advantage of new technologies available at the time as well as advances in molecular and cell biology made by the Human Genome Project and expanded knowledge of molecular and cellular responses to radiation and helped better understand biological responses at low doses of radiation. The program was terminated owing to BER's change of focus toward bioenergy and environmental research. National laboratories have traditionally been a vital component of DOE's research capabilities, but since termination of the low-dose radiation research program, they have been refocused on research areas other than low-dose radiation mechanisms and effects.

A separate office within DOE, the Office of Health and Safety, supports research programs mandated by Congress or required by international agreement, including the Japan program that supports studies of the Japanese atomic bombing survivors of Hiroshima and Nagasaki carried out at the Radiation Effects Research Foundation. The Office of Health and Safety does not have available funds to support competitive external grants and contracts. A few other federal agencies within the United States (primarily the National Aeronautics and Space Administration, the National Institutes of Health [NIH], the Centers for Disease Control and Prevention, and the Department of Defense) have programs that support or conduct research on low-dose radiation relevant to the agency's specific missions. Some offices within these agencies have relevant expertise but the research they support is primarily in higher doses and exposures.

> *Finding 9:* Impacted communities exposed to radiation as a result of activities carried out as part of the U.S. nuclear weapons program (1942–1991) have strongly objected to the Department of Energy's (DOE's) management of the low-dose radiation program. They assert that the agency's role in promoting nuclear technologies and its responsibility for management and cleanup of its nuclear sites conflict with its role as a manager of studies on low-dose and low-dose-rate radiation health

effects that may serve as the basis for exposure management decisions. This conflict, and the legacy of DOE's history of problematic community interactions, is a source of distrust of the agency by these communities.

Impacted communities in the context of this report include Indigenous communities; atomic veterans; nuclear workers; uranium miners, millers, transporters, and their families; and individuals or communities impacted by radioactive contamination or nuclear fallout due to nuclear weapons testing, offsite radiation releases from nuclear weapons production sites, and nuclear waste cleanup activities. Much of the distrust of these impacted communities toward DOE's management of the low-dose radiation program originates from DOE's and its predecessor organization's secrecy during the nuclear weapons program activities and cleanup operations. Based on the input from community representatives to the committee, it is apparent that there is continuing distrust toward the U.S. government, and there is a belief that the U.S. government has failed to accept responsibility for past radiation exposures and has failed to develop programs that adequately compensate all impacted communities.

Recommendation B: Agencies responsible for the management of the multidisciplinary low-dose radiation program should incorporate the following elements:
1. Programmatic commitment to developing and maintaining a long-term multidisciplinary low-dose radiation research program that leverages the advances in U.S. research infrastructure and health effects research.
2. Independent scientific advice and program evaluation by a trusted entity.
3. Transparent management of the research process.
4. A prioritized strategic research agenda developed with input from all relevant scientific, regulatory, and impacted stakeholder communities nationally and internationally.
5. Research sponsorship mechanisms that support competitive research and infrastructure development projects and employ transparent peer review to select projects that are aligned with the program's strategic research agenda.
6. Training and research support for scientists of all career levels and relevant disciplines that promote equity, diversity, and inclusion.
7. Commitment to engagement and communication with all relevant stakeholder communities.
8. Coordination across federal agencies and other national and international organizations that carry out low-dose radiation

research or have relevant expertise and entities that carry out relevant (non-radiation) research.

Long-term commitment to the low-dose radiation program is needed to address the research priorities discussed by the committee in this report and to take advantage of the continuing technological and biological advances. Congress has assigned the management of the low-dose radiation program to DOE, but congressional staff told the committee that other government agencies could initiate their own low-dose radiation programs, carry out research that is dedicated to low-dose radiation, or have a low-dose radiation research component. Because the only entity at this point that Congress has tasked with a focused low-dose radiation program is DOE, the committee saw a role for DOE in coordinating low-dose radiation research within the United States. However, the committee also recognized the concerns raised by members of impacted communities about DOE's inherent conflicts with leading low-dose radiation research and by the research community on DOE's shortcomings related to management of the previous low-dose radiation program. In addition, the research agenda proposed by the committee extends beyond any single agency's capabilities, and a partnership with an agency whose mission is to enhance health would be warranted.

Among various federal agencies with missions to enhance or protect health, NIH is widely trusted by the scientific community and members of the public and does not have any regulatory responsibilities related to setting or implementing radiation protection standards; therefore, it has no perceived conflict of interest with leading low-dose radiation research through a cross-institutional effort. In addition, it has well-established and transparent processes for soliciting, reviewing, and funding research. Within NIH, the National Institute of Allergy and Infectious Diseases' (NIAID's) Radiation and Nuclear Countermeasures Program (RNCP) could be suitable to support low-dose radiation research through a cross-institutional effort. Although RNCP currently supports research in moderate and high doses starting at about 1 gray and supports limited research on cancer (which is the primary focus of the National Cancer Institute [NCI]), the committee was impressed with the program management's commitment and transparency as well as engagement with its stakeholder communities. NCI has processes similar to NIAID's and by virtue of its mission it focuses on cancer research. The Advanced Research Projects Agency for Health (ARPA-H), a proposed agency tasked with building high-risk, high-reward capabilities to drive biomedical breakthroughs, could also contribute to innovative low-dose radiation research leadership.

DOE and NIH have traditionally supported most of the low-dose radiation research in the United States, and there is a precedent for a successful coordination by the two agencies to complete the Human Genome

Project. The committee supports a similar approach to be used to lead the coordination of low-dose radiation research, with DOE leading a portion of the strategic research agenda (e.g., on genome biology, computational, and modeling research, and support for facilities for low-dose and low-dose-rate exposures), and NIH, through a cross-institutional effort, leading the epidemiological and biological research, but with mechanisms in place to allow for integration of the different research lines.

The committee was not tasked with assessing the suitability of DOE to manage the low-dose radiation program or with recommending an alternative management structure. But congressional staff was interested in views and possible alternative options for the management of the low-dose program.

DOE does not currently meet important criteria for an effective managing agency, namely commitment to the program and absence of perceived conflicts with the research it supports. Among various federal agencies with experience with research funding, NIH is an example of a federal organization that meets these criteria.

The committee estimates that to initiate the new low-dose program, DOE could implement most of the essential elements identified by the committee within about 2 years given adequate funding. DOE's progress with implementing the essential elements needs to be formally and transparently assessed. For example, Congress may use the scheduled Government Accountability Office review of the low-dose program mandated in the Consolidated Appropriations Act, 2021, § 11001. This review is scheduled to take place in 2023, 3 years after the enactment of the law. If Congress finds that DOE failed to adopt the research agenda and implement the essential elements recommended by this committee, it may consider alternatives for placement and management of the low-dose radiation program, for example within NIH, likely as a cross-institutional effort, for example, by NIAID and/or NCI and/or the newly conceptualized ARPA-H.

1

Introduction

Ionizing radiation has a wide range of medical, industrial, military, and commercial applications. However, there are longstanding concerns about its potential to cause harm, even at low doses that may be delivered over long periods of time. A "low dose" of ionizing radiation (referred to as "radiation" in this report unless clarity is needed to distinguish from non-ionizing radiation) is generally taken to mean a dose below 100 milligray[1] (mGy; see Box 1.1 for basic radiation terms and units), and the term "low dose rate" is taken to mean a radiation dose rate of less than 5 mGy per hour. High doses of radiation can cause cell death promptly, and the damage may be extensive enough to adversely affect tissue or organ functions. Low doses of radiation delivered over long periods of time do not cause prompt tissue or organ damage but may cause cellular damage that increases an individual's long-term risk of cancer and hereditary disorders in a stochastic fashion.

Current radiation protection standards for low-dose and low-dose-rate exposure focus on protection against such stochastic effects. The risk of cancer following low-dose and low-dose-rate exposure is assumed to increase linearly with increasing dose and to increase after even very low-level exposures, albeit as very small excess risks. This assumption is based on biophysical observations regarding the stochastic nature of radiation energy deposition and resultant induction of DNA damage, as well as analysis of the shape of the relationship between radiation dose and cancer risk (referred

---

[1] The definition of low-dose radiation is in line with that of national and international advisory bodies and entities with radiation protection responsibilities. For comparison, the annual average dose due to background radiation in the United States is about 3 mSv.

to as the "dose-response curve") from epidemiological investigations. For low-dose and low-dose-rate exposures, scientific review committees have found that radiation is less effective per unit dose at causing cancer at low doses and low dose rates than at high doses and high dose rates. This difference in effectiveness is formulated by the application of a dose and dose-rate effectiveness factor when deriving risks at lower doses and dose rates from those observed at higher doses and dose rates (ICRP, 2007; NRC,[2] 2006a).[3]

Public perception and acceptance of radiation exposure is influenced by the context in which radiation is used (Slovic, 2012), but uncertainties associated with health effects attributed to low-dose radiation generally create communication challenges for every situation where exposure occurs. Some communication challenges recognized by radiation protection regulators include justifying regulating radiation to low levels in the presence of inconclusive scientific evidence of risk, addressing questions regarding a "safe" level of radiation exposure and about individual risks, and using appropriate risk comparisons.[4] Communicating about additional low-dose radiation exposures in relation to background natural radiation exposure levels also presents challenges.

Today, concerns about risks at low doses and low dose rates influence patient acceptance of medical diagnostic procedures, as well as U.S. government decisions and policies related to the future of nuclear power and clean energy policies, management of nuclear waste, and plans for and responses to radiological threats. Concerns about radiation risk also raise questions as to whether the public and workers are adequately protected from current environmental and occupational radiation exposures and from potential new sources of exposure such as rare earth element and lithium mining to support green energy and long-term energy policies in the United States.

In many communities directly impacted by past or current radiation releases,[5] decisions related to radiation protection policies as well as radiation research are viewed with skepticism and distrust. This distrust originates

---

[2] NRC stands for the National Research Council. As of July 2015, the name under which the three academies fulfill their mission of advising the nation and conducting related activities became the National Academies of Sciences, Engineering, and Medicine (the National Academies), and publications are referred to as National Academies publications.

[3] The International Commission on Radiological Protection (ICRP) is reviewing current science relevant to the estimation of risk at low doses and low dose rates and will provide recommendations on how this risk is estimated for radiological protection purposes.

[4] Jessica Wieder, Environmental Protection Agency, presentation to the committee on October 27, 2021.

[5] Impacted communities in the context of this report include Indigenous communities; atomic veterans; nuclear workers; uranium miners, millers, transporters, and their families; and individuals or communities impacted by radioactive contamination or nuclear fallout due to nuclear weapons testing, offsite radiation releases from nuclear weapons production sites, and nuclear waste cleanup activities.

BOX 1.1
Basic Radiation Terms and Units

Absorbed dose: The mean energy imparted by ionizing radiation to a medium per unit mass. The SI[a] unit for absorbed dose is joule per kilogram (J/kg) and its special name is gray (Gy) (ICRP, 2007).

Activity: The number of nuclear transformations of a radioactive material during an infinite time interval divided by its duration (s). The SI unit of activity is s^{-1} and its special name is becquerel (Bq) (ICRP, 2016a). The Bq corresponds to one disintegration per second. The conventional unit for activity is the curie (Ci) which corresponds to 3.7×10^{10} disintegrations per second. Radon concentrations in air are measured in (Bq/m^3). Some federal agencies in the United States still use the conventional units of picocuries per liter (pCi/L); $10 \text{ Bq/m}^3 = 0.27$ pCi/L.

Acute exposures: Exposures that result in individuals receiving a radiation dose within a brief period of time.

Cumulative dose/risk: The total dose/risk resulting from repeated or continuous exposures to ionizing radiation.

Dose rate: The radiation dose delivered per unit time and measured, for example, in grays per hour (ICRP, 2012). Low dose rate is generally taken to mean a radiation dose rate of less than 5 mGy per hour.

Effective dose: A weighted average of equivalent doses to organs or tissues, used for radiation protection purposes only. The averaging is performed over all organs and tissues of the human body for which radiation detriment can be quantified and for which tissue weighting factor values are assigned. The SI unit for effective dose is the same as for absorbed dose (J/kg) and its special name is sievert (Sv) (ICRP, 2015). For X-rays and gamma rays, 1 Sv = 1 Gy; 1 Sv = 1,000 millisieverts (mSv) and 1 mSv = 1,000 µSv. Some federal agencies in the United States continue to use the conventional unit for effective dose, the rem. 1 Sv = 100 rem (for reference: 1 mSv = 100 mrem and 100 mSv = 10 rem).

Equivalent dose: Dose calculated for individual organs and based on the absorbed dose to an organ, adjusted to account for the effectiveness of the type of radiation. Equivalent dose is expressed in millisieverts (mSv) to an organ.

Excess relative risk (ERR): The risk (or rate) of an outcome (e.g., cancer incidence or mortality) in an exposed population divided by the risk (or rate) of the same outcome in an unexposed population minus 1; that is, ERR = relative risk minus 1. By definition, the ERR is unitless but is often estimated per a unit difference in radiation dose (e.g., ERR per 100 mGy).

Interpolation: The committee uses the term *interpolation* to describe estimation of risks at low doses of radiation in studies that include observations for an unexposed or very low exposed group, and observations for a group exposed to intermediate or high doses of radiation. Examples of such studies include the atomic bombing survivors and many studies of medically, occupationally, and environmentally exposed populations. If studies predict risks at low doses of radiation based on a dose-response function estimated using only data at high doses,

continued

> **BOX 1.1 Continued**
>
> such that they are predicting risks beyond the range of observed data, then the committee uses the term *extrapolation*.
>
> **Low-dose radiation:** Doses below 100 mGy.
>
> **Protracted exposures:** Exposures that result in individuals receiving a radiation dose over longer periods of time. Protracted exposures can be episodic or chronic.
>
> **Stochastic effects:** Effects that occur by chance, generally occurring without a threshold level of dose, whose probability is proportional to the dose and whose severity is independent of the dose. In the context of radiation protection, the main stochastic effects are cancer and genetic effects.[b]
>
> ---
> [a] SI = International System of Units.
> [b] See https://www.nrc.gov/reading-rm/basic-ref/glossary/stochastic-effects.html.
> NOTE: The committee uses the radiation dose units as reported in the studies it references.

from the Atomic Energy Commission, was fostered by the Department of Energy's (DOE's) secrecy during the nuclear weapons program activities, and has persisted over multiple generations. Some impacted communities express continuing distrust toward the U.S. government because of their views on governmental unwillingness to accept responsibility for past radiation exposures and failure to develop programs that adequately compensate all impacted communities. (See discussion in Sections 2.1.6 and 6.7.)

This report argues that the increasing numbers of people exposed to radiation (primarily to medical radiation; see Chapter 2) and the improved capabilities to quantify health risks at low-dose and low-dose-rate exposures (see Chapter 5, specifically Sections 5.2 to 5.4) make it both urgent and feasible to improve the scientific understanding of the adverse human health effects from radiation exposures at doses and dose rates experienced by the U.S. population. This report also argues that a revitalized multidisciplinary low-dose radiation program that leverages advances in biotechnology, improved mechanistic understanding of disease processes, and research infrastructure, can provide evidence on risks from low doses of radiation for different health outcomes, thereby alleviating the need to rely on risk estimates interpolated from higher doses (see Chapter 5, specifically Sections 5.2 to 5.4). To assist with developing a low-dose radiation research strategy in the United States, this report sets priorities to guide research for a multidisciplinary coordinated low-dose radiation program that involves the broader U.S. research enterprise and extends beyond the resources of any one federal agency (see Chapter 5, specifically Sections 5.2 to 5.4). The recommended strategic agenda was developed to be neutral in terms of the impact of the proposed research on assessment of radiation health risks and consequently its potential impact on radiation protection policy and practice in the United States. This report also recommends essential elements (see Chapter 6) for a successful low-dose radiation program that achieves its scientific goals and which includes taking steps to mitigate the challenges of distrust toward some government-sponsored radiation research.

1.1 LOW-DOSE RADIATION EXPOSURES TO THE U.S. POPULATION

Agencies with radiation protection responsibilities including the Environmental Protection Agency and advisory bodies such as the National Council on Radiation Protection and Measurements communicate radiation exposures to the U.S. population in terms of average annual dose. However, there is notable variation among individuals and across populations in the types of sources of radiation and in the frequency, level, and duration of exposure (Simon and Linet, 2014), and therefore, these averages, although informative, do not identify individuals or communities that have received doses higher than the average and therefore are at higher risk.

The estimated annual average dose to members of the U.S. population is just over 6 mSv.[6] Half of the estimated average annual dose (about 3 mSv) comes from natural background radiation, primarily radon, and most of the remaining dose from medical diagnostic procedures (3 mSv; see Figure 1.1). Doses from industrial applications (including operation of nuclear power plants) and occupational exposures account for less than 0.1 percent of the average annual dose to the total U.S. population.[7] The contributions from other radiation sources to the average annual dose to the U.S. population such as from DOE's nuclear facilities and nuclear weapons testing is currently smaller (NCRP, 2009a). However, they are of concern to the impacted communities due to the disproportionate level of exposure compared to the general U.S. population and the higher past exposures (see Sections 2.1.6 and 2.1.7 for discussion and Table 2.1 for approximate sizes of currently exposed populations).

The global average annual radiation dose is about half that of the United States (about 3 mSv). This difference is primarily due to the lower global exposure from radon and the much lower global exposure from medical diagnostic procedures (see Figure 1.1), even in countries with similar health care levels as the United States.[8]

---

[6] See https://www.epa.gov/radiation/radiation-sources-and-doses.

[7] See https://www.epa.gov/radiation/radiation-sources-and-doses and Table 2.1 of this report for the estimated annual dose to nuclear workers and other occupationally exposed populations.

[8] For example, the average dose from medical diagnostic procedures to the population is about 2 mSv in Germany and less than 0.5 mSv in the United Kingdom (UNSCEAR, 2008). The United Nations Scientific Committee on the Effects of Atomic Radiation is in the process of updating these estimates.

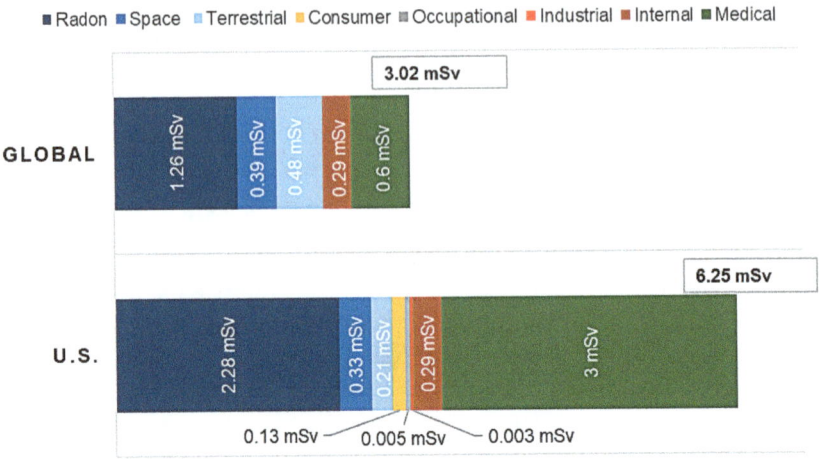

FIGURE 1.1 Estimated contributions to population exposure from different sources in the United States and globally.
NOTE: mSv = millisievert.
SOURCES: U.S. data from the Environmental Protection Agency, https://www.epa.gov/radiation/radiation-sources-and-doses, which subsequently uses NCRP (2009a); global data from UNSCEAR (2008).

Although some low-dose radiation exposures, natural or human-made, can be avoided or controlled (e.g., by limiting occupational exposures and those to members of the public from nuclear power plant routine operations and accidental releases or by remediating high radon levels in homes), others may be unavoidable (e.g., background radiation exposures from space and terrestrial radiation, or environmental contamination sources). To prevent adverse health outcomes caused by radiation during routine, accidental, or malevolent exposures to radiation, regulatory agencies within the United States and internationally have established radiation protection systems (see Chapter 3) that include exposure limits guidance that apply to a wide range of settings in which such exposure may occur to occupational workers and members of the public. Setting exposure limits and providing appropriate guidance requires an assessment of risks at low doses of radiation.

Cancer is the health outcome most commonly studied for its association with low doses of radiation. It is a common and heterogeneous disease in etiology and phenotype and is influenced by genetic, lifestyle, and environmental factors. Therefore, detecting the effects of low-dose radiation on cancer risk is challenging. Statistical estimates of low-dose cancer risk have become more precise as larger studies have been conducted. Fifteen years ago, when considering postnatal[9] exposure to radiation, a statistically significant estimate of the effect of radiation exposure on cancer was only directly detectable above about 100 mGy (NRC, 2006a; UNSCEAR, 2006a). Below that exposure level, risk estimates were derived from statistical models fitted to data derived from studies of populations that were exposed to higher doses of radiation, most notably the follow-up study of the Japanese atomic bombing survivors in Hiroshima and Nagasaki who received an average weighted absorbed colon dose of 200 milligrays (see Section 4.5.6). More recently, other cohort studies involving populations with medical, occupational, and environmental radiation exposures have allowed for direct estimates of the effect of radiation exposure on cancer risks following protracted exposures that are more relevant to the types of exposures received today by the U.S. population (Kitahara et al., 2015). These epidemiological studies have provided direct evidence that postnatal external exposure to radiation below 100 mGy is associated with elevated cancer risk. Evidence regarding low-dose internal exposures (aside from radon progeny) and different types of radiation is more limited (see, e.g., Schonfeld et al., 2013).

The quantitative relationship between postnatal exposure to radiation and cancer risk at the very low doses most commonly encountered by the U.S. population (e.g., below about 10 mGy) is not well established. There is also increasing evidence, some of which is summarized in this report, that low-dose radiation exposure may be associated with non-cancer health outcomes such as cardiovascular disease, neurological disorders, immune dysfunction, and cataracts. In epidemiological studies of populations exposed to higher doses of radiation, radiation-associated excesses of these non-cancer adverse health outcomes have been observed. In recent studies, such associations have been observed at doses lower than previously considered important for these effects (see Section 2.2). Therefore, elucidating their occurrence at low doses is of increasing interest. These other health effects are currently classified as "tissue reactions," and it is assumed that they do not occur below a certain threshold. However, this classification remains to be reassessed based on more recent studies of their induction at low levels of radiation (Clement et al., 2021; Little et al., 2021a).

Well-designed experimental studies in cells and animals or other models can supplement and redirect epidemiological studies in several contexts including where epidemiology has potential issues of inconsistency, bias, or lack of suitable cohorts. Experimental studies also provide mechanistic insights on the pathways leading to radiation-related cancer (NCRP, 2015a) and other diseases. Integration of information from radiation biology and epidemiology can be achieved by adding mechanistic information

---

[9] The association between low-dose radiation received prenatally by the fetus in utero and cancer risk is discussed in Section 2.2.1.

in cancer and other adverse health effects' risk models (Kaiser et al., 2014) or by using biological markers in epidemiological studies as described in Pernot et al. (2012) to enhance low-dose health risk assessment (NCRP, 2020a).

1.2 LOW-DOSE RADIATION RESEARCH IN THE UNITED STATES

Research focused on the mechanisms and outcomes from exposures to low-dose radiation can answer critical questions relevant to radiation protection of the U.S. population. A 2017 Government Accountability Office (GAO) report stated that between 2012 and 2016, DOE and the National Institutes of Health (NIH) were the two federal agencies primarily supporting low-dose radiation research in the United States. Within that period, the two agencies combined accounted for 98 percent of federal funding for low-dose radiation research, with the remaining 2 percent provided by other agencies including the Environmental Protection Agency, the U.S. Nuclear Regulatory Commission, the National Aeronautics and Space Administration (NASA), and the Centers for Disease Control and Prevention (GAO, 2017; see Figure 1.3).

DOE and its predecessor organizations, the Atomic Energy Commission (AEC) and the Energy Research and Development Agency (ERDA), have a long history of supporting research on radiation effects in academia, national laboratories, and elsewhere, in support of the U.S. nuclear weapons program. Starting in the 1940s, research supported involved human experiments[10] and the assessment of the effects of radiation on human health in the nuclear workforce (NRC, 2006b); studies of the effects of radiation on the Japanese atomic bombing survivors (Putnam, 1998); large radiobiology animal life-span studies (Brooks, 2012; NRC, 1998b; Zander et al., 2019);[11] elucidation of fundamental DNA damage and repair mechanisms (Bedford and Dewey, 2002); development of technologies including flow cytometry and sorting (Fulwyler, 1980; Van Dilla et al., 1969) and chromosome analysis to assess the effects of radiation in humans (Bigbee et al., 1997; Gray et al., 1992); and elucidation of the role of the microenvironment in carcinogenesis (Rizki and Bissell, 2004). This body of research made significant contributions toward understanding radiation health effects and radiation risk management. However, the management and use of the information by AEC, ERDA, and DOE have been criticized

---

[10] See https://ehss.energy.gov/ohre/roadmap/roadmap/index.html.

[11] Materials from the animals and detailed information are available at the Woloschak Laboratory website at Northwestern University (see janus.northwestern.edu/wololab). Archived data and tissues continue to be used today in laboratories in the United States and around the world.

for conflict and lack of transparency. In addition, human experiments and studies raised ethical concerns (DOE EHHS Openness, 1995).

In 1990, DOE initiated the Human Genome Project and co-managed it with NIH (Cook-Deegan, 1994; Patrinos and Drell, 1997) in recognition that detailed knowledge of the structure and function of the human genome can improve understanding of the health effects of DNA damage by radiation and chemicals (NRC, 1998b). The Human Genome Project generated the first publicly available reference genome and catalyzed many breakthroughs including inexpensive nucleic acid analysis technologies that have revolutionized biology, biotechnology, and drug development. The organizational rigor required to manage the Human Genome Project provided lessons learned to be applied in future programs (Gibbs, 2020).

DOE terminated the radiobiology life-span studies in the mid-1990s and, after some years of not supporting radiobiology research, initiated the low-dose radiation program in 1999 which continued until 2016. DOE's Low-Dose Radiation Research Program almost exclusively funded radiation biology studies and only supported one epidemiological study, the Million Person Study (Boice et al., 2022a),[12] toward the final years of its operation. The program took advantage of new technologies available at the time as well as advances in molecular and cell biology made by the Human Genome Project and expanded knowledge of molecular and cellular responses to radiation and helped better understand biological responses at low doses of radiation. For example, research supported by the Low-Dose Radiation Research Program (1) found that exposure to low-dose radiation resulted in both qualitatively as well as quantitatively different cellular and molecular responses when compared to higher doses; (2) provided evidence of systemic non-targeted effects of radiation, including bystander effects and genomic instability measured in cells not directly "hit" by the radiation; and (3) identified adaptive protective responses and molecular pathways activated by low-dose radiation (Brooks, 2012).

Over the course of the program, DOE provided an average of $14 million per year to universities and national laboratories for research on low-dose radiation. At its peak, in 2008, the program funded research at 45 institutions nationally and internationally. Just prior to its termination in 2016, it funded only two DOE-affiliated national laboratories—Pacific Northwest National Laboratory and Lawrence Berkeley National Laboratory (highlighted in yellow in Figure 1.2).

---

[12] More than 30 cohorts that fit in 7 broader groups make up the Million Person Study. The groups are DOE workers, nuclear weapons test participants, nuclear power plant workers, industrial radiographers, medical radiation workers, nuclear submariners and other U.S. Navy personnel, and radium dial painters. These groups were exposed to radiation from 1913 to the present (Boice et al., 2022a).

**Programs Funded By the DOE Low Dose Radiation Research Program 2008
45 Institutions, some with multiple awards.**

Columbia University	Medical College of Georgia	Thomas Jefferson University	Medical Research Council, UK
New Jersey Medical School	University of Chicago	University of Utah	Queen's University, UK
Colorado State University	University of California, Riverside	Northwestern University	Childrens Hospital, Oakland, Ca
University of Colorado	University of California, Irvine	Pacific Northwest National Laboratory	Memorial Sloan Kettering Cancer Center
Harvard University	University of California, San Francisco	Los Alamos National Laboratory	National Taiwan University
University of Texas	University of Massachusetts	Brookhaven National Laboratory	University of Lethbridge, Canada
Case Western University	Loma Linda University	Lawrence Berkeley National Laboratory	McMaster University, Canada
University of California Berkeley	Duke University	Lawrence Livermore National Laboratory	Simons Cancer Center
Washington State University, Tricities	University of Tennessee	Oak Ridge National Laboratory	High Throughput Genomics
University of North Carolina	Purdue University	NASA Johnson Space Center	Flinders University, Australia
University of Texas, Galveston	University of Rochester		
Texas Southern University	University of Maryland		
Texas A & M University	University of Iowa	Health Protection Agency, UK	

FIGURE 1.2 Support for low-dose radiation research by the Department of Energy's (DOE's) Low-Dose Radiation Research Program in 2008.
SOURCE: William F. Morgan, Pacific Northwest National Laboratory, presentation at a National Academies meeting on November 4, 2014, based on data provided by DOE.

The low-dose program was terminated because DOE's Office of Science Biological and Environmental Research (BER) program shifted its research focus to bioenergy and environmental research. BER's current mission is to "support scientific research and facilities to achieve a predictive understanding of complex biological, Earth, and environmental systems with the aim of advancing the nation's energy and infrastructure security."[13] In support of its mission, BER has remained at the forefront of genome biology research and has also produced computational infrastructure and modeling capabilities that are run on DOE's fastest supercomputers, among the most capable in the world.[14] However, as BER shifted its focus to bioenergy and environmental research, its interest and expertise in radiation research have markedly diminished. Despite suggestions from the Low Dose Radiation Expert Subcommittee of the Biological and Environmental Research Advisory Committee[15] for the scope of a small program on radiation health

---

[13] See https://www.energy.gov/science/ber/biological-and-environmental-research.
[14] See https://www.energy.gov/sites/default/files/2021-06/03%20BER%20Program%20Narrative%206_16_21.pdf.
[15] The Biological and Environmental Research Advisory Committee (BERAC) is tasked with advising the leadership of DOE's Office of Science on scientific and technical issues related to the BER program.

and an indication of promising research directions to pursue (BERAC, 2016), and a recommendation to create and lead an interagency coordinating mechanism for low-dose radiation research (GAO, 2017), DOE has maintained the position that it should not be leading low-dose radiation research and that low-dose radiation research does not align with current BER priorities (AIP, 2021; BERAC, 2016; GAO, 2017).

Federal support for low-dose radiation research dropped by about half between 2012 and 2016 following the termination of DOE's low-dose program in 2016 and parallel decline in funding by NIH (see Figure 1.3). According to DOE officials, decreases in funding for the program reflected the shift of research focus described above. At NIH, the decline in radiation research funding was not due to research priority changes but instead coincided with across-the-board budget cuts at federal agencies and a decline in the number of high-quality radiation proposals submitted to NIH as judged by NIH's peer-review process (GAO, 2017).

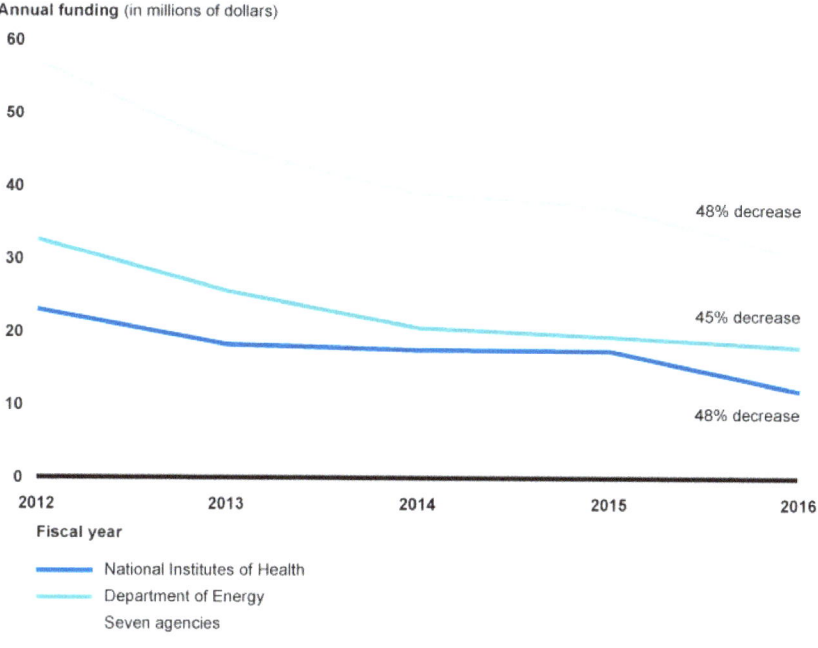

FIGURE 1.3 Funding for low-dose radiation research, 2012–2016.
NOTES: Funding from the Department of Energy (DOE) shown in the graph reflects that from the Biological and Environmental Research program in support of the low-dose program and from other DOE offices. The other five agencies that funded low-dose radiation research during that period were the U.S. Nuclear Regulatory Commission, the National Aeronautics and Space Administration, the Department of Defense, the Centers for Disease Control and Prevention, and the Environmental Protection Agency.
SOURCE: GAO (2017).

Today, a few federal agencies conduct or fund research in radiation topics that may also include low-dose radiation exposures, but none explicitly focuses on low-dose radiation research. This makes it difficult to assess the current effort and available funding dedicated to low-dose radiation research (see Chapter 4). Also, radiation research supported by these agencies lacks leadership and is generally fragmented, as it is set to respond to specific missions and not to an overarching strategic vision that aims to understand critical scientific issues relating to low-dose radiation. A much larger number of federal agencies, although they do not conduct or fund low-dose radiation research, use the research findings to meet their statutory responsibilities to set up radiation protection standards and guidelines, assist in the response to nuclear or radiological incidents, administer radiation compensation programs, or carry out other activities relevant to their missions that require knowledge of low-dose radiation risks (see Figure 1.4 and Chapter 3). Without good understanding of these risks, these agencies base decisions on potentially inaccurate information.

Attempts have been made in Congress to reestablish the low-dose radiation research program every year since its termination, in each case with DOE as the program-managing agency. In 2018, Congress passed legislation to resume the program (Department of Energy Research and Innovation Act, Public Law 115-246), and in 2021 it passed additional legislation (Consolidated Appropriations Act, 2021, Public Law 116-260; see Appendix A) that included directing the Secretary of Energy to enter into an agreement with the National Academies of Sciences, Engineering, and Medicine (the National Academies) to develop a long-term strategic and prioritized research agenda for low-dose and low-dose-rate research. The 2021 law states two goals for the program:

1. Enhance scientific understanding of, and reduce uncertainties associated with, the effects of exposure to low-dose and low-dose-rate radiation; and
2. Inform improved risk-assessment and risk-management methods with respect to such radiation.

The law also provides several clauses including coordination of the low-dose radiation program with the Physical Science Subcommittee of the National Science and Technology Council (NSTC) within the White House's Office of Science and Technology Policy (see Section 4.1.6 for its task) and an evaluation of the low-dose radiation program by GAO in 2023. Authorized funds for the low-dose program started at $20 million in 2021 and will reach $40 million in 2024 (see Appendix A). The appropriated funds in 2021 were $5 million.

Despite authorization to start the program and appropriation of limited funds, DOE has not reestablished a low-dose radiation program of the

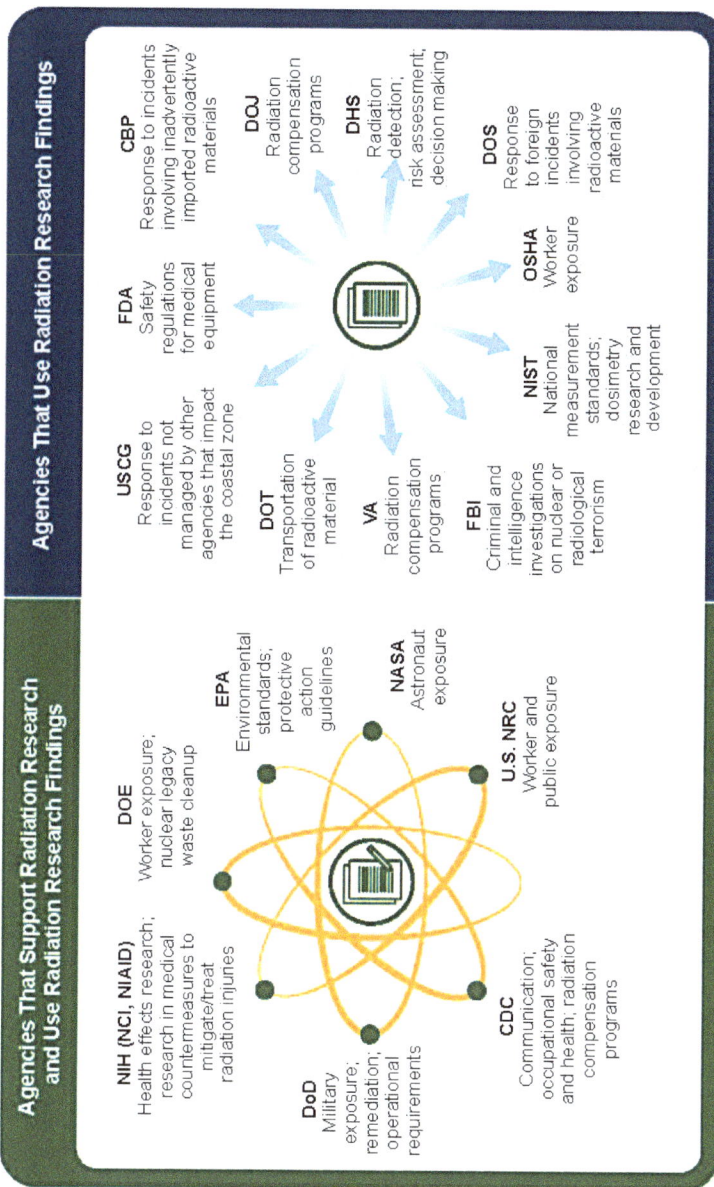

FIGURE 1.4 Federal agencies that support low-dose radiation health effects research and use the research findings (left panel) and agencies that use the findings of low-dose radiation research to accomplish their missions (right panel).

scale and scope defined in the Consolidated Appropriations Act, 2021.[16] In addition, BER did not direct the limited appropriated funds to support research focused on developing and testing new hypotheses that could provide foundational direction for the new program. Instead, DOE directed appropriated funds to support a project on artificial intelligence in cancer research carried out at three national laboratories (see Section 4.1.1).

1.3 STUDY TASK AND APPROACH

In response to the Consolidated Appropriations Act, 2021, the National Academies entered into an agreement with the Biological Systems Science Division in DOE's Office of Science/BER (referred to as DOE's Office of Science in the report) in April 2021. The charges agreed upon between DOE and the National Academies go beyond the original congressional charge to the National Academies as indicated in the Consolidated Appropriations Act, 2021. For example, in addition to developing a long-term strategic and prioritized research agenda for low-dose and low-dose-rate radiation research within DOE, the National Academies was also tasked by DOE with defining the health and safety issues that need to be guided by an improved understanding of low-dose and low-dose-rate radiation health effects and with identifying the essential elements of a low-dose radiation program as well as with addressing coordination with other entities. The complete Statement of Task is shown in Box S.1. A separate congressional directive (American Innovation and Competitiveness Act of 2017, Public Law 114-329) aims to develop a strategy for coordination of low-dose radiation research conducted across federal agencies and tasked NSTC with the coordination (see Section 4.1.6).

This study was carried out by the Committee on Developing a Long-Term Strategy for Low-Dose Radiation Research in the United States (referred to as "the committee" in this report), which was appointed by the president of the National Academy of Sciences. Brief biographies of the committee members and staff involved in this study are provided in Appendix B. The committee comprises experts in disciplines relevant to the study request, namely radiation biology, epidemiology, and biostatistics; radiation training and education; cancer and molecular research; health physics and dosimetry; risk assessment; economics; and scientific program development and management.

The committee collected the information it needed to write this report from July 2021 to February 2022. During that period, the committee received more than 80 presentations during 7 public meetings.[17] Invited

---

[16] Todd Anderson, DOE, presentation to the committee on January 24, 2022.
[17] All committee meetings took place via video-conferencing because of the COVID-19 pandemic and associated travel restrictions.

presenters included national and international subject-matter experts; congressional, federal, and state representatives; national laboratory staff; university researchers; and representatives from nongovernmental associations. The committee also invited presentations from members of and advocates for communities exposed to radiation as a result of the U.S. nuclear weapons program. These included officials and representatives of Indigenous communities; atomic veterans; nuclear workers; those individuals or communities impacted by radioactive contamination or nuclear fallout due to nuclear weapons testing or by radioactive fallout from nuclear weapons production sites (downwinders) and those impacted by nuclear waste cleanup activities. Appendix C provides the list of presentations the committee received during its information-gathering meetings, and these presentations and meeting recordings are posted on the National Academies website for open access.[18]

In addition to these information-gathering meetings, several committee members attended scientific meetings organized by other entities that addressed low-dose radiation issues including the Radiation Research Society's annual meeting and webinars organized by the National Council on Radiation Protection and Measurements, NASA's Human Research Program Space Radiation Quality Workshop, the International Society of Radiation Epidemiology and Dosimetry, the Electric Power Research Institute, and the National Academies. The committee also received written comments, both solicited and unsolicited, from government agencies, technical experts, and members of the public. Most of the commenters were based in the United States, but the committee also received comments from individuals and organizations concerned with radiation-related issues in Japan. These written comments were helpful in informing the committee about perspectives related to the study and for uncovering useful data sources and documents.

A number of the commenters were specifically concerned that the committee's report would reflect a pro-DOE bias because the study was funded by DOE. The National Academies study process is designed to protect the integrity and independence of the committee's work. To comply with the procedures implementing Federal Advisory Committee Act, Section 15, under which this committee operated, in the course of the study the information received by the committee was made available to the public upon request through the study's public access file.[19] Also, according to National Academies study processes, the committee kept an arm's-length relationship

---

[18] See https://www.nationalacademies.org/our-work/developing-a-long-term-strategy-for-low-dose-radiation-research-in-the-united-states.

[19] Inquiries and requests for the list of the public access file materials can be made to the National Academies' Public Access Records Office (see https://www8.nationalacademies.org/pa/managerequest.aspx?key=DELS-NRSB-21-02).

30   *REVITALIZE LOW-DOSE RADIATION RESEARCH IN THE UNITED STATES*

with the study's sponsor (DOE) in order to preserve its independence. For example, the sponsor did not have an opportunity to see the committee's draft findings and recommendations or otherwise appear to influence the content of the report.

1.4 REPORT ROADMAP

This report is organized in six chapters:

- Chapter 1 (this chapter) provides background information on low-dose radiation exposures to the U.S. population, the history of the low-dose radiation research program, and the study request.
- Chapter 2 discusses exposure sources that result or could result in low-dose radiation exposures to members of the U.S. population and the main health effects of concern associated with low-dose radiation exposures. This chapter addresses Charge 1 of the Statement of Task.
- Chapter 3 addresses the radiation protection framework in the United States and economic impacts of decisions related to changes in this framework. This chapter addresses Charge 7 of the Statement of Task.
- Chapter 4 addresses the status of low-dose radiation research in the United States. This chapter addresses Charge 3 of the Statement of Task and provides some background information to address Charge 6.
- Chapter 5 provides the committee's recommendation on the research priorities for the low-dose radiation program. This chapter addresses Charges 2 and 4 of the Statement of Task.
- Chapter 6 provides the committee's recommendation on the essential elements of the low-dose radiation program. This chapter addresses Charges 5 and 6 of the Statement of Task as well as parts of Charge 4 (on training and public engagement).

2

Low-Dose Radiation Exposures and Health Effects

This chapter addresses the first charge of the Statement of Task, which calls for defining the health and safety issues that need to be guided by an improved understanding of low-dose and low-dose-rate radiation health effects. To address this charge, the committee identified seven low-dose exposure sources relevant to members of the U.S. population. These are natural radiation sources, medical applications, occupational exposures, nuclear power routine operations and accidents, nuclear or radiological incidents, exposures from the nuclear weapons program, and nuclear waste. These sources are important in terms of low-dose and low-dose-rate exposures either because they contribute a large portion to the average annual dose to the U.S. general population or to specific populations (e.g., medical applications), or they are of concern to members of the public and impacted communities (e.g., nuclear waste management) or to current and future U.S. policies and plans (e.g., nuclear power operations). The relative contribution of these sources is displayed in Figure 2.1.

The seven low-dose exposure sources described in this chapter involve different types of ionizing radiation (e.g., alpha, beta, and gamma radiation), routes of exposure (internal and external), and durations of exposure (acute or protracted), as summarized in Table 2.1. For example, the type of radiation, route of exposure, and dose rate that are involved in releases from routine nuclear power plant operations are different from those from a medical computed tomography (CT) scan; therefore, the biological consequences of these two exposure sources may differ. Some members of the public may receive combined exposures from these different sources, both internally and externally, and over differing periods of time.

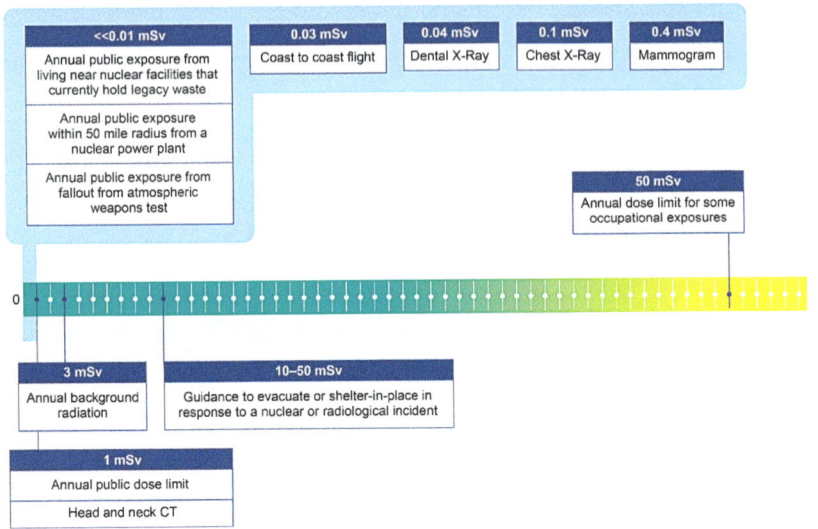

FIGURE 2.1 Typical or average current low-dose radiation exposures to the U.S. population. NOTE: CT = computed tomography; mSv = millisievert.

TABLE 2.1 Exposures to the General U.S. Population, Communities, Patients, or Workers, Following Different Exposure Sources

Exposure Source (exposed population)	Approximate Size of Exposed Population	Approximate Annual Effective Dose Today	Route of Exposure[a]
Natural Sources (general U.S. population)			
Terrestrial	Entire U.S. population	2.49 mSv[b]	Internal (inhalation, ingestion, absorption) and external
Space	Entire U.S. population	0.39 mSv[b]	External

Today, in the absence of a mechanistic understanding of different low-dose and low-dose-rate radiation sources and their direct health effects, estimation of risks and decisions related to exposures from substantially different sources often are made using the same generic approach—by relying on risks derived from higher, acute, external exposures to radiation, largely from the Japanese atomic bombing survivors, and applying appropriate correction factors in risk models.

In Section 2.2, the committee discusses current epidemiological evidence on health effects that are associated with low doses of radiation and identifies several knowledge gaps, particularly for health outcomes other than cancer, that are now being observed at lower doses than in the past.

2.1 LOW-DOSE RADIATION SOURCES AND EXPOSURES

The following sections illustrate common low-dose radiation sources and exposures to the U.S. population. The committee does not attempt to provide a complete review of the issues involved with these sources and exposures, but instead it uses some key references to the existing literature to indicate the current state of knowledge.

Types of Radiation[a]	Duration of Exposure (acute or protracted)	Typical Radioisotopes of Exposure[a] (not exhaustive list)	Radiation Protection and/or Policy Implications of New Low-Dose Radiation Information
Alpha, gamma	Protracted	Potassium-40; uranium-238 and -234 and the decay products of uranium, such as thorium-232, -230, and -228, radium-224 and -226, and radon-220 and -222	Decisions about housing and remediation; government radon mitigation programs; informing dose calculators for members of the public; decisions about air travel, space travel, and need for monitoring
Protons, neutrons, higher Z elements	Protracted	—	

continued

TABLE 2.1 Continued

Exposure Source (exposed population)	Approximate Size of Exposed Population	Approximate Annual Effective Dose Today	Route of Exposure[a]
Diagnostic Medical Exposures (patients)			
CT	74 million[c]	1.4–1.5 mSv[c]	External
Radiography and Fluoroscopy	271 million[c]	0.22 mSv[c]	External or internal (absorption)
Cardiac interventional fluoroscopy	3.6–4.1 million[c]	0.13 mSv[c]	External or internal (absorption)
Noncardiac interventional fluoroscopy	4 million[c]	0.13 mSv[c]	External
Nuclear medicine	13.5 million[c]	0.32 mSv[c]	Internal (injection, inhalation, ingestion, absorption)
Occupational Exposures			
Medical personnel, commercial nuclear workers, DOE facilities; industrial radiographers; mining and milling; other	3.86 million[d]	0.6–3.1 mSv[d]	External, internal (inhalation, ingestion, and absorption)
Aircrew	170,000[d]	3 mSv[d]	External

Types of Radiation[a]	Duration of Exposure (acute or protracted)	Typical Radioisotopes of Exposure[a] (not exhaustive list)	Radiation Protection and/or Policy Implications of New Low-Dose Radiation Information
X-ray	Acute	—	Benefit-risk balance for a procedure; need for regulation of patient doses or tracking of exposures; communications
X-ray	Acute	—	
X-ray	Acute	—	
X-ray	Acute	—	
Alpha, beta, gamma	Acute	Technetium-99; iodine-123, -125, -129, and -131; xenon-133; iridium-192; actinium-225; astatine-211; fluorine-18; gallium-67; yttrium-90; radium-223, -224, and -225; ruthenium-106; lutetium-177	
X-ray; alpha, beta, neutron, and gamma	Protracted	Potassium-40; uranium-238, -235, and -234; and the decay products of uranium, such as thorium-232, -230, and -228; radium-224 and -226; and radon-220 and -222	Revision of exposure limits for radiation workers; informing dose calculators for aircrews; setting exposure limits for aircrew; radiation compensation policies; communications
Galactic cosmic; solar particle events	Acute or protracted	—	

continued

TABLE 2.1 Continued

Exposure Source (exposed population)	Approximate Size of Exposed Population	Approximate Annual Effective Dose Today	Route of Exposure[a]
Nuclear Power Under Routine Operations (communities in vicinity)	1 million within 5 miles; more than 45 million within 30[e] miles	<<0.01 mSv	Internal (inhalation, ingestion) and external
Nuclear or Radiological Incident (impacted communities)	Varies depending on incident ranging from a few people to millions of people	Varies depending on incident	Internal (inhalation, ingestion, and absorption) and external
Nuclear Weapons Program (1942– 1991; impacted communities)	All areas of the United States received fallout but larger amounts over some parts of Utah, Colorado, Idaho, Nevada, and Montana[g]	<<0.01 mSv	Internal (inhalation, ingestion, and absorption) and external

Types of Radiation[a]	Duration of Exposure (acute or protracted)	Typical Radioisotopes of Exposure[a] (not exhaustive list)	Radiation Protection and/or Policy Implications of New Low-Dose Radiation Information
Alpha, beta, gamma	Protracted	Carbon-14; cobalt-60; tritium; iodine-129 and -131; krypton-85; xenon-135; cesium-137	Acceptability of nuclear power and current and new reactor technologies; decommissioning; implementation of permanent solution for nuclear waste storage and disposal; emergency planning zoning; communications
Alpha, beta, gamma	Acute and protracted depending on radiological incident	Incident-dependent but could involve americium-241; cesium-134 and -137; cobalt-60; iodine-129 and -131; plutonium-238, -239, and -240; polonium-210; strontium-90; uranium fission products; activation products[f]	Appropriate protective actions; remediation and reoccupation activities; communications
Alpha, beta, neutron, gamma	Acute and protracted	Uranium-238, -235, and -234; plutonium-238, -239, and -240; iodine-129 and -131; americium-241; strontium-90; tritium; cesium-137; carbon-14; fission products; activation products	Dose reconstruction; radiation compensation policies; communications

continued

TABLE 2.1 Continued

Exposure Source (exposed population)	Approximate Size of Exposed Population	Approximate Annual Effective Dose Today	Route of Exposure[a]
DOE Nuclear Waste Sites (communities in vicinity)[h]	3.8 million[i]	<<0.01 mSv	Internal (inhalation, ingestion, and absorption) and external

[a] Some information from https://www.epa.gov/radiation/radionuclides.
[b] See https://www.epa.gov/radiation/radiation-sources-and-doses.
[c] NCRP (2019).
[d] NCRP (2009a).
[e] NRC (2012).
[f] See https://www.nrc.gov/docs/ML0531/ML053130250.pdf.
[g] See https://www.cancer.gov/about-cancer/causes-prevention/risk/radiation/stateandcounty exposure.
[h] See U.S. NRC (2012).
[i] Based on population sizes in counties where the remaining 16 active sites are located.
NOTE: CT = computed tomography; DOE = Department of Energy; mSv = millisievert.

2.1.1 Natural Sources

The exposure of humans to radiation from natural sources is unavoidable. For the U.S. population, approximately half of the average annual dose (about 3 millisieverts [mSv]) is due to external exposure from terrestrial gamma and cosmic radiation and approximately half is due to internal exposure by inhalation of radon progeny and ingestion of radionuclides.[1] Radiation exposure from natural sources varies globally and within a country depending on the geology and altitude where people live. For example, in the United States, background radiation (excluding radon) can range from less than 0.1 mSv in low-elevation towns along the Gulf Coast to about 2 mSv in high-elevation towns in the Colorado Plateau.[2] Areas around the world where the annual

---

[1] Ingestion of radionuclides such as radioactive potassium-40 and radium-226 (present in plants and animals) or uranium and thorium (present in water) contribute to a dose of about 0.3 mSv to the average person in the United States.
[2] See https://www.epa.gov/radiation/calculate-your-radiation-dose.

Types of Radiation[a]	Duration of Exposure (acute or protracted)	Typical Radioisotopes of Exposure[a] (not exhaustive list)	Radiation Protection and/or Policy Implications of New Low-Dose Radiation Information
Alpha, beta, neutron, gamma	Protracted	Cesium-137; strontium-90; technetium-99; tritium; plutonium-238, -239, -240; curium-242; fission products; activation products (nickel-63)	Cleanup activities; communications

effective dose to the populations due to background radiation is above 20 mSv are considered high background areas (Hendry et al., 2009).

High Background Areas

Studies of the health of populations living in areas with high levels of background radiation conducted during the past 25 years are a potential source of information on the effects of low-dose protracted exposures that are also relevant to the U.S. population. These include descriptive studies in Guarapari (Brazil), Kerala (India), Ramsar (Iran), and Yangjiang (China), where levels of background radiation are high due to high concentrations of radioactive minerals in the soil. Overall, these studies have not found any associations between background radiation and cancer risk or other health problems arising from these high background radiation levels (Dobrzyński et al., 2015; Nair et al., 2009; Tao et al., 2012) although one study found that a higher level of background radiation was associated with a higher incidence of chromosomal aberrations (Hayata et al., 2004). These studies of high background areas have several design limitations including lack of individual estimates of doses to specific organs from internal and external exposures, lack of consideration of high-risk populations (e.g., children), which would increase statistical power to detect health effects, and lack of well-documented health statistics, in particular, organ-specific cancer rates (Hendry et al., 2009). Better designed nationwide registry-based studies of background radiation in the United Kingdom, France, Germany, and Switzerland have resulted in conflicting results with some showing an association of childhood leukemia and gamma radiation exposure (Kendall et al., 2013; Mazzei-Abba et al., 2021)[3] and others not showing an association (Berlivet et al., 2020; Spix et al., 2017). The German study found an association with incidence of central nervous system tumors in exploratory analyses (Spix et al., 2017). These studies also lacked information on children's individual exposure to radiation from natural and other sources. Participants of an international scientific workshop aimed to evaluate how epidemiological studies of background radiation and childhood cancer can best improve current understanding of the effects of low-dose protracted radiation. They determined that in the absence of individual cumulative doses, it is difficult to draw firm conclusions about risks. (For a summary of the discussions of the workshop, see Mazzei-Abba et al., 2020.)

Residential Radon

Initial information regarding cancer risks from radon came from observations following occupational exposures of underground miners in the 1950s and 1960s (Holaday and Doyle, 1964), when the average concentrations of radon progeny in uranium mines were high—approximately 92,000 becquerels per cubic meter (Bq/m^3) or approximately 2,500 picocuries per liter (pCi/L) due to poorly ventilated underground mines. These studies, conducted in Germany (Kreuzer et al., 2018), France (Rage et al., 2015), Canada (Navaranjan et al., 2016), Czech Republic (Tomásek, 2012), and the United States (Samet et al., 1991; Schubauer-Berigan et al., 2009), consistently showed a positive dose-response relationship between occupational exposure to radon decay products and lung cancer risk. These studies also demonstrated that radon and cigarette smoking have a synergistic effect on lung cancer rates, so that smokers are at higher risk from radon exposure (Grosche et al., 2006). Although early in the debate about radon-related risks it was questioned whether findings from high occupational exposures to radon could be used to understand risks from lower exposures

---

[3] These studies found a 4–12 percent excess relative risk of childhood leukemia per millisievert of cumulative red bone marrow dose from gamma radiation.

to radon in the home, studies on residential radon exposures (Cheng et al., 2021; Darby et al., 2005; Field et al., 2000; Krewski et al., 2006; Lorenzo-Gonzalez et al., 2019; Turner et al., 2011) provided consistent evidence that radon exposure presents an important environmental health hazard.

The Environmental Protection Agency (EPA) estimates that the average indoor radon concentration for homes is about 1.3 pCi/L, and nearly 1 out of every 15 homes in the United States is estimated to have an elevated radon level (4 pCi/L or more; EPA, 2018a); that is, more than 7 million houses need mitigation. Of those only about 2 million had radon mitigation systems installed, implying that about 5 million houses still have high indoor radon concentrations.[4] Based on risk models developed by the National Research Council's Biological Effects of Ionizing Radiation VI committee (NRC, 1999a), EPA estimates that radon is responsible for about 21,000 lung cancer deaths every year, making it the second-leading cause of lung cancer after smoking (EPA, 2003). Several programs and initiatives carried out by EPA and partners aim to reduce radon-induced lung cancer deaths by mitigating elevated indoor radon levels and adopting radon-resistant construction techniques.[5]

The effects of exposure to the low levels of radon decay products and health outcomes other than cancer are not well understood. One study of residential exposure suggested an association of radon with stroke (Kim et al., 2020). The Pooled Uranium Miner Analysis (PUMA) study is anticipated to provide additional insights on exposure to low levels of radon decay products and health outcomes other than cancer. PUMA is the largest study of uranium miners conducted to date that combines information from cohorts of uranium miners from North America and Europe. PUMA was designed to identify health effects of contemporary uranium miners employed in settings with mechanical ventilation where average concentrations are typically held below the range 500–1,500 Bq/m^3 (Rage et al., 2020). Comparisons of mortality rates in the PUMA cohort with those of the general population showed elevated risks for cancers of the lung, stomach, larynx, liver, and gallbladder but not for cardiovascular disease (Richardson et al., 2021). Analyses on the exposure-response relationships for different disease outcomes are not yet available.

Rare Earth Element and Lithium Mining

New natural radiation exposure sources are becoming of concern for populations in the United States, notably the possible pollutants or

---
[4] See https://cfpub.epa.gov/roe/indicator.cfm?i=27. The cost for radon mitigation depends on the size, layout, and foundation of the house. An average price is more than $1,000.
[5] See https://www.epa.gov/radon.

contaminants that could result from rare earth element (REE)[6] and lithium[7] mining. REEs have become increasingly important resources for modern technological applications including those that support clean energy transition such as cellular telephones, computer hard drives, electric and hybrid vehicles, flat-screen monitors and televisions, and permanent magnets used for motors and wind farm operations. Similarly, demand for lithium, a key component of batteries used in hybrid and electric cars, is also increasing (Graham, 2021). Availability of REEs and lithium is a high priority for green energy and long-term energy policies in the United States (Tracy, 2020).

China had been the major supplier of REEs until supply issues related to export restrictions arose in the past decade (Tracy, 2020), leading the United States and other countries to explore alternative economic REE deposits. The Mountain Pass deposit in California has produced most of the REEs mined in the United States since the late 1960s and resumed mine production in 2017 following a period of inactivity. Other potential domestic resources for REEs are located in Alaska, Nebraska, Texas, and Wyoming (Tracy, 2020). For lithium, roughly 70 percent of the world's deposits are located in salt flat regions in Chile, Bolivia, and Argentina. Chemetall in Nevada is currently practicing lithium extraction from brine, and Salton Sea in California is being explored as a possible lithium mining resource. Despite the benefits of mining REEs and lithium in support of clean energy transition, under normal operations, these mining activities may have adverse social and environmental impacts similar to other mining activities related to thorium present in REE deposits and chemicals used in the extraction process (Cheminfo Services Inc., 2012) which results in technologically enhanced naturally occurring radioactive material (TENORM wastes,[8] see Section 2.1.3). These mining activities also raise concerns related to contamination of groundwater and drinking water with radionuclides, during both normal operations and accidents (Cone, 1997; Penn and Lipton, 2021).

Space Radiation

Space radiation consists of high-energy charged particles of extraterrestrial origin that constantly bombard Earth and contribute a natural source of background radiation (about 0.4 mSv annually). Some of these particles come from the sun (solar particle events [SPEs]), but most are from deep

---

[6] There are 17 REEs, most of which have unique magnetic and optical properties and are not rare, as the name implies. These are lanthanum, cerium, praseodymium, neodymium, promethium, samarium, europium, gadolinium, dysprosium, holmium, terbium, thulium, ytterbium, lutetium, scandium, and yttrium.

[7] Lithium is a naturally occurring metal found in pegmatitic minerals, ocean water, and some brines and clays.

[8] See https://www.epa.gov/radiation/tenorm-rare-earths-mining-wastes.

space (galactic cosmic radiation [GCR]). Earth's atmosphere and magnetic shield protect against cosmic radiation, and only a low dose of low-energy ionizing radiation eventually makes it to sea level. Exposure to space radiation from SPEs becomes more relevant to airplane passengers, especially at higher altitudes and latitudes. Long-distance air travel can lead to low radiation exposures—about 0.03 mSv for a roundtrip airplane flight from New York to Los Angeles. Most people do not fly frequently enough to be exposed to high levels of radiation from space, but aircrew and frequent flyers could add a significant amount to their total radiation dose because of how often they fly. (For more information on aircrew exposures, see Section 2.1.3.) There is currently no radiation protection guidance for members of the public who are frequent flyers.

Space tourism (i.e., space travel for recreational or leisure purposes) became a reality in 2021 with three commercial companies commencing suborbital flights (Howell, 2021). Space travel is likely to expand in the current year and beyond, with additional suborbital flights and trips to the International Space Station initially and potential future space tourism experiences with destinations such as the moon, planets, and asteroids (Bushnell, 2020). The Federal Aviation Administration estimates that the risk to crewmembers on suborbital commercial spaceflights due to radiation exposure is comparable to that of air-carrier aircrews (average 3 mSv per year; NCRP, 2009a) but likely lower until space tourism flights become frequent and have durations similar to those of commercial aviation. There is currently no radiation protection guidance for members of the public who engage in space tourism.

2.1.2 Medical Exposures

Medical procedures that use ionizing radiation such as CT diagnostic examinations, nuclear medicine, and fluoroscopy-guided intervention have revolutionized medicine and improved medical decision-making and patient care. Their use contributes to diagnosis of disease and injury, informs appropriate care, and often allows patients to avoid more invasive procedures (Rubin, 2014). Between the 1980s and 2006, the average exposure of the U.S. population to radiation from medical diagnostic procedures increased sevenfold, primarily due to increased use of CT and nuclear medicine (NCRP, 2009a), making it the biggest human-made source for radiation exposure to the U.S. population. That increase in exposure plateaued in the last decade (NCRP, 2019), but exposure from medical diagnostic procedures remains the biggest human-made radiation source, contributing an estimated dose to the U.S. population of 3 mSv. Today, CT diagnostic procedures account for about 60 percent of the dose received by the U.S. population from medical diagnostic procedures (see Figure 2.2), with about 74 million CT procedures taking place in 2016 (Mettler et al., 2020).

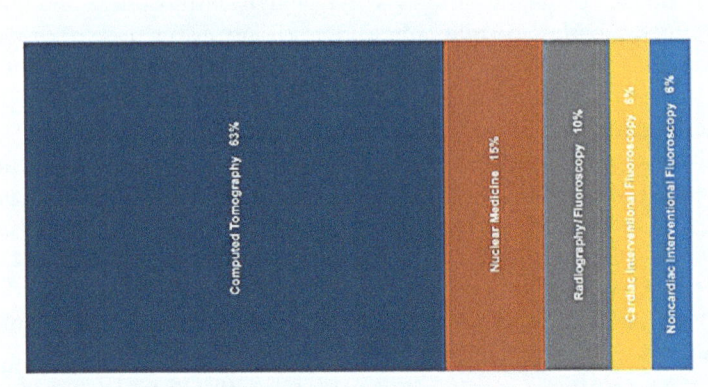

FIGURE 2.2 Contribution of different medical diagnostic procedures to the effective dose in the U.S. population. NOTE: mSv = millisievert. SOURCE: Recreated from NCRP (2019). With permission of the National Council on Radiation Protection and Measurements.

Effective radiation doses have been estimated for a number of typical diagnostic medical procedures, and they can range from about 1 mSv for a head and neck CT to 9 mSv for cardiac CT (NCRP, 2019). Although a single medical diagnostic procedure is within the low-dose range, some patients undergo multiple procedures, and their cumulative dose can exceed the low-dose range. Using data from multiple institutions in the United States, Rehani et al. (2020) found that more than 1 percent of patients were exposed to cumulative effective doses above 100 mSv, with a median cumulative effective dose of 130 mSv and a maximum effective dose of about 1,200 mSv. Patients who received these cumulative doses were typically older (>50 years of age), but a significant fraction (about 20 percent) was younger (Rehani et al., 2020). According to a different study, 80 percent of CT examinations in patients receiving cumulative effective doses above 100 mSv were related to evaluation or follow-up of a malignancy (Jeukens et al., 2021). Globally, it was estimated that 1 million patients per year are exposed to cumulative effective doses of more than 100 mSv due to medical diagnostic procedures (Brambilla et al., 2020).

Effective doses from diagnostic X-rays are much lower than from CT or nuclear medicine procedures, on the order of 0.1 mSv for a chest X-ray, and in the case of mammography on the order of 0.4 mSv (NCRP, 2019). Radiation therapy is another important medical use of radiation that benefits treatment of about half of the patients with cancer (Tyldesley et al., 2011). The intent of radiation therapy is to destroy cancer cells, and therefore the doses and dose rates utilized are much higher—on the order of hundreds or thousands of times higher than in the diagnostic procedures. Radiation therapy becomes relevant to the issues discussed in this report because of the lower doses to *tissues* outside the treatment field, some within the low-dose range (Lee et al., 2014).

A recent review noted that "the recurrent application of medical imaging procedures involving ionizing radiation are of concern, from the viewpoint of radiological protection" (Rühm et al., 2022). With the exception of mammography, radiation doses to patients are not regulated and limits do not apply. There are two guiding principles for the safe use of radiation in medicine: justification and optimization (ICRP, 1996). For justification, the expected benefit of the diagnostic procedure should exceed any expected harm. For optimization, exams should use the lowest dose possible to achieve the desired clinical outcome. Despite these principles and several campaigns that reinforce them, including the Image Wisely and Image Gently campaigns,[9] there are concerns about overutilization of medical diagnostic procedures such as CT scans. Approximately 20 to 50 percent of imaging exams are thought to yield little or no clinically useful information (Cremer et al., 2014; Litkowski et al., 2016), and some studies have shown highly variable and, in some cases, higher-than-needed doses to patients (Smith-Bindman et al., 2014, 2015). Another study found that use of CT during pregnancy increased almost fourfold during the period 1996 to 2016 in the participating medical sites in the United States and Canada (Kwan et al., 2019).

As older medical equipment is replaced with more modern equipment and post-imaging software for image quality improves, the radiation dose to the patient from diagnostic procedures is expected to decrease. However, both overutilization and lack of optimization may result in unnecessary and preventable radiation risks, particularly in potentially sensitive subpopulations such as children and pregnant women and the small percentage of the population with cancer predisposition syndromes (Brodeur et al., 2017; Reid and States, 2018).

Recent studies in pediatric populations have reported cumulative absorbed organ doses of about 50 milligrays (mGy) delivered with CT were associated with triple the risk of leukemia compared to doses below 0.5 mGy. Similarly, cumulative absorbed organ doses of 60 mGy delivered by pediatric CT were associated with triple the risk of brain cancer (Abalo et al., 2021; Bernier et al., 2019; Berrington de González et al., 2021; Hauptmann et al., 2020; Pearce et al., 2012), although confounding by some other factor or reverse causation[10] are arguments against concluding that this association is causal. However, systematic examination of this

---

[9] See https://www.imagegently.org and https://www.imagewisely.org.
[10] The CT scan may have taken place because of preexisting cancer and therefore not have been a cause (see Little et al., 2022a).

issue in key studies did not identify other factors (e.g., cancer predisposing conditions) that could account for the observed associations (Berrington de González et al., 2021). EPI-CT is a retrospective European multinational cohort of children and young adults subjected to CT from the 1970s to 2014. The study aims to include more than 1 million individuals, is facilitated by electronic record linkage, and uses an improved and standardized dosimetric approach; therefore, it has the potential to provide some insight on the impact of confounding by indication in medically exposed populations (Thierry-Chef et al., 2021). Results from EPI-CT are expected in the near term.

Large-scale studies of medically exposed populations facilitated by electronic record linkage have not yet been possible in the United States owing to the lack of a centralized health care system and fragmentation of patient services across multiple health care providers (NASEM, 2019c), although record linkage studies within single health care systems are common. At least three experts who briefed the committee noted that the lack of studies of medically exposed populations in the United States is a missed opportunity[11] and called for a national effort to collect the data needed for such a study. This effort would require long-term buy-in and commitment from both the research and medical communities. Currently there is a general resistance among medical professional organizations in the United States to track radiation exposures from medical diagnostic procedures for the purposes of patient dose and risk assessments (AAPM, 2021). The International Atomic Energy Agency's Safety Standard document, co-sponsored by eight international organizations including the World Health Organization (IAEA, 2018), and a more recent publication (IAEA, 2021) state that tracking individual patient exposures can support the process of justification and appropriateness of a procedure and provide information on collective dose to population and trends. The dilemma today appears to be that there is enough knowledge to be concerned that medical diagnostic procedures contribute significantly to the annual average dose to the U.S. population but not enough about the actual risk to act decisively. The debate of tracking exposures from medical diagnostic procedures to inform a patient's dose and risk assessment is likely to continue until risks at low doses are better understood.

---

[11] Armin Ansari, Centers for Disease Control and Prevention, presentation to the committee on September 24, 2021; Rebecca Smith-Bindman, University of California, San Francisco, presentation to the committee on October 26, 2021; and Jonine Bernstein, Memorial Sloan Kettering, presentation to the committee on November 17, 2021.

2.1.3 Occupational Exposures

Workers in a variety of occupations in the United States have potential occupational exposure to low doses of radiation. These occupations include, but are not limited to, physicians and dentists, radiology and nuclear medicine technologists, workers employed in the nuclear power and nuclear fuel cycle industry, industrial radiographers, and aircrews. In addition, countries with nuclear weapons programs such as the United States, United Kingdom, and France employed hundreds of thousands of workers over the past years who were exposed to radiation due to nuclear weapons production and testing activities. In general, occupational radiation exposures have declined over the years due to several radiation protection measures adopted in medical practices and in nuclear and other industries.

Ionizing radiation has been recognized as an occupational hazard for more than a century and as an occupational carcinogen for decades. Case reports of occupational injury related to work with ionizing radiation began to appear shortly after the discovery of X-rays, and included both prompt effects of burns as well as descriptions of malignant skin tumors caused by occupational external ionizing radiation exposure. By the 1950s, there was evidence of radiation-related excess mortality among radiologists in the United Kingdom and the United States (Court-Brown and Doll, 1957; Seltser and Sartwell, 1965). Major industrial cohort studies of radiation-exposed workers began after the Manhattan Project in the United States and have permitted quantitative analysis of health effects associated with occupational external radiation exposures that had been measured by personal dosimeters worn by employees on the job. These studies have been periodically updated, expanded, and refined since the 1970s, and national cohorts have been assembled that aggregate information on nuclear industry workers as well as workers in other industries and professions that require radiation monitoring and for whom registries of radiation workers have been assembled, such as medical radiology technicians, industrial radiographers, and commercial nuclear power workers. Table 2.2 lists some of the studies on occupationally exposed cohorts and cancer risks. Outcomes other than cancer following occupational exposures are discussed in Section 2.2. A brief discussion of health effects among uranium miners can be found in Section 2.1.1.

These studies are important because the doses received have been accumulated as many low doses of radiation over protracted periods, often many years (Rühm et al., 2022), and therefore are more relevant to public exposures compared to, for example, the higher and acute doses received by the Japanese atomic bombing survivors.

Occupational exposures to radiation also occur from TENORM, which includes radioactive materials that are found naturally but have been

TABLE 2.2 Summary of Some Occupational Cohort Studies and Cancer Risks

Study	Outcome	Sample Size	Cancer Cases	Mean Dose	ERR per 100 mGy	95% CI (90% CI)	Reference
Korean workers	Cancer mortality	79,679	134	6 mSv	0.72	−0.5 to 2.1	Ahn et al., 2008
Korean nuclear workers	Cancer incidence	16,236	203	20 mSv	0.21	−0.19 to 0.9	Jeong et al., 2010
Rocketdyne employees	Cancer mortality	46,970	647	14 mSv	0.02	−0.18 to 0.17	Boice et al., 2011
Japanese workers	Cancer mortality	200,583	2,636	12 mSv	0.13	−0.03 to 0.30	Akiba and Mizuno, 2012
Canadian workers	Cancer mortality	45,316	437	22 mSv	0.18	−0.04 to 0.53	Zablotska et al., 2014a
German nuclear workers	Cancer mortality	8,972	115	20 mSv	−0.1	−0.4 to 0.1	Merzenich et al., 2014
U.S. radiology technologists	Breast cancer	66,915	1,922	37 mGy	0.07	−0.005 to 0.19	Preston et al., 2016
U.S. nuclear workers	Cancer mortality	119,195	10,877	20 mSv	0.01	−0.02 to 0.05	Schubauer-Berigan et al., 2015
UK national registry of radiation workers	Cancer incidence	167,003	13,985	25 mSv	0.012	0.005 to 0.02	Haylock et al., 2018
French nuclear workers	Cancer mortality	59,004	2,536	26 mSv	0.04	−0.04 to 0.13	Fournier et al., 2016
INWORKS	Cancer mortality	308,297	17,957	21 mGy	0.05	0.018 to 0.079	Richardson et al., 2015
Million Person Study (analysis restricted to subpopulation of nuclear power plant workers)	Cancer mortality	135,193	8,445	52.6 mGy	0.01	−0.03 to 0.05	Boice et al., 2021

NOTE: CI = confidence interval; ERR = excess relative risk; INWORKS = International Nuclear Workers Study of nuclear industry workers in France, the United Kingdom, and the United States; mGy = milligray; mSv = millisievert.
SOURCE: Adapted and updated from NASEM (2019c).

concentrated or exposed to the accessible environment as a result of human activities such as manufacturing, mineral extraction, or water processing (EPA, 2008). Concentration of radioactive materials in the oil industry on the inside of pipes or in sludge has been well documented to lead to higher worker exposures and to wastes with relatively high radioactivity levels.[12] Enhanced exposure to radioactivity has recently been observed in unconventional shale gas drilling workers and to occur downwind of hydraulic fracturing (Li et al., 2020). The use of the term TENORM is generally not applied to activities specifically regulated under the Atomic Energy Act of 1946 such as nuclear energy or military uses.

Exposures to aircrews differ from the occupational exposures described thus far and are primarily due to galactic cosmic radiation and solar particle events. Studies of cancer mortality among aircrew members are inconsistent and generally complicated by the effects of occupational exposures other than radiation as well as circadian rhythm disruption from crossing multiple time zones. Although increased risk of malignant melanoma, brain cancer, and leukemia has been reported in some studies (Hammer et al., 2009; Sigurdson and Ron, 2004) and female flight attendants were more likely to be diagnosed with breast cancer (Lynge, 1996; Pukkala et al., 1995), several studies have observed statistically significant lower mortality from cancer and cardiovascular diseases among aircrew members compared with the general population (Blettner et al., 2003; Yong et al., 2014; Zeeb et al., 2010, 2012). These results likely reflect the healthy worker effect of the members of this occupationally exposed group, who, due to job requirements, are also under continuing medical surveillance to maintain fitness and health qualifications to fly (Sykes et al., 2012). The literature is sparse with respect to radiation health effects on flight crew and other health outcomes. A study found that exposure during the first trimester to cosmic radiation as low as 0.36 mSv may be linked to increased risk of miscarriage (Grajewski et al., 2015).

2.1.4 Nuclear Power Operations

The nuclear energy industry produces energy by initiating and controlling a sustained nuclear chain reaction. Radioactive sources from the life cycle of nuclear power plants stem from uranium mining, milling and mill tailings, power plant operation, and nuclear waste.[13] Nuclear energy facilities are subject to and must comply with multiple engineering, regulatory,

---

[12] See https://www.epa.gov/radiation/tenorm-oil-and-gas-production-wastes.

[13] Other (non-nuclear) industries of electricity production are also a source of radioactive exposure. For example, waste from coal-fired power plants and from oil and gas drilling contain radioactive material. Exposures to radiation from these other industries are not generally monitored or systematically reported (UNSCEAR, 2016). See also discussion on TENORM in Section 2.1.3.

and administrative measures to minimize unintentional releases and to ensure minimal exposures to the neighboring communities. Under normal power plant operations, only a small amount of radioactivity (a few curies to a few hundred curies) is typically released to the environment each year, contributing to a small portion of the average dose to the U.S. population. In the United States, effluent releases in airborne and liquid forms from nuclear plants must be controlled, monitored, and reported to the U.S. Nuclear Regulatory Commission (U.S. NRC) and other federal and state regulatory agencies. EPA sets the permissible annual dose equivalent to individual members of the public from a nuclear power plant at 0.25 mSv in a year but the U.S. NRC estimates that the average dose to members of the public living within a 50-mile radius of a nuclear power plant is much lower, about 0.0001 mSv.[14]

Populations living near nuclear facilities have expressed concerns about risks to their health from releases during routine operations of these facilities. To address these concerns, since 1985, several countries, including the United States, carried out epidemiological studies of cancer risks in populations near nuclear facilities. The majority of these studies investigated rates of cancer deaths or cancer occurrence in populations living in various-size geographic areas including counties and municipalities, zones of increasing distance, or zones based on models of dispersion of releases from the nuclear facilities (NRC, 2012). These studies have come to different conclusions, with some suggesting no associations (Heinävaara et al., 2010; Nuclear Safety Council and the Carlos III Institute of Health, 2009; White-Koning et al., 2004) and others suggesting positive associations between leukemia in children living in proximity to a nuclear facility (COMARE, 2016; Kaatsch et al., 2008; Sermage-Faure et al., 2012; Spix et al., 2008). Even studies that found positive associations have been unable to attribute them to radioactive releases from the facilities (Sermage-Faure et al., 2012).

In the United States, studies on risks to populations living near nuclear facilities are more than 30 years old. In 1991, the National Cancer Institute (NCI) compared cancer mortality rates in counties that contained nuclear facilities with rates in counties that were similar to the study counties in terms of population size, income, education, and other socioeconomic factors but did not contain nuclear facilities and found no differences in cancer rates (Jablon et al., 1991). The U.S. NRC requested that the National Academies reexamine risks around nuclear facilities and update the 1991 findings. The U.S. NRC request led to two National Academies studies that provided recommendations for the appropriate methods for assessing risks to populations around nuclear facilities (NRC, 2012) and information on

---

[14] See https://www.nrc.gov/about-nrc/radiation/related-info/faq.html.

piloting the study to validate the recommended methods (NRC, 2014). In 2015 the U.S. NRC decided to terminate the National Academies efforts due to budgetary constraints (U.S. NRC, 2015b). In the fiscal year 2022 Appropriations Bill, Congress "encourages" the Department of Health and Human Services to contract with the National Academies to carry out the pilot study.

In addition to concerns about health effects from nuclear power plant operations that need to be addressed, uncertainties about risks from low doses such as those resulting from routine nuclear power plant operations create major challenges to the U.S. government about the acceptability of nuclear power and its future in the country's energy mix. The risk and benefit perceptions regarding nuclear power have been dynamic, responding to changing context such as the cost and availability of clean energy and in relation to accidents that result in radiation releases (Gupta et al., 2019; see Figure 2.3). The 2011 Fukushima accident in Japan, triggered by the Great East Japan Earthquake and tsunami, revived the debate about the future of nuclear power globally and risks from unintentional releases of radiation. There were no immediate fatalities due to radiation releases from the accident and the average dose to a member of the public from releases from the accident was low (about 6 mSv to adult evacuees and 1–15 mGy to the thyroid of children; UNSCEAR, 2020b). Leukemia and thyroid cancers can manifest a few years after exposure, and other types of cancer can develop decades later. The Fukushima Prefectural Government offered thyroid ultrasound examination to children age 18 or younger. The examination revealed an unexpectedly large number of thyroid cancers among children screened that could not be explained by the relatively low doses received (NASEM, 2019b). The screening findings caused public anxiety about the health effects of radiation and raised concerns within the scientific and medical community about over-diagnosis following thyroid screening (IARC, 2018; NASEM, 2019b).

Evacuees and residents of Fukushima (Suzuki et al., 2015, 2018), similar to those from areas affected by the 1986 Chernobyl accident (Bromet, 2011, 2012, 2014; Bromet and Litcher-Kelly 2002), demonstrated high prevalence of psychological effects due to loss of life and social ties, homes, and employment; relocations; and the perceived health risk due to radiation exposure. The perceived risk and scientific uncertainty about the health effects of low-dose radiation exposures also fostered social problems. Many workers engaging in recovery operations following the Fukushima accident were likely to suffer from public discrimination resulting in general psychological distress and post-trauma. In addition, there are reports of school bullying of affected children and adolescents (Sawano et al., 2018), and many young women in Fukushima were afraid that they might be viewed negatively due to possible effects of radiation on future pregnancy

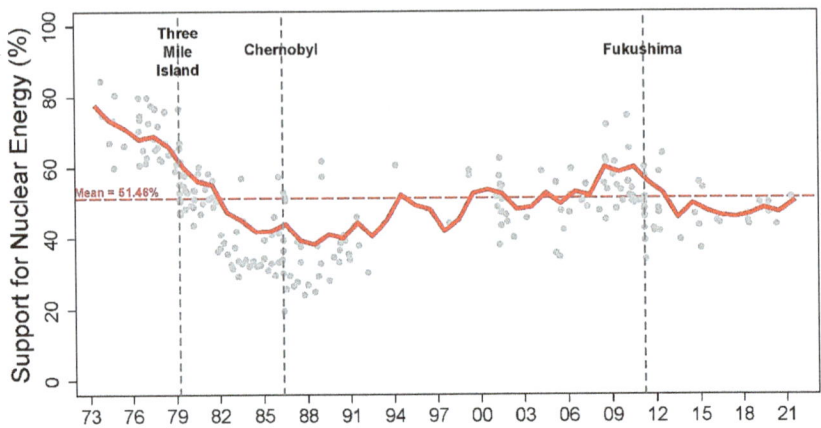

FIGURE 2.3 Support for nuclear energy over the past 50 years. SOURCE: Updated figure from Gupta et al. (2019), provided by Hank Jenkins-Smith, University of Oklahoma.

or transgenerational effects (Glionna, 2012; Save the Children, 2012). Social stigma and self-stigma are well-documented consequences of radiation exposure among survivors of the Fukushima accident as well as among the Japanese atomic bombing survivors (Amano et al., 2021) and those affected by the Chernobyl nuclear power plant accident in the former Soviet Union (Trichopoulos et al., 1987).

Scientific uncertainty about the health effects of low-dose radiation exposures also complicates government decision-making about decontamination of the plant and how to handle releases of radiation to the environment. In April 2021, the Japanese government approved the release of more than 1 million tonnes of contaminated water from the plant into the sea. According to an analysis, the resulting radioactivity in the sea will be below national regulatory standards and international guidelines (WNN, 2021). The release of the contaminated water into the sea was perceived unfavorably by environmental groups, fisheries organizations, and neighboring countries due to concerns about the possible environmental impact of the discharge (Normile, 2021).

Public attention to the Fukushima nuclear power plant accident and subsequent cleanup continues to influence the perceived balance of risk and benefit for nuclear energy (Jenkins-Smith et al., 2017). A main argument for the need for nuclear power in the world's energy mix is its contribution toward clean energy.[15] However, the operating nuclear power reactors in the United States are aging, and the number is declining. Barriers to a

---

[15] Nuclear power results in no direct CO_2 emissions; therefore, some see it as a promising energy production option for climate change mitigation. See, for example, Johnson (2019).

nuclear energy renaissance exist, among them high costs to build new reactor systems, safety concerns, and capacity for renewable energy sources to provide energy (Johnson, 2019). According to some, the general stringency in nuclear power regulation and the lack of a permanent solution for disposing of the accumulating volumes of high-level waste from more than six decades of nuclear power plant operations[16] are also affecting the extent to which nuclear power can contribute in the world's energy mix (Cohen, 1987; Cuttler and Pollycove, 2009; see also Batkins, 2016). Implementation of both clean energy and waste disposal solutions are affected by uncertainties in low-dose radiation health effects to the surrounding populations and future generations.

The Department of Energy's (DOE's) Office of Nuclear Energy, the office responsible for nuclear power sustainability, has announced large investments over the next few years to support the industry to further develop and deploy advanced reactors, including small modular reactors (DOE, 2020b).[17] Improved knowledge of low-dose radiation health effects can impact acceptability of these new technologies, safety assessments for reactor siting, and decisions about emergency planning zones for these new technologies (Smith et al., 2021; U.S. NRC, 2020a).

2.1.5 Nuclear or Radiological Incidents

The dose to affected populations and potential health impacts of a nuclear or radiological incident depend on a number of variables including the type of incident (i.e., a nuclear power plant accident, an unintentional radiation release from a radioactive source, or attack by terrorists using a radiological dispersal device [RDD] or an improvised nuclear device [IND]); form of the radioactive material; size of the exposed population; meteorological conditions; and protective and mitigation response actions. An RDD detonation, for example, is likely to occur in highly populated areas with the intent to cause disruption and widespread panic and fear of radiation. With possible exceptions, the doses to members of the public are expected to be low (NASEM, 2019b). Similarly, doses to members of the public from a nuclear power plant accident could be reduced if appropriate protective actions such as evacuations are taken. An IND, whether it involves a surface detonation or high-altitude burst, would have severe consequences in terms of immediate casualties from physical trauma and radiation and

---

[16] In the absence of a permanent repository for nuclear waste, federal facilities and nuclear power plants across the country store highly radioactive waste on site.

[17] Developers of small modular reactors claim that they provide scalability and flexibility and can be deployed quickly and cost-effectively. This type of reactor has not yet been deployed in the United States or elsewhere.

would expose large populations to moderate to low doses of radiation from the fallout (NASEM, 2019b). Emergency workers and workers involved in long-term cleanup activities are exposed to doses higher than those of the members of the public. For example, over the first 12 months after the Fukushima accident, emergency and cleanup workers received effective doses of about 13 mSv, but a small percentage of the workforce—less than 1 percent corresponding to fewer than 200 individuals—received effective doses higher than 100 mSv with a maximum effective dose of about 680 mSv (UNSCEAR, 2020b).

In the United States, several federal agencies have responsibilities for preparedness and response to a nuclear or radiological incident, and their roles and authorities depend on the type of incident (DHS, 2016). All federal agencies involved have published plans and guidance documents to assist with a coordinated response (see CDC, 2020, for a listing). Federal plans and guidance documents for a response to a nuclear or radiological incident are based on available scientific evidence for radiation risks and are informed by recommendations from national and international bodies such as the National Council on Radiation Protection and Measurements and the International Commission on Radiological Protection (ICRP). Because many incidents are likely to involve exposures to populations within the low-dose range, knowing what the risks are from these low-dose exposures is important for responders to make the appropriate risk-benefit evaluation before they make decisions (e.g., to evacuate populations from the area). Evacuations, although they can reduce the dose of radiation to affected communities, can also cause harm, particularly when made without adequate planning, as evidenced most recently by evacuations during the Fukushima nuclear power plant accident. In the absence of direct knowledge of risks at low doses, it is not possible to optimally balance the risks and benefits of evacuations.

Vulnerable populations such as residents of nursing homes are often the most affected by evacuations, as was the case following the Fukushima accident (Nomura et al., 2013). In the Fukushima Prefecture, about 165,000 people who lived near the nuclear power plant were evacuated at the directive of the Japanese government because the annual cumulative doses would be highly likely to exceed 20 mSv after the accident, which is the standard limit for radiological protection in emergency exposure situations. Murakami et al. (2015) used the loss-of-life-expectancy measure to compare the risks of evacuation with the risks of radiation exposure caused by staying among nursing home residents and the staff members who cared for them following the Fukushima accident. They showed that the mortality risk associated with rapid evacuation without sufficient preparation was about 400 times higher than that of radiation exposure associated with staying in the nursing home for 3 months after the disaster and concluded that evacuation planning needs to be balanced with the tradeoffs against radiation-related risks (Murakami et al., 2015). The risks of staying in the contaminated area due to damaged infrastructure, interruptions in food and medical supplies, human assistance, and other factors were not considered in this analysis.

Evacuations following the Fukushima accident also resulted in long-term displacement of large populations. Today, in Fukushima Prefecture, decontamination of prefectural land has been completed in all areas except for the zone referred to as the "difficult-to-return zone," where annual doses are higher than 50 mSv. Still, out of the about 165,000 people who evacuated, about 35,000 remain under evacuation orders and about an equal number of evacuees has chosen not to return due to concerns about risks from radiation.[18] Although the Government of Japan aims to lift the remaining evacuation restrictions by 2023 (FPG, 2021), it is likely that a considerable number of evacuees will never return because they have relocated permanently elsewhere (Budgen, 2021).

Recent radiological incidents that involved small releases of radiation and low risks to affected people, because protective actions were taken promptly, resulted in complex response to the incidents and in significant economic costs to achieve remediation at the applicable standards. One such incident is the release of a small amount of cesium, estimated to be about 1 curie (Ci) (37 gigabecquerels), during the recovery of a sealed cesium-137 source from the Harborview Research and Training Facility in Seattle, Washington, in 2019. The incident resulted in contamination (internal and external) of 13 individuals who received effective doses no greater than 0.55 mSv. Contamination of the facility forced more than 200 researchers and laboratory staff to relocate until recovery operations were complete, with direct effects on funded research programs. The projected costs for response, recovery, remediation, and reconstruction will exceed $100 million (NASEM, 2021b).

Effective communications and engagement with the impacted communities at all stages of the response to a nuclear or radiological incident are recognized by the U.S. government to be crucial as they can build credibility, inspire confidence, and ultimately contribute to an effective response. Similar to other aspects of preparing for a nuclear or radiological incident, a series of documents and tools is available.[19] Although different incidents present their

---

[18] Letter from Hisako Sakiyama, Kuniko Takagi, Yoshiyuki Segawa, Akiko Okumura, Yasuko Nagasoe, Noriko Nonaka, Tomio Negishi, and Akiko Ohashi to the committee, on February 12, 2022. According to the letter, the Government of Japan raised the public dose limit in the Fukushima Prefecture from 1 mSv per year to 20 mSv per year and stopped providing housing support to evacuees who refuse to return. The evacuees, however, especially those with small children, are concerned about risks associated with radiation exposures. The letter also states that several lawsuits have been filed by evacuees against the Japanese government claiming legitimacy of their evacuation and compensation for damages.

[19] Communication resources from different federal agencies are listed on EPA's website. See https://19january2021snapshot.epa.gov/radiation/pag-public-communication-resources_.html.

own communication challenges, questions about radiation risks (immediate and long term) from radioactive releases are expected to be central to all scenarios. Disagreement within the radiation community about health risks at low doses of radiation and the generally complicated terms and units used by experts to describe exposure may give the appearance of inconsistent public messaging and ultimately lead to loss of trust in those who deliver it (NASEM, 2019b). Communication about radiation risks with first responders, who typically only have basic training and understanding of radiation health effects, is also complicated. The Department of Homeland Security representative who briefed the committee noted that first responders are risk averse when it comes to radiation, and this aversion appears most often to derive from a lack of understanding or preconceptions about radiation effects and risks.[20]

2.1.6 Nuclear Weapons Program

The Manhattan Project (1942–1946) and the Cold War (1947–1991) involved activities related to nuclear weapons production and testing conducted under the auspices of the Atomic Energy Commission (AEC) and later DOE. Nuclear weapon production activities were carried out with a sense of urgency and under policies that demanded immense secrecy. At Hanford Nuclear Site, a site built in the 1940s to produce plutonium for nuclear weapons, volatile gases from fuel processing were vented directly into the atmosphere, and reactor cooling water contaminated with chemicals, metals, and radioactive materials was discharged into subsurface soil, groundwater, and the Columbia River, exposing populations in the surrounding areas to radiation. It was not until later that DOE released previously unavailable or classified documents about past operations. For example, in the mid-1980s, as a result of repeated Freedom of Information Act public requests and media stories, DOE released information on past operations at the Hanford Site. The released information showed that large amounts of iodine-131 (about 740,000 Ci or 2.73×10^{16} Bq; see Heeb et al., 1996; Napier, 2002) and other radioactive materials were released into the air from Hanford from 1944 through 1957.

In July 1945, the United States conducted the world's first atomic bomb test at the Trinity site south of Los Alamos, New Mexico. Soon after that, U.S. bombers dropped atomic bombs on Hiroshima and Nagasaki as part of a strategy to end World War II. After the war's end, the Cold War led to new national defense priorities and prompted the government to initiate a program of nuclear weapons testing. More than 1,000 atomic weapons tests took place between 1945 and 1992, the majority of which were conducted at the Nevada Test Site. Tests were also conducted in other places

---

[20] Jonathan Gill, Department of Homeland Security, presentation to the committee on October 27, 2021.

within the United States and the Marshall Islands, primarily on Bikini and Enewetak atolls, which were then designated as United Nations Trust Territory governed by the United States. Although most tests were underground tests, some were atmospheric tests in which the atomic weapons exploded at or above ground level, resulting in radioactive material being released into the atmosphere, some of which reached ground as nuclear fallout. In contrast to nuclear weapons production operations, nuclear tests were generally not a secret. The tests were considered events or spectacles announced in advance, and the public and test-site workers observed the events often with encouragement to do so at the expense of personal safety or protection (NRC, 2005). In 1955, the AEC distributed a booklet outlining the testing procedures (AEC, 1955) and generally underplayed the risks to the exposed populations. All areas of the United States received fallout from at least one nuclear weapons test, but larger amounts of I-131 from the Nevada Test Site fell over some parts of Utah, Colorado, Idaho, Nevada, and Montana.[21] The radioactive fallout from those tests represents a source of continuing exposure even today, albeit at very low levels (UNSCEAR, 2008).

The nuclear weapons program also resulted in radiation exposures to people employed in uranium mining and milling enterprises and their families from inhaled radon progeny and other hazards in the mines. People of the Navajo Nation worked the mines, often living and raising families in close proximity to the mines and mills. Navajo miners have reported that they were not educated about the hazards of uranium mining and were not provided with protective equipment or ventilation (Dawson, 1992). Today the mines are closed, but a legacy of uranium contamination remains, including more than 500 abandoned uranium mines as well as homes and water sources with elevated levels of radiation.[22] Disparities in tribal infrastructure, social and behavioral risk factors for disease, and complex environmental stressors are known to exacerbate risks for disease to Indigenous people (Lewis et al., 2017). These disparities also raise important health questions, for example, whether these communities are at higher risk of developing disease from low-dose radiation exposures and social questions regarding environmental injustice.

A variety of legal, political, and social actions taken by groups representing downwinders, test-site workers, veterans, and uranium workers pressured the government to accept liability for its actions and offer compensation for the damage. As a result, several compensation programs emerged, which are described in congressional testimony (U.S. Congress, House, 2021) and briefly in Box 2.1 in order of enactment.

---

[21] See https://www.cancer.gov/about-cancer/causes-prevention/risk/radiation/stateandcounty exposure.

[22] See https://www.epa.gov/navajo-nation-uranium-cleanup/abandoned-mines-cleanup#

Based on the input from community representatives to the committee, it is apparent that there is continuing distrust toward the U.S. government, and there is a belief that the U.S. government has failed to accept responsibility for past radiation exposures and has failed to develop programs that adequately compensate all impacted groups.[23] These groups include downwinders who resided in geographic areas outside those designated by the Radiation Exposure Compensation Act (RECA), uranium workers who worked in mines after 1971, and servicemen who were involved in the cleanup of Enewetak Atoll. The Radiation Exposure Compensation Act Amendments of 2021 (H.R. 5338) aim to extend and expand RECA to include several of these groups, but without further congressional action, RECA will expire in July 2022.

Distrust toward the U.S. government also continues within the Marshallese government and impacted atoll communities. The U.S. government officially returned the atolls to the Republic of the Marshall Islands in 1986. Today, all the atoll islands and the lagoon are accessible except for Runit Island, which contains a structure with radioactively contaminated soil and debris and therefore remains quarantined. Recently, concerns about the leaking structure and the rising sea level around the Marshall Islands led Congress to request that DOE provide a plan to repair the structure, evaluate the environmental effects on the lagoon over the next 20 years, and assess the potential risk to the people who live near it. DOE (2020a) found "no evidence to suggest that the containment structure represents a significant source of radiation exposure relative to other sources of residual radioactive fallout contamination on the atoll." The Marshallese government rebutted DOE's finding and noted that the agency is "downplaying" the risks and is declining to take responsibility for Runit Dome and its leaking contents.[24]

Human health studies on the impacts of nuclear weapons program activities are generally few and have inherent uncertainties, having been conducted decades after the initial exposures occurred when critical data on releases and exposures were often missing or were unreliable because of

---

[23] Stakeholder engagement panel discussion with President Jonathan Nez, Navajo Nation; Jill Jim, Navajo Nation Department of Health; Mary Dickson, representative of downwinders of U.S. nuclear tests; Keith Kiefer, National Commander of the National Association of Atomic Veterans; Benetick Maddison, Marshallese Educational Initiative (pre-recorded presentation); Arjun Makhijani, Institute for Energy and Environmental Research; Trisha Pritikin, Hanford Downwinder, author of *The Hanford Plaintiffs: Voices from the Fight for Atomic Justice*; and Beata Tsosie-Peña, Environmental Health and Justice Program at Tewa Women United in New Mexico (pre-recorded presentation) on October 28, 2021.

[24] Benetick Maddison, Marshallese Educational Initiative, pre-recorded presentation to the committee on October 28, 2021.

BOX 2.1
Radiation Compensation Programs Related to the U.S. Atomic Weapons Program

The Veterans Dioxin and Radiation Exposure Compensation Act administered by the Department of Veterans Affairs was enacted in 1984 to provide compensation for service-connected death or disability based on a veteran's exposure to ionizing radiation from the detonation of a nuclear device either in connection with testing or the American occupation of Hiroshima or Nagasaki, Japan. Exposure determination is made based on the estimated dose of radiation the veteran received while in service. Using this estimated dose and epidemiological formulas for radiation risk assessment established by the National Cancer Institute, the probability that a given veteran's medical condition was caused by his or her estimated dose of radiation is calculated. If this probability of causation is 50 percent or greater, benefits are awarded based on the level of disability.

The Radiation-Exposed Veterans Compensation Act (REVCA, origin 1988; amended 1992, 1989, 2004), also administered by the Department of Veterans Affairs, was established to some extent because veterans expressed concerns about the difficulty in receiving compensation under the 1984 law. Under REVCA, any veteran who participated in a specified radiation-risk activity and has one of the specified cancers is presumed to have a service-connected condition and is eligible for disability compensation.

The Radiation Exposure Compensation Act (RECA, origin 1990; amended 2000, 2002) administered by the Department of Justice provides compensation to civilian onsite participants who were involved in aboveground nuclear weapons tests at various U.S.-owned test sites in the United States and overseas; downwinders who at the time of the tests lived in parts of Nevada, Utah, and Arizona designated by RECA; and uranium miners, millers, and ore transporters who worked from 1942 to 1971, the last year of the federal government's procurement of uranium for atomic weapons. Eligibility of downwinders to the RECA program is based on whether the claimant has been diagnosed with any of the cancers or other diseases recognized as radiation related under the law and geographic location, but not on modeling the probability of causation.

The Energy Employees Occupational Illness Compensation Act (EEOICPA) was enacted in 2000 and is administered by the Department of Labor. It provides compensation to eligible Department of Energy nuclear weapons workers (including federal employees, contractors, and subcontractors) and compensation to certain eligible survivors. Many workers at the U.S. nuclear weapons production and testing sites have been defined under EEOICPA as Special Exposure Cohort status and do not have to undergo dose reconstruction to prove causation. Workers under this special status must be diagnosed with any of the radiogenic cancers or other diseases on the list within EEOICPA, and must have worked at the site in question for a minimum period of time.

Although not a formal compensation program, the federal government also provided payments and other forms of assistance to residents of the Marshall Islands.

inadequate recordkeeping and monitoring. A sample of these health studies and their conclusions are listed in Box 2.2. Many of these studies recognize the great uncertainty in the estimates of radiation doses and caution that the number of cancer cases possibly attributed to the exposures are also uncertain. Radiation from fallout from atmospheric weapons tests has been dramatically reduced by radioactive decay and weathering (NCRP, 2009a).

BOX 2.2
Sample of Studies on Health Impacts of Nuclear Weapons Program Activities

- A study of a small number of veterans involved in atmospheric testing who received doses up to about 30 millisieverts showed increased risk of leukemia compared to other servicemembers (Caldwell et al., 1980).
- A study of cancer mortality found a statistically significant increase in leukemia deaths among adults and children living downwind from the Nevada Test Site in southwestern Utah compared to those living in other parts of the state (Machado et al., 1987).
- A study of children exposed to radioactive iodine from nuclear weapons testing at the Nevada Test Site from 1951 through 1962 found an increased risk of thyroid neoplasms and autoimmune thyroiditis up to 30 years after exposure. The average dose to the thyroid in this study was 120 milligrays (mGy) (Lyon et al., 2006).
- A study estimated that the Nevada atomic weapons tests during the 1950s resulted in an average cumulative thyroid dose from iodine-131 fallout of 20 mGy for the U.S. population collectively and an average cumulative dose of 100 mGy for a large part of the population that was under age 20 at time of exposure. The report also cites that testing at the Nevada Test Site could have caused between 11,000 and 212,000 thyroid cancer cases, with a point or central estimate of 49,000 cases (NCI, 1997).
- A study of thyroid disease among people who were exposed to radioactive iodine from the Hanford Nuclear Site in Washington State, funded by the Centers for Disease Control and Prevention and carried out by the Seattle-based Fred Hutchinson Cancer Research Center, found no associations between Hanford's iodine-131 releases and thyroid disease (Davis et al., 2002). The National Academies, at the request of the Centers for Disease Control and Prevention, provided an independent assessment of the Hanford Thyroid Disease Study and concluded that it was well designed but that researchers reported the findings as more conclusive than they were (NRC, 2000). A community-participatory health study suggested an excess of illnesses among Hanford Downwinders (Nussbaum et al., 2004).
- A study showed that the 1945 New Mexico Trinity Test resulted in doses <0.1 mGy for the vast majority of the population in the surrounding area and could be linked with 250 to 1,000 cancers due to radiation exposure from the fallout (Cahoon et al., 2021; Simon et al., 2020).

2.1.7 Nuclear Waste Management

As the Cold War came to a close in 1991, the United States shifted its focus from nuclear weapons production to remediation of nuclear weapons production facilities. Management of nuclear weapons legacy waste is often used as a demonstration that the federal government is making large expenditures of taxpayer funds to address uncertain and in some cases potentially low or non-existent risks to current and future generations due to exposures to low doses of radiation (Blush and Heitman, 1995). Others have stated that the assumption that even low doses of radiation carry risks make radiation contamination cleanup goals stricter, resulting in extraordinary cleanup costs (Cardarelli and Ulsh, 2018) and misallocation of scarce national resources. Implementation of less stringent regulatory measures and cleanup criteria could accelerate cleanup and result in billions of dollars in savings.

Cleanup of nuclear weapons legacy waste is primarily the responsibility of the DOE-Environmental Management (EM) cleanup program. The program was established in 1989 and has cleaned up 91 sites at a cost of about $170 billion (GAO, 2019). However, the largest and most complex sites—the Hanford Site in Washington, the Savannah River Site in South Carolina, the Oak Ridge Reservation in Tennessee, the Idaho Site, and the Portsmouth Site in Ohio—still require remediation. At all these sites, radioactive and other hazardous contaminants are present in soil, waste burial grounds, groundwater, or surface water. DOE-EM projects related to cleanup of the remaining 16 sites will continue for at least another 50 years (until 2070 or beyond) at an estimated cost of $406 billion (GAO, 2021). DOE's cleanup responsibilities are almost certainly underestimated because many of the cleanup technical challenges have not yet been sufficiently characterized and costs have not been estimated (NASEM, 2019a).

Doses to the populations living near nuclear facilities that currently hold legacy waste are considered to be very low. According to the National Council on Radiation Protection and Measurements (NCRP, 2009a), the annual exposure to a maximally exposed individual (MEI)[25] ranges from a few microsieverts (μSv) to a fraction of a μSv. For example, the annual exposure to the MEI is estimated to be 8.5 μSv for the Portsmouth Gaseous Diffusion Plant and 0.1–0.6 μSv for the Hanford Site. Still, the lives of communities living near the nuclear waste sites are disrupted by cleanup activities and decisions about these activities, with Indigenous communities being disproportionately impacted. At Hanford, environmental contamination of the land and Columbia River (see Figure 2.4) has presented a health risk to

---

[25] DOE defines an MEI as a hypothetical individual who because of proximity, activities, and living habits would receive the highest radiation dose, taking into account all pathways, from a given event, process, or facility. See https://www.directives.doe.gov/terms_definitions/maximally-exposed-individual.

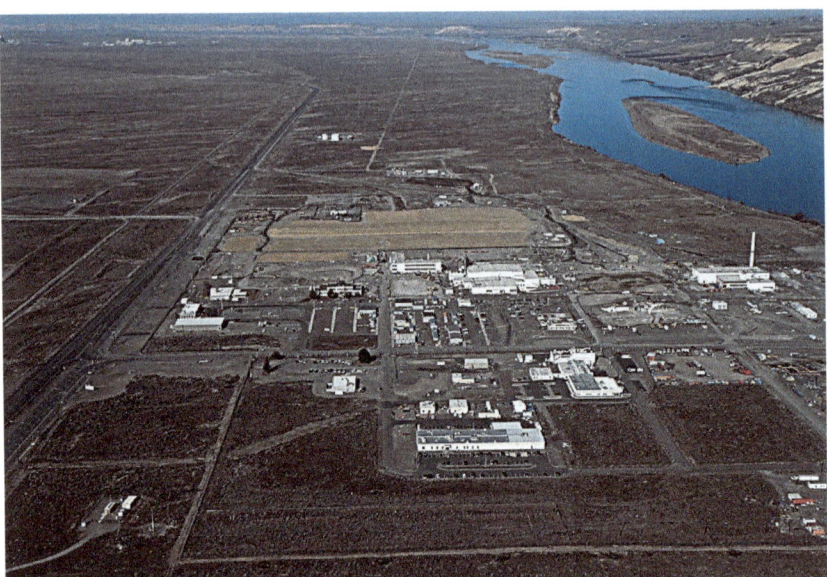

FIGURE 2.4 Area at Hanford Site (known as 300 Area) at one time dedicated to uranium fuel fabrication operations. Six small-scale nuclear reactors were located in this area, which is adjacent to the Columbia River. SOURCE: Department of Energy, https://www.hanford.gov/page.cfm/RL/RiverCorridor.

members of the Yakama Indian nation, the Umatilla Tribe, the Wanapum, and the Nez Perce Tribe, and has impacted their cultures as they can no longer use the land for farming, hunting, fishing, or ceremonial purposes.[26] Many of the impacted tribes are engaged with the federal government to develop strategies to restore the habitat of the Columbia basin, but unmet milestones and violated agreements[27] create issues of distrust.

Concerns about health effects from legacy waste continue to be raised by other communities near nuclear facilities that hold legacy waste and are still in the process of remediation. For example, the 2019 discovery of trace amounts of neptunium-237 near the Zahn's Corner Middle School in proximity to the Portsmouth Gaseous Diffusion Plant prompted the closing of the school and attracted national media attention. The news stories highlighted the local community's distrust of DOE, which was exacerbated

---

[26] See https://www.atomicheritage.org/history/native-americans-and-manhattan-project.

[27] Cleanup schedule milestones and endpoints are described in legally enforceable agreements with states and regulators that govern the work to be done. Most of DOE's major sites have more than one agreement in place. For example, DOE, EPA, and the State of Washington Department of Ecology signed a cleanup and compliance agreement (known as the Tri-Party Agreement) in 1989 for cleanup work to be carried out at the Hanford Site. See https://www.atg.wa.gov/hanford for legal actions related to unmet milestones of the Tri-Party Agreement.

by the delayed release of the 2017 environmental report that first detected the contamination (Ali, 2019). There has been an ongoing discussion about independent examination of the contamination and risks. Concerns about health effects have also been raised by communities near nuclear facilities where cleanup activities have been completed, such as Rocky Flats in Colorado (Tabachnik, 2019).

The lingering mistrust of DOE's nuclear waste cleanup program is at least partly due to the agency being relatively slow in stakeholder involvement and risk communication for its cleanup program. In 1978, DOE established the New Mexico Environmental Evaluation Group (EEG) to conduct an independent technical evaluation of the potential for radiation exposure to people near the Waste Isolation Pilot Plant (WIPP) Project which became operational in 1999 for the disposal of transuranic radioactive wastes generated by the national defense programs (Neill et al., 1996). EEG was defunded in 2004. Among the last activities conducted by EEG was a workshop on technical issues regarding some of the high-level waste tanks at the Hanford Site and whether some of the wastes could be disposed of at WIPP.[28]

Based on the recommendation of the National Research Council (NRC, 1994) to involve academia to provide more trust in cleanup activities, DOE began to fund university-based programs. The Consortium for Risk Evaluation with Stakeholder Participation (CRESP), a partnership among university researchers, has been a major recipient of the funding and has been working with DOE through cooperative agreements since 1995. Research goals of these agreements have been largely based on eliciting community concerns and on helping DOE-EM make cleanup decisions by reducing significant uncertainty about risks at the nuclear waste sites that interferes with or delays implementation of cleanup.

CRESP aims to better address citizens' concerns and needs by engaging with stakeholders and integrating their input into the research process from problem formulation, to analysis of data, to dissemination of research findings (Goldstein et al., 1999). An example of CRESP's approach is the involvement of the Aleut people in testing radionuclide levels in biota, subsistence foods, and commercial fish on and around Amchitka Island in southwest Alaska, a site of three underground nuclear tests from 1965 to 1971. CRESP's participatory approach resulted in acceptance of the testing results by the impacted communities and termination of DOE's managerial responsibility for the site (Burger et al., 2009). Despite this and other examples that demonstrate the effectiveness of CRESP in engaging with

---

[28] See http://www.sric.org/nuclear/eeg.php.

communities around nuclear sites, some have expressed concerns about CRESP's independence from DOE.[29]

2.2 CURRENT EPIDEMIOLOGICAL EVIDENCE ON LOW-DOSE RADIATION HEALTH EFFECTS

This section summarizes some epidemiological evidence of low-dose radiation health effects. Similar to Section 2.1, the committee does not make an attempt to provide a complete review of the existing literature. The primary focus of the section is on most recent studies on the adverse health effect discussed to indicate the current state of knowledge.

Cancer is the most well-established and most studied adverse health effect following exposure to radiation (Section 2.2.1). Recently, associations of other adverse health outcomes including cardiovascular disease (Section 2.2.2), neurological disorders (Section 2.2.3), immune dysfunction (Section 2.2.4), and cataracts and other lens opacities (Section 2.2.5) have been observed at doses lower than previously considered important for these effects. Heritable genetic effects (Section 2.2.6) are also a concern following low-dose radiation exposures. As a result, there is increasing interest in the radiation research and radiation protection communities to better understand the risks and mechanisms of radiation effects at low doses and low dose rates. Research into the mechanisms of low-dose radiation effects has the potential to contribute to improved understanding of risks of adverse health outcomes in humans and into the factors that modulate these risks. Some proposed mechanisms for the radiation-linked health effects are also discussed in this section.

2.2.1 Cancer

Cancer is the most well-established adverse health effect following exposure to radiation, and, accordingly, the extensive literature on this topic is reviewed in a number of publications (Berrington de González et al., 2017; Hauptmann et al., 2020; Kitahara et al., 2015; Little et al., 2022b; Rühm et al., 2022; UNSCEAR, 2006a). The following subsections briefly describe the state of knowledge regarding radiation-related cancer risks following postnatal exposure and exposure in utero, focusing on low-dose exposures.

Postnatal Exposures

Radiation-related cancer risks differ by organ or tissue. The most radiosensitive tissues are the bone marrow, brain, thyroid, skin, and breast,

---
[29] Letters to the committee from impacted community members and members of advocacy groups on January 6, 2022, and February 1, 2022.

although cancer risks have been demonstrated following radiation exposure for nearly every tissue and organ in the body. Cancers that have not been convincingly or consistently linked to low-dose radiation include chronic lymphocytic leukemia, Hodgkin's and non-Hodgkin's lymphoma, and melanoma (Boice et al., 2022b). Compelling evidence based on results from various exposure scenarios supports that, for a given dose, cancer risks are higher among individuals exposed at younger ages. Sex has also been shown to modify the radiation dose-response relationship, and in some cases higher risks are reported for women compared to men (ICRP, 2007; see additional discussion in Chapter 5).

The key data on these observations derive from the Japanese atomic bombing survivor cohorts for individuals of all ages (see Section 4.5.6) and from medical exposures (particularly CT scans, as reviewed in Section 2.1.2), natural background radiation (Section 2.1.1) in childhood, and occupational exposures (Section 2.1.3) in adulthood. The evidence from these studies is also generally consistent with a linear relationship between radiation dose and cancer risk across the dose ranges investigated, even <100 mGy, albeit with different magnitudes of risk for different sexes and tissues. However, a nonlinear relationship at low doses cannot be ruled out. Although substantial data have been presented on the modification of radiation-related risks by age at exposure, data on other potential modifiers of risk are sparse and generally inconsistent.

In Utero Exposures

Overall, in utero exposure studies have revealed that the risk of developing cancer following radiation exposure is no greater than that following exposure during early childhood. The association between low doses of ionizing radiation received by the fetus in utero from diagnostic radiography and the subsequent risk of cancer in childhood was initially reported in the 1950s when the frequent use of abdominal X-ray for pregnant women in the United Kingdom was common. At the time and until about 1975, the frequency of abdominal X-raying of pregnant women accounted for 10–15 percent of all pregnancies and >90 percent during the third trimester. The *Oxford Survey* of Childhood Cancers (OSCC) was the first and largest in utero exposure study to provide risk estimates with reasonable precision. The fetal dose received was around 10 mGy of X-rays, and the excess absolute risk coefficient at this level of exposure is approximately 6 percent per gray (Doll and Wakeford, 1997; Wakeford and Little, 2003). OSCC found an almost uniformly raised relative risk for nearly all types of cancer that are most frequent in children. This uniformity in cancer risk is the most notable argument against the observed associations being causal. A recent study compared the results found in OSCC with those of all other case-control and case-cohort studies (Wakeford and Bithell, 2021). The study found that the meta-analysis of the case-control and case-cohort studies also showed consistent and clear elevations of risk for all types of childhood cancer combined, all leukemia, and all cancers except leukemia combined. The expert who briefed the committee, who was also the author of the study, noted that on the balance of the evidence, it seems likely that this association has a cause-and-effect interpretation, but greater understanding of biological mechanisms is required for definitive conclusions to be drawn for specific types of cancer.[30]

In the Japanese atomic bombing survivor cohorts, individuals exposed in utero received a range of doses with an estimated mean dose of 122.9 mGy, but about half received less than 5 mGy (using maternal uterine dose as a proxy; Sugiyama et al., 2021). Early studies of the atomic bombing survivors showed impaired physical and mental development among children exposed in utero. Associations between in utero exposure and excess cancer mortality or incidence were not observed until later when there was sufficient accumulation of data that accompanied the aging of the cohort (Ozasa et al., 2018). The magnitude of the risks was comparable to those observed in survivors who were exposed at young age (Preston et al., 2008). The most recent update found that atomic bomb radiation was associated with mortality from solid cancer for females but not males (Sugiyama et al., 2021). Only a small portion (14 percent) of the survivors exposed in utero had died at the end of follow-up, so this cohort is expected to continue to provide valuable information on the effects of in utero exposure and cancer mortality later in life. Long-term excess occurrences of leukemia following in utero exposure in the atomic bombing survivor cohorts have not been observed, but these results need to be interpreted cautiously due to the shorter latency period between radiation exposure and leukemia compared with solid tumors.

2.2.2 Cardiovascular Disease

The heart and vasculature have long been recognized as potential targets for the adverse effects of radiation exposure at high doses (see, e.g., HPA, 2010; ICRP, 2012). A substantial body of evidence relating to the effects of radiation on the heart comes from studies following breast cancer patients after radiotherapy, where doses to the heart are on the order of 1–2 Gy and disease presents 10–20 years after exposure (ICRP, 2012). Risk from lower and more protracted exposures has also been observed, for example, in studies of the Japanese atomic bombing survivors

---

[30] Richard Wakeford, University of Manchester, United Kingdom, presentation to the committee on November 16, 2021.

(Ozasa et al., 2012) and in occupational exposure studies (Azizova et al., 2018; Gillies et al., 2017). In 2012, ICRP issued a statement that "medical practitioners should be made aware that the absorbed dose threshold for circulatory disease may be as low as 0.5 Gy to the heart or brain" (ICRP, 2012). Since the ICRP statement was issued, several analyses and meta-analyses of low-dose radiation epidemiological studies have been published (e.g., Azizova et al., 2018; Gillies et al., 2017; Little et al., 2012, 2021a; Ozasa et al., 2012; Rajaraman et al., 2016; Tran et al., 2017; Zhang et al., 2019). Some of the analyses and meta-analyses indicate an elevation of risk at doses less than 500 mGy (e.g., Little et al., 2012; Tran et al., 2017) and that risk of circulatory disease may follow a linear dose-risk relationship at doses below 500 mGy (Little et al., 2012). Other findings include a reduction in risk with increasing time since exposure (Tran et al., 2017) and an inverse dose-fractionation association in ischemic heart disease mortality in the Canadian Fluoroscopy Cohort Study (Zablotska et al., 2014b). Given the high prevalence of cardiovascular disease, if these associations are confirmed, the estimates of overall radiation-related mortality would approximately double compared with the current estimates based on cancer alone (Little et al., 2012). Many of the epidemiological studies have not fully controlled for potential confounding exposures, notably tobacco smoking and alcohol consumption, and therefore explanations for the observed increased risk in cardiovascular disease other than radiation are plausible (Wakeford, 2019).

2.2.3 Neurological Disorders

The adverse effects of high-dose radiation (Armstrong et al., 2010; Chen et al., 2015) and of radiation exposure prenatally (Black et al., 2019; NCRP, 2013; Otake and Schull, 1998) on neurological disorders are well established. However, the effects of postnatal radiation exposure on neurological disorders including cognitive impairment at low doses and low dose rates are poorly characterized in part because of the difficulty in exploring cognitive deficits in experimental animals and because of the difficulty in discerning the subtle changes that need to be measured at low doses.

Studies funded by the National Aeronautics and Space Administration documented some evidence of cognitive dysfunction in rodent systems, predominantly following high linear energy transfer (LET) GCR exposures to brain tissue (Jones et al., 2020; Perez et al., 2020), including possible inflammatory responses in the central nervous system (Rola et al., 2005). Cognitive decline is likely the result of damage in multiple neural cell types due to vascular changes, glial and neuronal cell function, decreased neurogenesis, and an enhanced inflammation in the central nervous system (Hladik and Tapio, 2016).

In population studies that involve low-LET radiation, Chernobyl cleanup workers were reported to have some cognitive impairment related to effects on the hippocampus, and the effects were evident among workers with doses above 100 mSv, particularly among those with doses above 500 mSv (Bazyka et al., 2015). Blomstrand et al. (2014) noted few cognitive effects following low-dose irradiation of the infant brain in a population-based cohort study in Sweden. More recently, Azizova et al. (2020) demonstrated a linear association of Parkinson's disease incidence within the Mayak Worker study[31] with cumulative dose from external radiation exposure to the brain above 100 mGy, and the risk estimate increased with increasing dose. The Million Person Study is also addressing the issue of low-dose and low-dose-rate exposures and the impact on dementia, Alzheimer's disease, Parkinson's disease, motor neuron disease, and cognitive impairment, with some unpublished data suggesting the presence of an effect for some of these adverse health outcomes (Boice et al., 2021).

A recent review of the literature on possible cognitive impairment at low doses of radiation concluded that both biological and epidemiological research provide evidence for an effect, but a better characterization of the effects and improved understanding of the mechanisms are needed (Pasqual et al., 2021).

2.2.4 Immune Dysfunction

A comprehensive review of available data on radiation effects on the immune system was published by the United Nations Scientific Committee on the Effects of Atomic Radiation (UNSCEAR, 2006b) and recently updated with a focus on low-dose radiation effects (UNSCEAR, 2021). This and subsequent evidence indicate that radiation at low doses can significantly alter immune homeostasis by changing the balance within the immune system, its functional integrity, and overall resilience (Lumniczky et al., 2021). Epidemiological, clinical, and experimental studies at low doses in this field tend to report rather subtle changes compared with the more dramatic effects of high-dose exposures, where cytotoxicity plays a major role in immune response, and the clinical effects of this immune dysfunction remain poorly understood.

There is some clinical and experimental evidence that low-dose radiation can drive the functional profile of CD4$^+$ T cells toward a Th2

---

[31] The study follows workers, both men and women, who during the period 1948–1982 were employed at the Mayak Production Association, the first nuclear complex in the former Soviet Union. Workers were exposed to external gamma rays and to internal exposures from plutonium inhalation which were relatively high during the early years of operations of the nuclear complex.

phenotype.[32] CD8+ T-cell damage tends to be less consistent, perhaps because of variation in radioresistance, which may be associated with activation status. A rise in rare double negative CD4−CD8−, alpha/beta T cells has also been reported (Kusunoki et al., 2003; Kyoizumi et al., 2010), which in a non-radiation setting has been associated with lymphadenopathy and splenomegaly, autoimmunity, and autoimmune lymphoproliferative syndrome (Bleesing et al., 2002). Dose-dependent increases in T-cell receptor (TCR) mutant frequency were noted in Chernobyl cleanup workers (Saenko et al., 2011) while the TCR repertoire seems more limited, at least in atomic bombing survivors, which may be associated with low-grade inflammation later in life that involves myeloid cells, known as inflammaging, or defective thymic output (Denkinger et al., 2015; Franceschi et al., 2019; Fulop et al., 2018; Kusunoki and Hayashi, 2008; Kyoizumi et al., 2010).

Epidemiological evidence generally points to the peripheral lymphocyte balance shifting in favor of B cells with increased serum immunoglobulin (Ig) levels and some degree of humoral immune enhancement, even when some individuals seem more prone to certain bacterial infections. However, a dose-dependent decrease in B cells, activation of T cells, and increase in cytokine interleukin (IL)-1 levels can also be seen in individuals externally exposed to whole-body doses below 100 mSv in Chernobyl studies (Ilienko et al., 2018).

Experimental studies of the functional effects of low-dose radiation on humoral immunity are few but stimulatory effects are also generally seen on natural killer (NK) cells. Although these studies are often short term and performed in vitro, Oradovskaia et al. (2011) studied a cohort of cleanup workers who developed malignant disease, and they identified reduced CD3+CD4+ T-cell levels, increased CD8+ T-cell levels, a reduced CD4/CD8 ratio, and a prevalence of NK T cells over conventional NK cells 1–3 years before the manifestation of cancer. Radiation exposure increased the frequency and counts of monocytes in a dose-dependent fashion, and this increase was more evident after 60 years, showing a possible acceleration of age-dependent clonal hematopoiesis (Yoshida et al., 2019). However, among the elderly atomic bombing survivors, response to vaccination did not appear to be impaired by radiation exposure early in life (Hayashi et al., 2018). The perturbed lymphocyte homeostasis, especially at the level of the TCR and the skewing toward memory over naïve subsets, combined with the myeloid shifts that can alter the antigenic epitopes that are presented,

---

[32] A Th2 profile is indicative of T helper cell differentiation toward production of interleukin (IL)-4, IL-5, IL-9, or IL-13 and has been historically seen as a sign of an immune system skewed toward B-cell activation and antibody production. The Th2 profile is often seen in diametrical opposition to the TNF-alpha, IFN-gamma, and GM-CSF pro-inflammatory Th1 profile needed for macrophage and cytotoxic T-cell activation during cell-mediated immunity and delayed-type hypersensitivity.

provide the framework for induction of symptomatic immune dysfunctions that are clinically relevant such as infections, allergies, autoimmunity, and immunoproliferative diseases. Although it is tempting to relate some of these observations to the anti-inflammatory effects of low-to-moderate doses of low- and high-LET radiation that have frequently been reported to improve the clinical symptoms in individuals with local inflammatory conditions (Donaubauer et al., 2021; Micke et al., 2017; Trott and Kamprad, 1999), long-term observations of cohorts exposed to acute or chronic low doses of radiation indicate a pro-inflammatory immune profile, which might contribute to chronic immune dysfunction and disease.

2.2.5 Cataracts

Cataracts are defined as the opacity or clouding of the lens of the eye, a process that is typically associated with aging (Hamada et al., 2020). It is the leading cause of visual impairment in the world and can be repaired through surgery and replacement with an artificial lens. Classification of cataracts falls into three major categories: cortical, nuclear, and posterior subcapsular (PSC), with PSCs and cortical associated directly with radiation exposure (Hamada et al., 2020). The eye lens is considered one of the most radiosensitive tissues; biological and mechanistic studies in in vitro and in vivo studies have determined that DNA damage and repair mechanisms, extracellular matrix effects, membrane damage, dysregulation in protein and gene expression, and oxidative damage and intercellular communication are some of the processes contributing to lens opacity and cataract development (Ainsbury et al., 2021, 2022; Hamada et al., 2020). Morbidities and environmental exposures other than radiation can also contribute to cataract development.

For more than 50 years, cataracts were considered a tissue reaction with a threshold of absorbed dose to the eye of 2 Gy and annual dose limits to the lens were set at 150 mSv. As more sensitive detection methods for cataracts emerged, the threshold was reduced to 500 mGy (Neriishi et al., 2007), resulting in further reduction of the equivalent dose limits to the lens of the eye for occupational exposures to 20 mSv averaged over 5 years, not to exceed 50 mSv in 1 year (ICRP, 2012; see also discussion in Section 3.3 for NCRP, 2016 recommendation). Shore (2016) reviewed epidemiological data reported since the 2012 ICRP publication and suggested that there could be a dose threshold somewhere between a few hundred mGy and 1 Gy, with little or no excess risk below 100 mGy. Another review by Thome et al. (2018) that included data from the Japanese atomic bombing survivors, Chernobyl cleanup workers, medical workers, and radiotherapy patients suggested that the evidence of an increase in cataract formation at doses below 500 mGy was inconclusive.

New studies continue to provide evidence of radiation-induced cataract at lower doses. The Mayak worker study has shown that the risk for cataracts increased linearly with chronic cumulative effective dose from external gamma rays at ≥250 mSv (Ainsbury et al., 2021). The U.S. Radiologic Technologists cohort study, on the other hand, suggested that radiation exposure at lower doses (<100 mGy) and low dose rates (<0.0005 Gy/h) can indeed lead to cataract development (Ainsbury et al., 2021; Little et al., 2020a,b, 2021a). In general, epidemiological evidence supports a lack of a clear dose-rate effect, with more data needed for a decision on dose-rate dependence (Ainsbury et al., 2021). Regarding high-LET radiation, there is clear evidence of cataract development in astronauts, although collection of epidemiological data was discontinued in 2012 (Hamada et al., 2020). Interventional cardiologists also show an increased risk for PSC opacities (Elmaraezy et al., 2017), seen also in populations living in high background areas, such as in the area of Yangjiang, Guangdong, China (Ainsbury et al., 2021).

2.2.6 Heritable Genetic Effects

A main concern of populations exposed to radiation, including the Japanese atomic bombing survivors, those exposed to radiation from the Chernobyl and Fukushima nuclear power plant accidents (Suzuki et al., 2018), and cancer survivors who undergo radiation therapy, has been the induction of heritable genetic effects due to damage to the DNA of germ cells in the gonads that can cause gene mutations. These mutations, in contrast to mutations in somatic cells, can be transmitted from generation to generation. Heritable genetic effects can include, but are not limited to, malformations, metabolic disorders, chromosome aberrations, and other effects. Although early experimental findings in fruit flies (Muller, 1927) and mice (Russell, 1951) have indicated that ionizing radiation causes heritable genetic effects, human data have not replicated the early experimental findings and often have had limited statistical power owing to small sample size, low gonadal dose, lack of dosimetry information, or inadequate comparison groups (Boice and Miller, 1999; Lim et al., 2015; Signorello et al., 2010).

Among the first studies of the atomic bombing survivors to explore possible heritable genetic effects were studies of untoward pregnancy outcomes such as major congenital malformations, stillbirths, or neonatal deaths, among births to both maternal and paternal survivors. Past analyses of untoward pregnancy outcomes among the survivors (Neel and Schull, 1956; Otake et al., 1990; Schull et al., 1981) generally showed a positive association between total parental dose and the frequency of untoward pregnancy outcomes, but they did not identify significant associations. Researchers updated the latest analysis to account for malformations that were not included in the 1990 analysis due to different inclusion/exclusion criteria and for updated estimates of gonadal dose (Yamada et al., 2021). The updated analysis showed that parental exposure to radiation was associated with increased risk of major congenital malformations and perinatal death, but the estimates were imprecise for direct radiation effects, and most were not statistically significant. The mean maternal, paternal, and conjoint doses were 30 mGy, 20 mGy, and 50 mGy, respectively (Yamada et al., 2021). The investigators discuss that harsh living conditions and the limited socioeconomic resources available to heavily exposed atomic bombing survivors after the war might have led to an overestimate of genetic effects of radiation and suggest that additional insights on radiation and reproduction might be gained by using contemporary genomic methods to compare the DNA of parents irradiated by the bombings with that of their children (Yamada et al., 2021).

Studies of the offspring of the atomic bombing survivors (F1) also aim to understand the potential heritable genetic effects of radiation by addressing whether radiation-induced mutations that might have been passed to the children of the survivors alter cancer and non-cancer incidence and mortality rates. These studies showed no increase in the children's mortality rates in relation to parental gonadal exposure (Grant et al., 2015). In addition, earlier molecular analyses of the F1 cohort for possible heritable genetic effects of radiation showed no changes in the sex ratio of births, no increases of chromosomal aberrations among children of exposed parents (Neel, 1998), and no changes in mutation rates at microsatellite loci (Kodaira et al., 2010). Planned genetic analysis of 1,000 parent–child trios, in which parents received varied levels of radiation exposure due to the bombings and children were conceived after the bombings, could help better understand the overall effects of preconception exposure to radiation on this population and on humans in general.[33]

Trio studies have been conducted using samples from individuals exposed to radiation from the Chernobyl accident. In 2021, NCI and collaborators published the findings of a study that highlighted how advances in DNA sequencing technology and comprehensive genomic analysis in well-designed epidemiological studies can enable addressing questions related to hereditary effects of radiation (Yeager et al., 2021). Investigators analyzed the complete genomes of 130 individuals born between 1987 and 2002 (i.e., between 46 weeks and 15 years after the accident) to parents exposed to radiation from the 1986 Chernobyl accident and their 105 mother–father pairs. The parents were exposed because they were either cleanup workers or residents who had been evacuated because they lived in close proximity

---

[33] Robert Ullrich, Radiation Effects Research Foundation, presentation to the committee on January 24, 2022.

to the accident site. The study found no evidence that radiation exposure to parents resulted in new genetic changes (de novo mutations) being passed from parent to child regardless of cumulative preconception gonadal paternal (mean dose 365 mGy) or maternal (mean dose 19 mGy) exposure to radiation.

Survivors of childhood cancers and their children are the largest group of people exposed to high doses of radiation for therapeutic purposes before reproduction and can provide insights on the potential heritable genetic effects of radiation. The Childhood Cancer Survivor Study provided evidence that the children of cancer survivors are not at significantly increased risk for congenital anomalies due to their parent's exposure to radiation or other mutagenic cancer treatments. The mean ovarian radiation dose in this study was 1.19 Gy and the testicular radiation dose was 0.48 Gy (Signorello et al., 2012). Tawn et al. (2011) also reported no increases in mutation rates among children born to survivors of childhood cancer who had received radiotherapy.

2.3 CHAPTER SUMMARY AND FINDING

The U.S. population is exposed or could potentially be exposed to low-dose and low-dose-rate radiation from a number of different sources including natural radiation sources, medical applications, occupational exposures, nuclear power routine operations and accidental releases, nuclear or radiological incidents, the nuclear weapons program, and nuclear waste management. These sources are important in terms of low-dose and low-dose-rate exposures either because they contribute a large portion to the average annual dose to the U.S. general population or to specific populations (e.g., medical applications), or they are of concern to members of the public and impacted communities (e.g., nuclear waste management) or to current and future U.S. policies and plans (e.g., nuclear power operations).

These low-dose radiation sources involve different types of radiation (e.g., alpha, beta, or gamma), routes of exposure (internal or external), and duration of exposure (acute or protracted). Today, in the absence of a mechanistic understanding of different low-dose and dose-rate radiation sources and their direct health effects, estimation of risks and decisions related to exposures from substantially different sources are often made using the same generic approach—by relying on risk estimates derived from higher, acute, external exposures to radiation, largely of the Japanese atomic bombing survivors, and applying appropriate correction factors.

Finding 1: A coordinated multidisciplinary low-dose radiation research program in the United States can improve understanding of adverse human health effects from exposures to radiation at doses and dose rates of relevance to the U.S. population. In addition, this program can identify mechanisms for induction of these health effects, develop improved risk models for doses and dose rates at which direct measurement of risks is not currently possible, and ultimately develop more individualized risk estimates.

3

Scientific Basis for Radiation Protection

This chapter provides background information on the radiation protection framework in the United States (Section 3.1) and the agencies with radiation protection responsibilities (Section 3.2), and it discusses how new science is incorporated in the radiation protection framework (Section 3.3). This chapter also attempts to address the seventh charge of the Statement of Task, which asks the committee to identify and, to the extent possible, quantify potential monetary and health-related impacts to federal agencies, the general public, industry, research communities, and other users of information produced by such a research program. The committee explains why it cannot provide a quantitative assessment of the economic impacts. Instead, the committee offers its assessment of whether knowledge from low-dose radiation research can affect the decision-making frameworks in the federal regulatory system and how (Section 3.4).

3.1 THE RADIATION PROTECTION FRAMEWORK

Governments around the world manage health, safety, and environmental risks from radiation through regulations and guidance that shape radiation protection systems. In the case of human health, these systems aim to avoid tissue reactions and keep stochastic effects (cancer and hereditary effects) to a level as low as reasonably achievable (ALARA)[1] by considering the estimated risks and the benefit to the individual or society derived from the use of the

---

[1] Based on the ALARA principle, even a low-dose exposure below the regulatory limit or proposed guideline needs to be avoided. See https://www.nrc.gov/reading-rm/basic-ref/glossary/alara.html.

particular application (ICRP, 2007). The basic approaches to radiation protection are consistent globally. Low-dose radiation protection standards have been developed to be applied for prospective planning purposes, and the associated regulation and guidance and, more specifically, dose limits are derived on the basis of a notional sex- and age-averaged person and are therefore not indicative of the outcome to any one individual. Radiation protection systems have evolved and will continue to evolve as scientific knowledge increases and the applications of radiation change in nature and scope (Clement et al., 2021).

Exposures to low levels of radiation may carry low levels of risk to an exposed individual; nonetheless they are a high priority for the radiation protection system, and the vast majority of regulations and guidance in the radiation protection system tend to address low-dose radiation exposures. In the absence of clear evidence of risks at low doses of radiation, radiation

---

BOX 3.1
Current Assumptions of the Radiation Protection System

The radiation protection system does the following:

1. Estimates cancer risks resulting from low-dose and low-dose-rate exposures based on interpolations from health effects observed in populations that were exposed to higher doses of radiation and to types of radiation that are different from those that may be of most relevance to the general population.
2. Assumes that there are hereditary effects following low-dose exposures, despite minimal evidence to date of such effects in humans. Estimates of risks for hereditary effects for protection purposes are based on animal experiments.
3. Assumes that cancer stochastic effects persist at exposure levels below those for which there currently exists direct evidence from epidemiological studies.
4. Assumes that stochastic effects are limited to cancer, despite accumulating evidence of effects on non-cancer outcomes including circulatory diseases, neurological disorders, immune dysfunction, and cataracts[a] following low-dose and low-dose-rate exposures in human studies.
5. Derives risk estimates from population averages that do not account for the known or potential variation in sensitivity among individuals due to genetic, lifestyle, and environmental factors.
6. Does not specifically consider more recently discovered mechanisms for tissue, cellular, and genetic regulation, such as epigenetic modification, cellular senescence, and aging.

---

[a] Cataracts have historically been included in radiation protection frameworks but have been regulated as a tissue reaction rather than a stochastic effect.

protection systems are based on certain assumptions about the possible risks (see Box 3.1).

The standard model used by regulatory agencies to describe the relationship between radiation dose and cancer risk is the *linear no-threshold* (LNT) model. This relatively simple model assumes that the excess risk of cancer from exposure to low doses of radiation is not zero regardless of how small the dose is (i.e., there is no threshold below which there is no effect) and that the excess risk is proportional to the dose of radiation (i.e., the risk increases as the dose increases). While a linear association between radiation dose and cancer risk has been established at moderate to high doses, linearity at low doses is typically assumed based on models that fit over the full dose range.

The LNT model has provided an adequate fit to the data from several major epidemiological studies of cancer risk following radiation exposures, including the Life Span Study of the Japanese atomic bomb survivors. Although no alternative model has convincingly been shown to provide a better fit to these data (Hauptmann et al., 2020; NCRP, 2018a; UNSCEAR, 2020a), recent analyses of the Life Span Study data have suggested a linear-quadratic association[2] of radiation dose with cancer risk when considering all solid cancers together, although such a nonlinear association could arise due to different associations of radiation dose with risk for different types of cancer (Brenner et al., 2022).

The use of the LNT model to describe risks in the low-dose range is also supported by biophysical arguments regarding the stochastic nature of ionizing radiation energy deposition. At least two biological processes have been identified in vitro which suggest a nonlinear induction of radiation effects at low doses. These are bystander effects observed in the vicinity of cells irradiated with alpha particles and adaptive response of cells exposed to low doses of ionizing radiation (Hamada et al., 2011; Morgan, 2003a,b; Rühm et al., 2017). Still, the use of the LNT model for radiation protection purposes is often justified as being "conservative" (Puskin, 2009).

LNT has been used in radiation protection as a regulatory model for more than 40 years and is also used in regulating chemical carcinogens (see Clewell et al., 2019, for review). For regulatory purposes it is assumed that the burden of proof for a model other than LNT is on those who suggest a different model. In addition to the LNT model (curve "a" in Figure 3.1), four other basic model options might be considered to describe risks following low doses of radiation (but not equally plausible, based on current knowledge): downward curving (decreasing slope, curve "b"), upward

---

[2] That means that at higher doses and dose rates, risk increases more sharply than at lower doses and dose rates, such that risks due to low-dose exposure are considered to be lower than estimated based on a simple linear dose-response model.

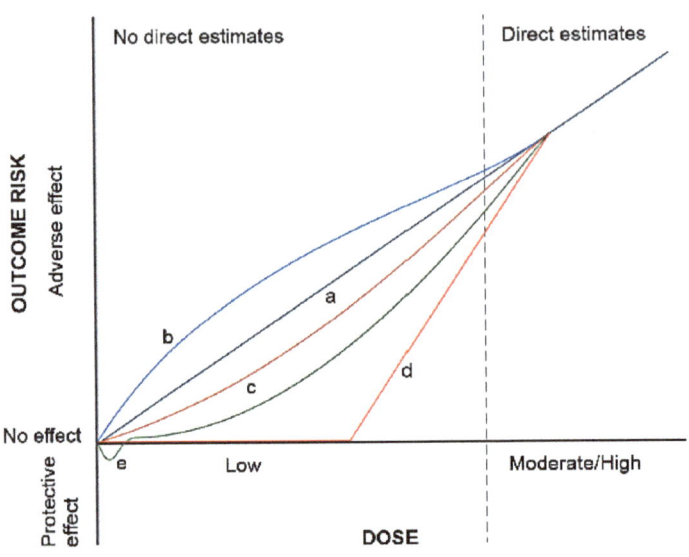

FIGURE 3.1 Plausible options for dose-response models to describe low-dose radiation risks: (a) linear, (b) downward curving (decreasing slope), (c) upward curving (increasing slope), (d) threshold, and (e) adaptive extrapolations. The dose-response relationships may differ across health outcomes and may be influenced by changes in medical care or the presence of response-modifying factors. The dotted vertical line indicates the dose below which there is an absence of direct estimates of the effect of radiation exposure on human health. The dose below which direct estimates exist is typically based on epidemiological data and varies depending on the health outcome. High doses that result in cell killing are excluded from this figure. SOURCE: Modified from Brenner et al. (2003).

curving (increasing slope, curve "c"), threshold (curve "d"), and adaptive response (curve "e"; see Figure 3.1). The only dose-response curve that predicts more risk at low doses than the linear model is curve "b." Any divergences from the LNT model imply that the current radiation protection system either overestimates or underestimates risks at low doses.

A broadly accepted illustration (see Figure 3.2) of the approximate magnitude of the risk from low-dose radiation based on the LNT model is that if 100 individuals (all circles in Figure 3.2) were each exposed to 100 millisieverts (mSv) in their lifetime, then approximately 1 of them (red circle) would develop a radiation-induced cancer over their lifetime, whereas around 42 (blue circles) would develop cancer from other causes (NRC, 2006a). Although the magnitude of risk from low doses of radiation can be considered to be small compared to the risk from all other causes

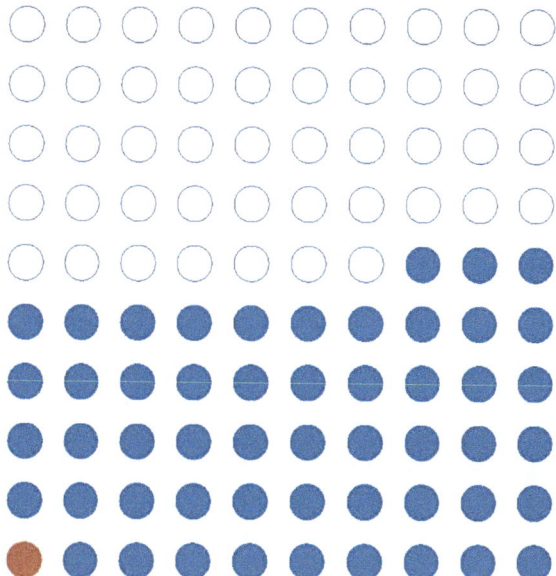

FIGURE 3.2 Illustration of the approximate magnitude of the risk from low-dose radiation (100 millisieverts [mSv]) based on the linear no-threshold model. If 100 individuals (all circles) were each exposed to 100 mSv in their lifetime, then approximately 1 of them (red circle) would develop a radiation-induced cancer over their lifetime, whereas around 42 (blue circles) would develop cancer from other causes. SOURCE: Modified from NRC (2006a).

combined, if large numbers of individuals are exposed to even small doses, then the magnitude of the radiation-induced health effects can become important at the population level and in terms of burdens on health care systems (Brenner, 2014). Notably, radiation-induced cancers cannot currently be distinguished from cancers of the same type initiated by other causes because no unique signature of radiation-induced damage in tumors has been identified to date (Behjati et al., 2016; Kocakavuk et al., 2021; Morton et al., 2021). One study found an excess of small deletions and balanced inversions (Behjati et al., 2016), but radiation dose estimates were not available in that study.[3]

---

[3] As discussed in Chapter 5, genome sequencing studies have identified genomic signatures in cancers that suggest specific, non-radiation causative agents for individual tumors (Alexandrov et al., 2020). These genomic signatures can be excluded from consideration in an assessment of radiation-induced carcinogenesis.

3.2 AGENCIES WITH RADIATION PROTECTION RESPONSIBILITIES IN THE UNITED STATES

In the United States, several federal agencies, and in some instances states, administer radiation protection standards. The Environmental Protection Agency (EPA) is the lead federal agency responsible for establishing human health and environmental radiation standards for air, surface water, drinking water, uranium mill tailings sites, and deep geologic repositories.[4] Various laws authorize other federal agencies to set regulatory limits and issue guidelines to protect the public and workers from exposure to ionizing radiation. The authority of a federal agency to administer those limits and guidance is rooted in statute and tends to vary depending on the setting in which radiation exposure occurs.

EPA issues Protective Action Guides (PAGs; EPA, 2017)[5] for use during a nuclear or a radiological emergency and suggests that public safety measures such as evacuation to minimize or prevent radiation exposure during an emergency be triggered when the projected dose to an individual is 10 to 50 mSv over 4 days. EPA also provides guidelines for drinking water interdiction. EPA has also developed guidance on establishing protective cleanup levels for radioactive contamination at sites managed under the Comprehensive Environmental Response, Compensation, and Liability Act (CERCLA or "Superfund"). When not based on other environmental standards that are Applicable or Relevant and Appropriate Requirements (ARARs), these cleanup levels correspond to acceptable lifetime excess cancer risk levels of 1 in 10,000 to 1 in 1,000,000 due to exposure to a site-related carcinogen but can vary across sites because of land use, exposure scenarios, and the statutory requirement for cost-effectiveness. EPA discourages decision-makers from using dose-based guidance[6] when developing cleanup levels and encourages using the CERCLA risk range instead for consistency with guidance for chemical carcinogens. According to EPA, dose assessments should only be conducted under CERCLA where necessary to demonstrate compliance with ARARs. For this purpose, EPA has defined protective dose-based standards as 0.12 mSv per year or below (EPA, 2014). This cleanup level is considerably lower than that recommended by the U.S. Nuclear Regulatory Commission (U.S. NRC) and the Department of Energy (DOE), as discussed below.

The U.S. NRC regulates worker exposure to radiation for specific radioactive materials for which it issues licenses. The U.S. NRC limits occupational doses to 50 mSv per year for workers in commercial nuclear facilities

---

[4] See https://www.epa.gov/radiation/radiation-regulations-and-laws.
[5] PAGs consider the risks to individuals from exposure to radiation and the risks and costs associated with a specific protective action such as evacuation or sheltering in place.
[6] Guidance that estimates risk from a given dose.

such as nuclear power plants, industrial radiography, and nuclear medicine[7] and the annual dose to the lens of the eye at 150 mSv (equivalent dose).[8]

DOE sets occupational dose limits for workers at DOE facilities. Similar to the U.S. NRC, it limits occupational doses to 50 mSv per year and public dose limits, including from cleanup of radioactive waste at DOE sites, to 1 mSv. Many contaminated DOE sites are being regulated by CERCLA authority (DOE and EPA, 1995), which requires the sites to clean up on the basis of acceptable risk ranges calculated by methods defined by EPA and state laws.

The Occupational Safety and Health Administration (OSHA) sets radiation limits for workers from exposure to radiation sources that are not regulated by the U.S. NRC or other federal agencies, such as X-ray equipment, some accelerators, and some naturally occurring radioactive material. OSHA's limits for workers vary by industry.[9]

The Department of Defense is responsible for military exposure and remediation as well as for setting requirements to operate in environments that could expose personnel to low doses of ionizing radiation.

The National Aeronautics and Space Administration (NASA) sets radiation limits for career exposure to astronauts but these limits are above the doses of interest for this report. The career limit was set at 3 percent risk of exposure-induced cancer death at 95 percent confidence level from fatal cancers, which corresponds to approximately 180 mSv for a 30-year-old female and approximately 700 mSv for a 60-year-old male astronaut. Following a recommendation by the National Academies (NASEM, 2021c), NASA revised the limit to 600 mSv career exposure for astronauts of all ages and sexes (NASA, 2022).

Other federal agencies apply radiation protection guidance and requirements (see Figure 1.4). These include the Federal Aviation Administration, which recommends limits to aircrews (a 5-year average effective dose of 20 mSv per year with no more than 50 mSv in a single year; FAA, 2003) and provides computer software for estimating the amount of galactic cosmic radiation received on a flight; the Food and Drug Administration, which issues radiation safety regulations for medical equipment (e.g., for mammography, these are based on the Mammography Quality Standards Act; FDA, 1998); the National Institute of Standards and Technology within the Department of Commerce, which maintains and disseminates the national

---

[7] The International Commission on Radiological Protection (ICRP) recommends limiting the annual exposure to radiation workers to 20 mSv (ICRP, 2007).

[8] ICRP recommends limiting exposure to the lens of the eye to 20 mSv averaged over 5 years, not to exceed 50 mSv in one year (ICRP, 2012) and the National Council on Radiation Protection and Measurements (NCRP) recommends a limit of 50 mSv in 1 year (Dauer et al., 2017; NCRP, 2016).

[9] See https://www.osha.gov/ionizing-radiation/standards.

measurement standards for ionizing radiation, carries out research in dosimetry, disseminates air kerma and absorbed dose standard data, and provides calibration services; the Department of Homeland Security, which is responsible for coordinating the federal response to a nuclear or radiological incident; the Department of Veteran Affairs and the Department of Justice, which manage radiation compensation programs; the Customs and Border Protection, which responds to incidents involving inadvertently imported radioactive materials; the Department of State, which coordinates the response to foreign incidents involving radioactive materials, if assistance from the United States is requested; and the United States Coast Guard, which responds to incidents not managed by other agencies that impact the coastal zone.

Representatives of agencies with radiation protection responsibilities are members of the Interagency Steering Committee on Radiation Standards (ISCORS). The goal of ISCORS is to improve consistency in federal radiation protection programs. Specific objectives relevant to this report include facilitating consensus on acceptable levels of radiation risk and promoting consistent risk-assessment and risk-management approaches in setting and implementing standards for radiation protection.[10] However, experts who briefed the committee noted that ISCORS does not provide a centralized radiation science and policy leadership within the U.S. government.[11] Individual agencies set the regulatory frameworks that are appropriate for their jurisdictions.

3.3 SCIENCE BEHIND RADIATION PROTECTION

Most U.S. radiation protection regulations and guidelines are informed by and are broadly consistent with the recommendations of ICRP; NCRP; and the International Atomic Energy Agency's Basic Safety Standards for Radiation Protection that are published jointly with the World Health Organization, the International Labour Organization, and the Organisation for Economic Co-operation and Development's Nuclear Energy Agency. ICRP and NCRP recommendations are based on scientific consensus publications such as the National Academies' Biological Effects of Ionizing Radiation (BEIR) committee reports and reports issued by the United Nations Scientific Committee on the Effects of Atomic Radiation (UNSCEAR). Both the National Academies and UNSCEAR periodically review the available scientific literature of epidemiological and mechanistic studies of radiation exposure and develop models for calculating

---

[10] See http://www.iscors.org.
[11] Vincent Holahan, U.S. NRC, and Mike Boyd, EPA, presentation to the committee on August 26, 2021.

risks of radiogenic cancers following low doses of radiation. Models and approaches recommended by the National Academies and UNSCEAR and extensions and modifications to them have been foundational in the radiation protection systems worldwide.[12] Both the National Research Council's BEIR reports (NRC, 2006a) and the UNSCEAR reports (UNSCEAR, 2006a) have supported the use of LNT and application of a dose and dose-rate effectiveness factor for solid cancers but have used a linear-quadratic model for leukemia. The BEIR VII committee notes that the difference between the linear and linear-quadratic models in the low-dose ranges is small relative to the uncertainty in the risk estimates (NRC, 2006a). A pooled analysis of leukemia risk following low-dose exposures in childhood, published over a decade after the BEIR VII and UNSCEAR reports, did not find strong evidence for departure from a linear model (Little et al., 2018).

A strong scientific underpinning for radiation protection is critical to adequately and appropriately protect people from exposure to radiation while making the most effective use of resources. Uncertainties in low-dose radiation risks raise questions about whether dose limits and guidance levels are set appropriately or whether they are set too high and therefore do not sufficiently protect workers and members of the public or too low and therefore result in unnecessary costs to reduce radiation exposure. Federal agencies have been formally challenged by members of the public about the use of LNT to set radiation protection standards at least twice in the recent past.

In 2015, the U.S. NRC received three petitions proposing that the agency raise its occupational and public dose limits so that higher exposures become permissible compared to those allowed today (U.S. NRC, 2015a). The U.S. NRC denied these petitions for rulemaking in 2021 and stated that "the LNT model continues to provide a sound regulatory basis for minimizing the risk of unnecessary radiation exposure" to both members of the public and radiation workers (U.S. NRC, 2021). Also in 2021, following a complaint that alleged that EPA is not following the best-available science regarding low-dose radiation because of its reliance on the LNT model, EPA's Office of Inspector General began an evaluation to examine EPA's process for updating federal radiation policies and guidance, specifically those that rely on the LNT model (EPA, 2021). The investigation found that although EPA does not have a formal process for updating its federal radiation guidance, the agency has taken steps to ensure that its radiation guidance, including that regarding low-dose

---

[12] For example, in 2011, EPA updated its estimates of cancer incidence and mortality risks due to low doses of ionizing radiation based on the 2006 BEIR VII recommendations.

radiation exposure, is updated and informed by the best-available and peer-reviewed science (EPA, 2022).

EPA states that "new science on radiation health effects" would affect its approach to protecting the public from radiation exposure (EPA, 2018b). Although state-of-the-art science is the essential ingredient in improving radiation regulations and guidance, regulations and guidance are not automatically updated when new scientific recommendations occur. For example, the U.S. NRC's regulations for protection against radiation (known as *10 CFR Part 20*) are still based primarily on scientific publications issued in the 1970s (ICRP, 1977, 1979) despite these publications being superseded by newer ones (ICRP, 1991, 1994, 1995, 2007). An example of differences between scientific consensus and U.S. radiation protection regulations relates to the allowable exposure to radiation workers and to the lens of the eye. ICRP recommends limiting the annual exposure to radiation workers to 20 mSv (ICRP, 2007) and made a substantial revision to the equivalent dose limit to the lens of the eye for radiation workers and reduced it from 150 mSv per year to 20 mSv per year (ICRP, 2012). The U.S. NRC regulatory limit for the annual exposure to radiation workers is 50 mSv total effective dose equivalent, with an additional limit for the lens of the eye at 150 mSv per year. According to the U.S. NRC, these requirements and adherence to the principle of ALARA result in occupational exposures that are generally below these newer ICRP recommendations.

3.3.1 The Regulatory Development Process

When a change in standards requires a new regulation or a change in an existing regulation, the process typically involves the following steps:[13]

1. Agency develops proposed regulation and supporting analysis.
2. Office of Management and Budget (OMB) reviews the proposed regulation and supporting analysis, if applicable.[14]
3. Agency publishes preamble and proposed rule in the *Federal Register*, placing supporting technical documents in the regulatory docket, and requests public comments.
4. Agency develops, OMB reviews (if applicable), and agency publishes final rule and supporting documents.

---

[13] Lisa Robinson, Harvard T.H. Chan School of Public Health, presentation to the committee on October 27, 2021.

[14] The U.S. NRC is excluded from OMB review because it operates independently of the White House, like the Federal Reserve Board or the Consumer Product Safety Commission.

5. Congress reviews rule under the Congressional Review Act, if applicable.
6. Federal courts review the rule, if applicable, for example, when an agency is sued by one or more stakeholders.

3.3.2 Decision-Making Frameworks for Radiation Protection

Risk-based regulation is a particular strategy or set of strategies that regulators use to target their resources at those sites and activities that present threats to their ability to achieve their objectives.

Economic analysis of the impacts of the proposed change (Step 1 in the regulatory development process described in the previous section) is required if the regulation is economically significant or the regulation is issued by an executive branch agency, such as EPA, and cabinet agencies that report to the President. Agencies may also choose to assess the impacts of less significant regulations, and independent agencies such as the U.S. NRC typically follow the analytical requirements voluntarily. Central to the analysis of proposed changes to regulations is an understanding of the risks with and without regulation. The expert who briefed the committee[15] noted that such risk assessments, and the benefit-cost analyses they support, motivate detailed examination of impacts, and important discoveries are typically made during the process. These discoveries may include a better understanding of the preferences of those affected by the regulation; the key sources of uncertainty; the magnitudes of the costs and benefits; the effectiveness of alternative policies; the distribution of the impacts across types of organizations and advantaged and disadvantaged individuals and groups; sources of support and opposition; and otherwise unanticipated consequences. Comparison of alternative regulatory and nonregulatory alternatives is desirable to identify the most appropriate use of resources.

Typically these regulatory benefit-cost analyses inform rather than determine a decision. Decision-makers also consider legal and political issues, budgetary constraints, and ethical ramifications and community sentiments. Independent of the outcome, this type of analysis can assemble and integrate relevant evidence to support complex decision-making in transparent ways.

Several federal agencies have published extensive guidance on regulatory analysis (see, e.g., DOT, 2021; EPA, 2010 [with updates; undergoing revision]; HHS, 2016; U.S. NRC, 2017 [draft update]). In radiation protection regulations, the usefulness and acceptability of an analysis depends

---

[15] Lisa Robinson, Harvard T.H. Chan School of Public Health, presentation to the committee on October 27, 2021.

on how well its scientific evidence and underlying assumptions and their implications are understood by those planning to use its results. A crucial element of regulatory analysis is a characterization of the risk of the disease caused by the level of radiation the regulation aims to limit. This is often called the baseline risk; the residual risk is the amount of risk expected to remain after the regulatory limit is implemented.

3.3.3 Characterization of Risk in the Regulatory Development Process

Lave (1981) identified the different frameworks used by regulatory federal agencies, arranged them in a typology, and described the informational requirements that each framework places on those responsible for managing risk. Each framework seeks to answer the same question: How safe is safe enough? The committee simplified Lave's typology into four basic frameworks—negligible risk, lowest feasible risk, net risk, and cost-benefit balancing—and discusses each framework briefly below. Although these frameworks are only part of the radiation protection risk governance, this discussion illustrates the importance of low-dose radiation knowledge and therefore research in low-dose radiation health effects to inform radiation protection regulation and guidance. Each aspect of a risk-based framework involves a complex set of decisions that regulators need to take including selecting the methods they will use to assess those risks; managing the implementation of the risk-based framework; justifying and communicating about it; responding to changes; and, ultimately, setting the level of acceptable risk.

Negligible Risk

When protecting the public from exposure to ionizing radiation, the most ambitious goal might be to eliminate exposure in its entirety and thereby accomplish zero risk. However, accomplishing zero risk from radiation is impractical and in fact impossible due to background radiation that constitutes about half of the annual exposure to the U.S. population today. As a step toward practicality, regulators developed the concept of *negligible risk*, also called "de minimis risk."[16] Whether a risk is negligible depends on multiple factors such as the incremental probability of harm, the severity of the harm, whether the risk of harm is assumed voluntarily or involuntarily by those exposed, and the number of people exposed to the potential harm. Regulators could either consider that no safety measures need to be taken to address a negligible risk or regulate it in a more permissive way than a non-negligible risk.

---

[16] *Monsanto Co. v. Kennedy*, 613 F.2d 947 (DC Cir. 1979); see, generally, Whipple (1987).

There is no general agreement on how small a risk must be for it to be considered negligible; the most common approach in cancer risk management, where exposures are often involuntary and the harm can be premature death, is to define a threshold probability that is sufficiently small above which risks are addressed and below which risks may be accepted. The number of people exposed may also be considered.

The concept of negligible risk originated in food law where exceptions were needed to allow minute concentrations of chemical additives or contaminants in food or animal feed that pose at most a negligible risk of cancer to the public. In food law the threshold for fatal cancer was defined as a 1 in 1,000,000 chance on a lifetime basis when an LNT model is used to compute risk (FDA, 1977). For comparison, the risk of dying from cancer is 1 in 5 (ACS, 2020). An incremental risk might be considered negligible if it increased that background risk of cancer death to no more than 1.00001 in 5.

Another way to comprehend such a small risk of death is to compare it to another involuntary risk of death that people experience routinely. Commercial aviation poses an involuntary risk of fatality to people on the ground as well as a voluntary risk to passengers and crew. According to one rough calculation, the lifetime probability that a person on the ground in the United States will be killed by a crashing airplane is about 4 in 1,000,000. The risk to groundlings is larger for people living near airport runways, and some measures are taken to protect those groundlings. This comparison has for decades been used in risk communication (Goldstein et al., 1992).

Negligible-risk concepts also have a place in the history of federal radiation protection policies, especially at the U.S. NRC and EPA. In 1986, the U.S. NRC adopted a variety of qualitative and quantitative safety goals for the operation of nuclear power plants. For example, the risk of latent cancer fatalities from living within 10 miles of such plants should not exceed "one tenth of one percent" or 0.001 of the sum of cancer fatality risks resulting from all causes (U.S. NRC, 1986). Assuming a baseline fatal cancer risk of 1 in 5 (ACS, 2020), this translates into a safety goal for cancer death risk of 2 in 10,000 per year, or 140 in 10,000 per lifetime, assuming the standard lifetime assumption at the time, which was 70 years.

Under both the Clean Air Act and the Superfund program for cleanup of hazardous wastes, EPA uses a negligible-risk range for fatal cancer of 1 in 10,000 to 1 in 1,000,000 per lifetime. The most exposed individual must be protected against risks at the higher end of the range, and as many exposed people as possible must be protected against the smaller risk level of 1 in 1,000,000.[17] Inherent in EPA's risk formulation is that at any such

---

[17] *Natural Resources Defense Council v. EPA*, 838 F.2d 1224 (D.C. Cir. 1987).

risk level, the size of the exposed population will determine the number of cases that will occur during any given time period. For example, consider the risk of cancer due to long-lived radionuclides in nuclear waste near a community with a population of 10,000. Assuming a stable population and an average 85-year life span, a lifetime risk of 1 in 100,000 would result in one additional cancer every 850 years. Weinstein et al. (1996) reported that such formulations for lower-level risks are of less concern to the public.

In the early 1990s, the U.S. NRC and EPA engaged in a harmonization effort on radiation risk management because EPA's negligible-risk range under the Clean Air Act appears more protective than the U.S. NRC's negligible-risk level for community exposure (GAO, 1994, 2000). These discrepancies in the standards arise because of their different regulatory applications and different technical methodologies to derive them. The agencies acknowledged that EPA tends to set stringent risk limits but then permits variances or exemptions for facilities on a case-by-case basis where compliance is not practical. The U.S. NRC's risk-based limits on radiation doses appear less stringent, but the U.S. NRC requires licensees to consider additional measures ("reasonably demonstrated technology") to drive exposures as far below the risk limits as reasonably achievable. Thus, the net impact of the two agencies' regulatory practices is more alike than one would assume by simply comparing the numerical risk levels of negligible risk (Sadowitz and Graham, 1995). Despite decades of dialogue, the two agencies have not accomplished complete harmonization of radiation risk management methodologies.

The level of negligible risk for a worker is typically different—and larger—than for a community resident, presumably because risk to the worker arises from a contractual relationship (and therefore financial benefit) and the size of the exposed worker population may be smaller than the size of the exposed community population. Concerning fatal cancer risk, OSHA has not precisely defined a level of negligible risk but has indicated that cancer death risk levels above 1 in 1,000 for a career are "significant" enough to justify rulemaking, and risks below 1 in 100,000 might be considered safe (Sunstein, 2002). This "significant" risk threshold emerged from litigation (discussed below) surrounding OSHA's 1980 benzene standard (Graham et al., 1988).

Decision theorists have raised some thorny normative problems with the concept of negligible risk (Lundgren and Stefánsson, 2020). For example, if it is inexpensive to eliminate negligible risks, why not eliminate them? If a person is exposed to 100 negligible risks from different sources, is the cumulative overall risk still negligible? The concept of negligible risk survives, however, due to tradition and practicality considerations.

Net Risk

In a setting where a regulation would reduce some risks but increase other risks, the regulator could compare the risks and ensure that the regulation is designed to reduce net risk (Graham et al., 1995). The risk-tradeoff concern emerged at EPA under the Safe Drinking Water Act where the chlorination—and alternative processes (e.g., ozonation)—of drinking water is associated with both health benefits and health risks. In the Safe Drinking Water Act amendments of 1996, Congress required EPA to weigh such "health-health tradeoffs" when setting maximum contaminant levels (Sunstein, 2002). The tradeoff analysis ensures that reducing exposure to one contaminant to benefit health does not cause unacceptably large increases in risk from exposure to a different contaminant.

The net-risk framework may be applicable to decisions about whether to evacuate or relocate communities following a nuclear or radiological incident. As discussed earlier in this report (see Section 2.1.5), recent research following the 2011 Fukushima nuclear power plant accident suggests that evacuations intended to avoid radiation exposure may trigger both immediate and longer-term risks in the impacted communities. At the same time, the risks of staying in the contaminated area due to damaged infrastructure, interruptions in food and medical supplies, human assistance, and other factors have not been sufficiently quantified. A net-risk decision framework would require the risk manager to analyze and weigh these risk tradeoffs.

Lowest Feasible Risk

The feasibility standard in risk management has roots in the Occupational Safety and Health Act of 1970. Congress stipulated that OSHA, when setting health standards, "shall set the standard which most adequately assures, to the extent feasible, on the basis of the best available evidence that no employee will suffer material impairment of health or functional capacity even if such employee has regular exposure to the hazard dealt with by such standard for the period of his working lifetime" (Occupational Safety and Health Act § 6(b)(5)). What did Congress mean by the word "feasible"?

Based on a series of rulemakings and judicial decisions from 1970 to 1979, OSHA defined two dimensions of feasibility: technological capability to reduce worker exposures and financial capability of the industry to reduce worker exposures. OSHA argued that the health standard should be as health protective as possible for workers unless no technology is available to meet the standard or the standard would be so costly that it would bankrupt a substantial segment of the affected industry (OSHA, 1977). According to this definition of feasibility, OSHA did not need to conduct a quantitative risk assessment or perform a cost-benefit analysis to support a new health standard. Instead, a qualitative determination of hazard is sufficient to support rulemaking, and the stringency of rule is based on the industry's financial capability to reduce worker exposures.

Industry challenged OSHA's definition of feasibility in litigation about new standards to limit worker exposure to benzene and cotton dust. Industry argued that OSHA should be required to support a new health standard with a quantitative risk assessment of worker exposures and with a cost-benefit analysis of alternative standards.

The U.S. Supreme Court rejected OSHA's complete reliance on the affordability test and in the benzene case (1980), vacated OSHA's new benzene standard. In a plurality opinion, Justice John Paul Stevens explained, based on "reasonably necessary" language in the preface of the Act, that OSHA had not demonstrated that benzene exposure at the prevailing standard was a "significant risk" and that the lower standard would "significantly reduce that risk."[18] In response to this decision, OSHA now supports new health standards with quantitative risk assessments.

In the cotton dust case (1981), the court affirmed OSHA's new cotton dust standard. Writing for a court majority, Justice William Brennan reasoned that "feasible" means "capable of being done," which does not entail a cost-benefit analysis. Brennan reaffirmed the court's previous reasoning concerning significant risk.[19]

In the 40 years since the court's cotton dust decision, two developments have limited the Brennan reasoning to the OSHA context (Masur and Posner, 2018). First, feasibility-like concepts also appear in environmental laws such as the Clean Air Act and the Clean Water Act. Recent judicial interpretations of those concepts (e.g., "best available technology"), where the policy objective is protection of the public, have tended to permit cost-benefit considerations (Noe and Graham, 2020; Sunstein, 2017). Second, presidential executive orders since 1981 have required agencies to prepare cost-benefit analyses of economically significant rulemakings. The findings from such analyses may not be used to override statutory requirements (Carey, 2014). This "cost-benefit balancing" is discussed in the next section.

Feasibility-like concepts influence radiation protection at the U.S. NRC, but they have evolved differently from those at OSHA and EPA. The U.S. NRC's safety goals for the design of nuclear power plants call for a first level of risk-based protection (regardless of costs) plus additional protection based on "reasonably demonstrated technology" to protect the residents living within 50 miles of the plant. Technically, this approach has been

---

[18] *Industrial Union Department, AFL-CIO v. American Petroleum Institute*, 448 U.S. 607 (1980).

[19] *American Textile Manufacturers Institute v. Donovan*, 452 U.S. 490 (1981).

SCIENTIFIC BASIS FOR RADIATION PROTECTION 91

defined to reduce radiation exposures to ALARA, subject to a favorable ratio of benefits to costs. The U.S. NRC's approach, including use of cost-benefit analysis, is also discussed in the next section.

Cost-Benefit Balancing

In the laws governing consumer product safety, toxic substances, and pesticides, Congress has called for prevention of "unreasonable" risks, which means weighing the costs and benefits of regulatory alternatives and choosing the alternative with the most favorable balance of benefit to cost. Where Congress is silent or ambiguous about the applicable decision-making framework, presidential executive orders require agencies to support new regulations with an analysis of benefits and costs.

In some laws, Congress expressly uses cost-benefit language. In the Safe Drinking Water Act Amendments of 1996, Congress directed EPA to establish a drinking water standard for radon based on a novel cost-benefit approach. Since control of radon in drinking water can be costly, Congress authorized EPA to allow states and water systems to offset high levels of radon in drinking water with programs to reduce indoor air radon levels. Based on a National Academies report on radon (NRC, 1999a), EPA estimated that radon is responsible for about 21,000 lung cancer deaths every year (EPA, 2003), only 160 of them due to inhalation of radon that evaporated from drinking water. In its 1999 proposed rule, which allowed states to focus on indoor air radon levels instead of waterborne radon, EPA estimated $362 million in benefits due to reductions in the number of cancers compared to a best estimate of $121 million in costs related to engineering costs of treatment systems, with a range of cost estimates from $60 million per year to $408 million per year (EPA, 1999). The EPA rulemaking is still pending.

The U.S. NRC staff conduct a regulatory analysis, including cost-benefit analysis, of any changes to the agency's radiation protection guidance. To compare the monetary costs of radiation protection measures to health benefits, the U.S. NRC uses a "dollar per person-rem"[20] conversion factor of $5,200 in 2014 dollars (U.S. NRC, 2022).[21] The number results from the multiplication of the U.S. NRC's $9 million value of a statistical life (VSL) by a mortality risk coefficient of 5.8×10^{-4} per person-rem.[22,23]

---

[20] The U.S. NRC continues to use the conventional unit "rem."

[21] The U.S. NRC recently reassessed its dollar per person-rem conversion factor policy (U.S. NRC, 2022). The dollar per person-rem conversion factor used by the U.S. NRC until recently was $2,000 (U.S. NRC, 1995).

[22] Letter from John Tappert, U.S. NRC, to Ourania Kosti, National Academies, on October 8, 2021.

[23] The U.S. NRC adopted the EPA cancer mortality risk coefficient that is based on the 2006 BEIR VII committee report (NRC, 2006a) and is specific to the U.S. population.

VSL is an economic value used to approximate society's willingness to pay for reductions in mortality risks. Because mortality risk reduction is most often the basis for the justification for government policies, VSL is an important component of the benefit-cost analyses that are part of the regulatory process in the United States. The U.S. NRC's VSL value of $9 million is consistent with the values used at other federal agencies. For example, EPA and the Department of Transportation use VSL values around $9–$10 million (Viscusi, 2018).

A literature review discussed in the U.S. NRC's recent white paper (U.S. NRC, 2020b) indicated that federal agencies vary considerably in how they monetize nonfatal health effects. Moreover, since the U.S. NRC's VSL measure is based primarily on studies of fatal injury in the workplace, the U.S. NRC may consider a cancer premium on the basis that public willingness to pay to prevent a cancer death could be larger than a death from occupational injury. As knowledge of low-dose radiation health effects advances to quantify non-cancer health effects (e.g., cardiovascular effects, neurological disorders, and other effects), monetization techniques will also be necessary for those health effects.

When radiation protection measures are analyzed in medicine, the VSL approach to monetization is rarely used (IOM, 2006). Instead, clinical strategies are compared with cost-effectiveness ratios, where the numerator of the ratio is the net cost of the clinical strategy (gross costs of technology and labor minus any savings in health care costs from less disease) and the denominator is the number of life years saved or the number of quality-adjusted life years (QALYs) saved, which accounts for morbidity and other quality-of-life factors. Decision-makers then use a critical threshold for the ratio to help determine whether the clinical strategy is worthwhile. There is no consensus among experts as to what the critical threshold needs to be (Menzel, 2021).

One of the advantages of using the QALY approach is that health-utility tools have already been developed to estimate the quality-of-life decrements attributable to contracting cancer and other chronic diseases. Thus, if radiation science quantifies cardiovascular as well as carcinogenic effects, the two health outcomes can be combined with the QALY metric. A disadvantage of the QALY method is that it is not grounded rigorously in welfare-economic theory, which is the intellectual foundation for cost-benefit analysis (IOM, 2006).

One of the limitations of cost-benefit balancing is that it can be seen as disrespectful of fundamental human rights as defined by the United Nations (UN, 2021). Some commentators argue that there is tragedy when premature deaths are not prevented due to cost-benefit considerations (Tallarita, 2020). Others argue that cost-benefit analysis can strengthen the case for protection of human rights (Aceves, 2018).

SCIENTIFIC BASIS FOR RADIATION PROTECTION 93

3.4 POTENTIAL ECONOMIC IMPACTS OF THE LOW-DOSE RADIATION RESEARCH PROGRAM

Costs for complying with radiation protection standards and guidelines, administering radiation compensation programs, or for using technologies that utilize radiation in medical and other applications are balanced with the health, societal, and other benefits based on current scientific understanding of low-dose radiation exposures. These costs are substantial. For example,

- Costs for mitigating the 5 million houses in the United States that have high indoor radon levels exceed $5 billion (see Section 2.1.1).
- Medical costs for radiology services for computed tomography scans alone (see Section 2.1.2) exceed $74 billion assuming cost per scan of $1,000 (Jiang et al., 2022).
- Annual costs to the nuclear industry to comply with regulatory standards (see Section 2.1.4) are about $16 billion (Batkins, 2016; Batkins et al., 2017).
- Costs to respond to nuclear or radiological incidents (see Section 2.1.5) vary significantly depending on the incident. The costs for cleanup of the Fukushima nuclear site, for example, are estimated to reach 35 trillion to 80 trillion yen (approximately $290 billion to $670 billion) over 40 years (JCER, 2019).
- Future liability for compensation program payments will cost billions of dollars. For example, Energy Employees Occupational Illness Compensation Act payments (see Section 2.1.6) alone have been estimated to be about $43 billion (Gross, 2021).
- Cleanup of nuclear waste sites will cost hundreds of billions of dollars over several decades (see Section 2.1.7) and the costs per site accelerate the more restrictive the protection levels (GAO, 2000). For example, although decades old, past analysis of cleanup options for plutonium contamination at the Nevada Test Site estimated $35 million in costs to achieve a 1-mSv/year level. The costs were three times higher to achieve a 0.25-mSv/year level, six times higher to achieve a 0.15-mSv/year level, and 28 times higher to achieve a 0.5-mSv/year level (GAO, 2000).

To the committee's knowledge, comprehensive estimates of overall costs to federal agencies and society to comply with current radiation protection standards and guidelines are unavailable. Similarly, comprehensive estimates for the overall cost savings for protecting the U.S. population's health by implementing these standards and guidelines are also unavailable. Without these current estimates as a starting point, preparing comprehensive estimates of overall costs to comply with prospective radiation protection standards or guidelines is not possible. In addition, the committee judges that it would be inappropriate to speculate what the new scientific information might be or how it may be used by radiation protection agencies; therefore, it cannot quantitatively estimate the potential economic impacts of the low-dose radiation research program. When adjustments in radiation protection standards and guidance are proposed based on new information, agencies can estimate the economic impacts of the changes and perform benefit-cost and cost-effectiveness analyses of alternative measures. These analyses can also be informed by econometric studies of the social impacts of low-dose radiation exposures on health or other endpoints (e.g., education) which have provided plausibly causal economic loss estimates associated with these exposures (Almond et al., 2009; Black et al., 2019; Danzer and Danzer, 2016). Although the committee does not provide a quantitative estimate of the potential economic impacts of the low-dose radiation program, it assesses whether knowledge from low-dose radiation research can affect the decision-making frameworks in the federal regulatory system and how.

The committee's review of decision-making frameworks in the federal regulatory system reveals that knowledge from low-dose radiation research plays a central role in three of the four frameworks. The negligible-risk, net-risk, and cost-benefit frameworks require estimates of low-dose radiation risks to be implemented. Only the lowest-feasible-risk framework, as implemented by OSHA in the 1970s, did not require knowledge of low-dose health effects, since standard setting could proceed based on a qualitative determination of possible hazard and the stringency of standards was determined entirely by engineering and industrial-affordability considerations. However, the Supreme Court's decision in the 1980 benzene case required OSHA to perform quantitative risk assessment in the standard-setting process, which in turn required OSHA to estimate benzene-related low-dose health effects. OSHA then justified a new benzene standard as necessary to protect against leukemia and quantified the risk of leukemia to workers on the basis of the LNT model.

Feasibility-like concepts are also employed by EPA and the U.S. NRC, but those concepts typically permit or require cost-benefit analysis as part of the feasibility determination. Thus, the committee concludes that advances in knowledge of low-dose radiation effects will be inherently useful for federal agencies in radiation protection decisions and likely by some agencies charged with compensating impacted communities for damage suffered due to radiation exposures (see Box 2.1).

New knowledge that emerges from the low-dose program can inform the radiation protection regulations and guidance in several ways: by improving understanding of adverse human health effects from exposures at doses and dose rates experienced by the U.S. population, identifying mechanisms for induction of these health effects, developing improved risk models for doses and dose rates at which direct measurement of risks is not possible, and ultimately developing more individualized risk estimates.

This new information can help address specific concerns raised by patients, workers, members of the public, and communities because of their medical, occupational, and environmental low-dose and low-dose-rate radiation exposures. This new information can also inform national policies such as the future of nuclear power, response to nuclear or radiological incidents, nuclear waste management, and radiation compensation programs.

New findings on health effects emerging from the low-dose radiation program will provide evidence on whether current (primarily cancer) risk estimates at low doses are accurate, underestimated, or overestimated. This evidence may impact radiation protection by confirming that current regulations and guidance sufficiently protect human health or by supporting either more restrictive or less restrictive regulations and guidance. Importantly, new findings will inform radiation protection for health outcomes currently not considered in radiation protection systems or radiation compensation programs.

In some setting(s), anti-backsliding provisions in agency statutes preclude changes to current regulations unless changes provide for greater protection of the health of persons. In any case, a challenge for the federal government agencies with radiation protection responsibilities will be reaching consensus on how new findings on health effects emerging from the low-dose radiation program need to inform or alter radiation protection regulation and guidance and achieve harmonization of risk goals.

3.5 CHAPTER SUMMARY AND FINDINGS

Exposures to low levels of radiation may carry low levels of risk to an exposed individual; nonetheless, they are a high priority for the radiation protection system. The vast majority of regulations and guidance in the radiation protection system tend to address low-dose exposures. In the United States, several federal agencies, and in some instances states, administer radiation protection standards and guidelines.

A strong scientific basis for radiation protection is critical to ensuring adequate and appropriate protection of the U.S. population from the use of radiation while making the most effective use of resources. Uncertainties in low-dose radiation risks raise questions about whether dose limits and guidance levels are set appropriately or whether they are set too high and therefore do not sufficiently protect workers and members of the public or too low and therefore result in unnecessary costs to reduce radiation exposure. The regulatory development process to update standards is a multistep process that requires a supporting analysis that involves an understanding of the risks without the proposed regulation and risk-reduction improvements of the proposed regulation. Advances in knowledge of low-dose radiation effects will be inherently useful for federal agencies in radiation protection decisions and in decisions in support of radiation compensation programs.

Costs for complying with radiation protection standards and guidelines, administering radiation compensation programs, or for using technologies that utilize radiation in medical and other applications are balanced with the health, societal, and other benefits based on current scientific understanding of low-dose radiation exposures. These costs are substantial but to the committee's knowledge, comprehensive estimates of overall costs to federal agencies and society to comply with current radiation protection standards and guidelines are unavailable. Similarly, comprehensive estimates for the overall cost savings for protecting the U.S. population's health by implementing these standards and guidelines are also unavailable. Without these current estimates as a starting point, preparing comprehensive estimates of overall costs to comply with prospective radiation protection standards or guidelines is not possible.

Finding 2: Comprehensive understanding of adverse human health effects emerging from the multidisciplinary low-dose radiation program will enable better assessment of whether current risk estimates (primarily for cancer) at low doses and low dose rates are accurate, underestimated, or overestimated and provide improved risk estimates for other adverse health outcomes. This assessment may impact radiation protection by confirming that current regulations and guidance sufficiently protect human health or by supporting either more restrictive or less restrictive regulations and guidance.

Finding 3: The committee is unable to quantify the low-dose radiation program's economic impacts because comprehensive estimates of overall costs to comply with current radiation standards are unavailable. Additionally, any changes to the current estimates will depend on new information on adverse health effects that will be generated by the low-dose radiation research program. When adjustments in radiation protection standards and guidance are proposed based on new information, agencies can estimate the economic impacts of the changes and perform benefit-cost and cost-effectiveness analyses of alternative measures.

4

Status of Low-Dose Radiation Research

This chapter addresses the third charge of the Statement of Task, which calls for an assessment of the status of current low-dose radiation research in the United States and internationally. This chapter also provides background information to address the sixth charge of the Statement of Task on coordination of low-dose radiation research, which is explicitly addressed in Section 6.8 of this report as one of the seven essential elements of the low-dose radiation program.

The committee discusses the status of low-dose radiation research within the U.S. government (Section 4.1), national laboratories (Section 4.2), universities (Section 4.3), other U.S.-based entities (Section 4.4), and internationally (Section 4.5). The committee notes that currently within the United States there is no dedicated entity to lead, conduct, or otherwise support low-dose radiation research. Instead, a few entities as described in the following sections support research with low-dose radiation components or support research on higher doses of radiation but have expertise that is relevant to low-dose radiation research.

4.1 LOW-DOSE RADIATION RESEARCH IN THE U.S. GOVERNMENT

A few federal agencies within the United States have programs that support or conduct research on low-dose radiation relevant to the agency's specific missions. However, these programs are not explicitly low-dose radiation research programs (see Table 4.1); therefore, estimating the relative commitment to low-dose radiation research and allocated funds is not a straightforward task. A 2017 Government Accountability Office (GAO) report indicated that between 2012 and 2016, the Department of Energy (DOE) and the National Institutes of Health (NIH) were the two agencies supporting most of the low-dose radiation research in the United States. Within that period, the two agencies combined accounted for 98 percent of federal funding for low-dose radiation research. In 2016, the total funding for low-dose radiation research was about $35 million (GAO, 2017).

This section summarizes information on government agencies that support or conduct research on low-dose radiation or whose research is primarily focused on higher doses but have radiation subject-matter expertise. The information summarized below is primarily based on briefings representatives of these agencies provided to the committee during the September 24, 2021, and January 24, 2022, meetings or in follow-on written communications. In addition to the agencies described in this section, the committee also invited the National Institute of Environmental Health Sciences (NIEHS) to provide a briefing but was told that NIEHS does not currently conduct any research related to radiation health. The committee also asked for information in writing from the National Science Foundation (NSF) about its role in low-dose radiation research but did not receive a response. To the best of the committee's knowledge, NSF does not support or conduct research in radiation health.

4.1.1 Department of Energy

Two offices within DOE have historically supported research in low-dose radiation: the Office of Science and the Office of Health and Safety.

Office of Science

The history of the Office of Science Biological and Environmental Research (BER) program's management of the low-dose radiation program (1999–2016) and its current mission are described in Section 1.2. As noted, in support of its mission, BER has remained at the forefront of genome biology research and has also produced computational infrastructure and modeling capabilities that are run on DOE's fastest supercomputers, which are among the most capable in the world (DOE, 2021b). BER supports three DOE Office of Science user facilities: the Atmospheric Radiation Measurement Climate Research Facility, the Environmental Molecular Sciences Laboratory, and the Joint Genome Institute. Additionally, four DOE Bioenergy Research Centers were established to pursue early-stage research on bio-based products, clean energy, and next-generation bioenergy technologies.

TABLE 4.1 Federal Agencies That Support Low-Dose Radiation Research or Have Relevant Expertise

	Low-Dose Radiation Research[a]	Considerable Radiation Health Expertise
Department of Energy		
Office of Science	Not explicitly	No
Office of Health and Safety	Not explicitly	Yes
National Aeronautics and Space Administration	Not explicitly	Yes
National Institutes of Health		
National Cancer Institute		
Radiation Epidemiology Branch	Not explicitly	Yes
Radiation Research Program	No	Yes
National Institute of Allergy and Infectious Diseases	No	Yes
National Institute of Environmental Health Sciences	No	No
Centers for Disease Control and Prevention		
National Institute for Occupational Safety and Health	Not explicitly	Yes
Radiation Studies Section	Not explicitly	Yes
Department of Defense		
Defense Threat Reduction Agency	Not explicitly	Yes
Armed Forces Radiobiology Research Institute	No	Yes
Intelligence Advanced Research Projects Activity	Not explicitly	No
National Science Foundation	No	No

[a] Some agencies define "low dose" as a dose below 1 gray, which is not a low dose for the purposes of this report.

Despite authorization to start a low-dose radiation program and appropriation of funds, DOE's Office of Science has not reestablished a low-dose radiation program of the scale and scope defined in the Consolidated Appropriations Act, 2021. Notably, the Biological Systems Science Division, the division within DOE's Office of Science tasked with establishing the low-dose radiation program, issued its strategic planning report in April 2021 (DOE, 2021a) and did not mention the mandate from Congress to reestablish the low-dose radiation program.

In 2020, DOE's Office of Science received $5 million in appropriations funds for low-dose research and directed it to three national laboratories (Argonne National Laboratory [ANL], Brookhaven National Laboratory [BNL], and Oak Ridge National Laboratory [ORNL]) for "the exploration of the potential for artificial intelligence [AI] and machine learning to advance low-dose radiation biology research."[1] The RadBio-AI project built on models and methods used by the DOE-National Cancer Institute (NCI) collaborative project CANDLE (CANcer Distributed Learning Environment), which aims to develop deep learning methods on computing platforms to support cancer research and enable precision medicine (Peterson and Cooke, 2019). DOE has reported that researchers are adapting models and methods from CANDLE for low-dose radiation research in three areas:[2]

1. Discovering, detecting, and characterizing molecular signatures of radiation damage in biological tissues and determining the potential differentiation of any signatures from radiation types, doses, and exposure patterns.
2. Extracting from the literature and medical records information that can estimate dosing, exposure, and radiation types an individual has been exposed to as well as associated comorbidities.
3. Searching for new methods that can be used to enhance detection sensitivity of molecular signatures, evidence of exposure, and outcomes.

In 2021, the same three DOE national laboratories received an additional $4.5 million to continue work on the RadBio-AI project.[3] In both years, the grants to the national laboratories to support this project were non-competitive, non-peer reviewed, and solicitation was not made to the broad scientific community.

Office of Health and Safety

The mission of the Office of Health and Safety includes establishing DOE worker safety and health policy; conducting health studies to determine worker and public health effects from exposure to hazardous materials associated with DOE operations; implementing medical surveillance and screening programs for current and former workers; and supporting the operation and maintenance of several registries including the Comprehensive Epidemiologic Data Resource, the U.S. Transuranium and Uranium Registries, and the Beryllium-Associated Worker Registry.[4] The Office of Domestic and International Health Studies, within the Office of Health and

---

[1] Email communication from Todd Anderson, DOE, to Ourania Kosti, National Academies, on September 21, 2021.
[2] Email communication from Todd Anderson, DOE, to Ourania Kosti, National Academies, on September 21, 2021.
[3] At the time of this writing (February 2022) publications from this project were not available.
[4] See https://www.energy.gov/ehss/domestic-health-studies-and-activities.

Safety, also supports research programs mandated by Congress or required by international agreement. These include[5]

- The Marshall Islands Program, which provides annual medical surveillance and care, environmental monitoring and characterization, and dose assessment for the peoples of four atolls that were impacted by the U.S. nuclear testing.
- The Russian Health Studies Program, which supports epidemiological studies, radiation dose reconstruction studies, and a tissue repository focused on workers at the Mayak Production Association (Mayak), and on the residents of the communities surrounding this facility, specifically the population living near the Techa River.
- The Japan Program, which supports studies of the Japanese atomic bombing survivors of Hiroshima and Nagasaki carried out at the Radiation Effects Research Foundation (RERF; see Section 4.5.6).

The Office of Health and Safety does not have available funds to support competitive external grants and contracts.

A representative of the Office of Domestic and International Health Studies who briefed the committee did not describe a formal coordination of efforts with the previous low-dose program. However, both the DOE Office of Science and the Office of Environment, Health, Safety and Security supported the Million Person Study at different time periods and interacted during program meetings.[6]

4.1.2 National Aeronautics and Space Administration

The National Aeronautics and Space Administration's (NASA's) primary interest in radiation research is to characterize and mitigate the risk to astronauts' health from space radiation. Space radiation is comprised primarily of galactic cosmic rays, solar particle events, and trapped radiation, making it both quantitatively and qualitatively different from terrestrial radiation (see NASEM, 2021c). The doses received over an astronaut's career tend to be within the moderate-dose region and are expected to be higher (exceed 1 Sv) for long-duration Mars missions. However, low-dose radiation research is highly relevant for some NASA space missions, for example, to the International Space Station. Furthermore, the health outcomes of interest and the scientific approaches to understand the effect of radiation are consistent across the low- and moderate-dose regions.

---

[5] See https://www.energy.gov/ehss/international-health-studies-and-activities.
[6] Anthony Pierpoint, DOE, presentation to the committee on August 26, 2021.

NASA supports three research programs that investigate the effect of radiation on health (NASEM, 2019c):

1. The Human Research Program (HRP), which aims to investigate and mitigate the risks to astronauts' health and performance in support of exploration missions. HRP utilizes an Integrated Research Plan to identify research activities and approaches to address known risks to astronauts' health (NASA, 2021), and these activities are undertaken by one of five HRP Elements.[7] The main focus of the Space Radiation Element is the characterization and mitigation of radiation risk.
2. The Space Biology Program, which examines how plants and animals regulate and sustain their growth in space.
3. The Space Station Research and Technology Program, which conducts research on a large array of different experiments from biology and biotechnology to human health research relevant to exploration missions.

NASA has developed several databases and repositories for human and non-human data and samples to enable future experiments. The Lifetime Surveillance of Astronaut Health repository contains astronaut medical data for clinical use; the Life Science Data Archive contains data from astronauts collected by HRP for research purposes; the Ames Life Sciences Data Archive (ALSDA) contains data from mammalian and microbial experiments; and GeneLab contains space-related -omics data. According to the NASA representative who briefed the committee,[8] usage of FAIR (findable, accessible, interoperable, and reusable) data principles (Wilkinson et al., 2016) for GeneLab and ALSDA help optimize the reusability of archived datasets and transform multiple databases to a knowledge-based system for risk modeling and risk assessment and for meta-analysis (see Figure 4.1).

Collaboration between NASA and DOE started with NASA's support for operations of the Princeton Particle Accelerator and the Lawrence Berkeley National Laboratory (LBNL). Following the closing of the LBNL Bevalac accelerator, NASA and DOE signed agreements to ensure that beams of high-energy heavy ions continued to be available to simulate space radiation for physics and radiobiology research. NASA also had significant programmatic engagement with DOE's low-dose program, likely more than any other federal agency. In 2002, DOE's Office of Science and NASA's Office of Biological and Physical Research under the Space Biology Program signed a memorandum of understanding (MOU) to establish

---

[7] See https://www.nasa.gov/hrp/elements.
[8] Sylvain Costes, NASA, presentation to the committee on September 24, 2021.

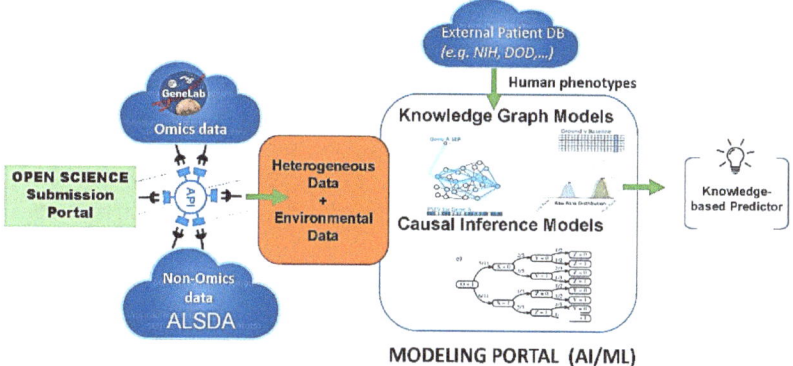

FIGURE 4.1 The National Aeronautics and Space Administration's (NASA's) knowledge-based system integrates information from multiple databases. The committee did not examine the effectiveness of the system.
NOTE: AI = artificial intelligence; ALSDA = Ames Life Sciences Data Archive; API = application programming interface; DB = database; DoD = Department of Defense; ML = machine learning; NIH = National Institutes of Health.
SOURCE: Sylvain Costes, NASA, presentation to the committee on September 24, 2021.

"formal scientific collaboration in understanding and predicting the effects and health risks resulting from low-dose and low-fluence radiation" (Schimmerling, 2011). Areas of common interest included relation between endogenous oxidative damage and low-dose radiation-induced damage, adaptive responses, bystander effects, and individual genetic susceptibility to low-dose radiation (Schimmerling, 2011). From 2003 to 2010, NASA and DOE jointly funded more than 50 projects that led to critical data generation and training of radiobiologists. The two agencies also co-funded workshops with international partners including RIKEN, Japan's research institution in physics, engineering, chemistry, and computational science. According to the expert who briefed the committee, the reduction of funds at NASA for radiobiology research after 2010 along with the termination of DOE's low-dose program eliminated opportunities for joint projects at that time.[9]

---

[9] Francis Cucinotta, University of Nevada, Las Vegas, presentation to the committee on August 26, 2021.

4.1.3 National Institutes of Health

The committee received information on two programs within NCI and one within the National Institute of Allergy and Infectious Diseases (NIAID) that conduct or support research in low-dose radiation or have relevant expertise. The NCI programs on which the committee received information are the Radiation Epidemiology Branch (REB) within the Division of Cancer Epidemiology and Genetics, which is part of NCI's intramural research program; and the Radiation Research Program within the Division of Cancer Treatment and Diagnosis, which is part of NCI's extramural research program.[10] The program within NIAID is the Radiation and Nuclear Countermeasures Program (RNCP), which is also an extramural program. The committee is also aware that NCI's Environmental Epidemiology Branch within the Division of Cancer Control and Population Sciences supports extramural projects on low-dose chronic radiation exposures but did not have the opportunity to hear directly on that office's research portfolio.

Radiation Epidemiology Branch, NCI

REB's mission is to identify and quantify the risk of cancer in populations exposed to medical, occupational, or environmental radiation, and to advance understanding of radiation carcinogenesis. Some priority research areas within REB are quantifying the magnitude of the cancer risk at low doses and the impact of dose and dose rate, identifying the most radiosensitive populations, understanding the dose response for cardiovascular disease or cataracts, and pairing epidemiological studies with molecular studies to understand the mechanisms of radiation-related carcinogenesis.

REB has collaborated with several government agencies on low-dose radiation research. For example, together with DOE, it co-funded studies of health effects of the Japanese atomic bombing survivors and studies of workers employed at the Mayak Production Association, the first plutonium production plant in the former Soviet Union. REB has also collaborated with the National Institute for Occupational Safety and Health (NIOSH) on research studies such as the U.S. flight attendant cohort, and with the Environmental Protection Agency to co-fund events such as the National Academies' Gilbert W. Beebe symposia, which aim to bring together the radiation science and radiation protection communities to discuss issues of radiation health. REB also collaborates in several studies with national and international academic and other organizations. For

---

[10] Intramural NCI research is carried out by NCI employees, and extramural research is carried out by universities and research centers across the United States and in some foreign countries by investigators who have been awarded grants through the NCI grant program.

example, the UK-NCI computed tomography scan study with the University of Newcastle (Pearce et al., 2012); the U.S. Radiologic Technologists with the University of Minnesota (Kitahara et al., 2018; Little et al., 2020b, 2021b; Velazquez-Kronen et al., 2020); the Ukrainian Trios Study (Yeager et al., 2021) and the Ukrainian liquidators case-control studies (Gudzenko et al., 2022) with the National Research Center for Radiation Medicine of the National Academy of Medical Sciences of Ukraine; and the U.S. interventional radiology physician cohort with the American Medical Association (Linet et al., 2017).

Radiation Research Program, NCI

The Radiation Research Program is responsible for management of NCI's research support for radiation science spanning clinical trials, combined-modality radiotherapy, experimental therapeutics, radiation treatment planning, radiobiology, physics, and technology. A "low dose" for radiation oncology programs is defined as a dose in the lower end of the therapeutic range, generally at least 1–2 gray (Gy). The program did not have formal collaboration with the previous low-dose radiation program but had informal interactions at professional scientific meetings.

Radiation and Nuclear Countermeasures Program, NIAID

NIAID's RNCP supports basic research, preclinical development, and advanced development related to medical countermeasures, biodosimetry, and decorporation following radiation public health emergency scenarios (e.g., detonation of a nuclear bomb or improvised nuclear device, a nuclear power plant accident or attack, and radionuclide exposures). RNCP's short-term focus is on triage and treatment of life-threatening, high-dose radiation exposures, and its long-term focus is on delayed effects of acute radiation exposure with limited focus on cancer (which is the primary focus of NCI). That is, through its mandate, RNCP typically researches the effects of doses higher than 1 Gy delivered acutely or cumulatively with low dose rate and has a limited portfolio on internal emitters for decorporation and biodosimetry purposes.

The representative who briefed the committee[11] said that RNCP collaborates and shares funding with other government agencies including the Office of the Assistant Secretary for Preparedness and Response, the Armed Forces Radiobiology Research Institute (AFRRI), the Biomedical Advanced Research and Development Authority, the Centers for Disease Control and Prevention (CDC), the Food and Drug Administration, NASA, and the

---

[11] Andrea DiCarlo-Cohen, NIAID, presentation to the committee on September 24, 2021.

National Institute of Standards and Technology. NIAID also collaborates with other NIH institutes. For example, it funded the development of a computer program for individual organ dose calculations from radiological accidents or terrorist events and retrospective biodosimetry research at NCI (McKenna et al., 2019). NIAID also collaborates with nongovernmental and international organizations including the Radiation Injury Treatment Network, the World Health Organization's Radiation Emergency Preparedness Action Network Collaborating Center, and many industry partners.

RNCP has hosted 26 scientific meetings since 2005, bringing together government agency representatives (funding agencies and regulators), researchers, and industry representatives, and shares the outcomes of these meetings through peer-reviewed publications. Some recent topics and publications included growth factors and cytokines for radiation injuries (Perez Horta et al., 2019), cutaneous radiation injuries (DiCarlo et al., 2020), neutron radiobiology and dosimetry (Stricklin et al., 2021), and polypharmacy approaches for acute radiation syndrome (Taliaferro et al., 2021).

RNCP has not had formal collaborations with DOE's low-dose program but has had informal interactions at DOE and professional society meetings.

4.1.4 Centers for Disease Control and Prevention

The committee received briefings from two offices within CDC that support low-dose radiation research: NIOSH and CDC's Radiation Studies Section.

National Institute for Occupational Safety and Health

NIOSH's mission is to develop new knowledge relevant to occupational safety and health and to transfer that knowledge into practice. Two divisions within NIOSH conduct or support radiation research: (1) the Division of Field Studies and Engineering, Field Research Branch, conducts epidemiological studies of the health effects of occupational exposure to radiation and evaluates exposures to radiation and other chemical and physical exposures; (2) the Division of Compensation Analysis and Support reconstructs the occupational radiation dose for certain workers with cancer who file claims under the Energy Employees Occupational Illness Compensation Act (see Box 2.1). NIOSH radiation research priorities include quantifying and controlling for sources of uncertainty affecting dose-response relationships; improving individual exposure assessment; evaluating cancer incidence and non-cancer mortality and incidence; expanding research on neutrons, tritium, and plutonium; and investigating potential synergistic effects between radiation and other agents.

Starting in 1990, NIOSH supported (both in intramural and extramural programs) epidemiological studies of workers at DOE nuclear facilities. This work was carried out under a MOU between DOE and the Department of Health and Human Services (HHS), which was put in place because of concerns about DOE's independence and objectivity in conducting research related to radiation health effects (epidemiological studies and radiation exposure assessments). The MOU named DOE as the administrator and funding source for the radiation health effects research while HHS conducted the research (see NRC, 2006b, for more details). The MOU also included clauses for sharing of employment and dosimetry records on Atomic Energy Commission/DOE workers.[12] An independent advisory board, the Advisory Committee for Energy-Related Epidemiologic Research (ACERER), was created to provide advice and strategic direction in conducting the program (see Section 6.2). The reports, peer-reviewed publications, and presentations were summarized and evaluated in a National Academies report (NRC, 2006b) and were distributed to workers and the public to increase transparency. Despite the expiration of the MOU between DOE and HHS, NIOSH continues to conduct radiation research, albeit on a more limited scale. This research includes epidemiological studies of aircrews (Grajewski et al., 2018; Pinkerton et al., 2018), uranium miners (Anderson et al., 2021), and DOE workers (Leuraud et al., 2021; Schubauer-Berigan et al., 2015). NIOSH also participates in analyses of international occupational cohorts including the Pooled Uranium Miner Analysis and the International Nuclear Workers Study and funds extramural research on low-dose radiation.

Radiation Studies Section

The mission of CDC's Radiation Studies Section (formerly Radiation Studies Branch) is to assess radiation-related hazards of public health concern; develop evidence-based environmental public health strategies and interventions to protect the public from radiation-related hazards; and disseminate and translate best practices guidance, training, tools, and information to professional and lay audiences. Exposures to radiation of public health interest include medical exposures, environmental exposures, occupational exposures, and exposures from accidents or acts of terrorism. The Radiation Studies Section carries out work to find out what information

---

[12] The shift of the responsibility for epidemiological studies of radiation health effects from DOE to HHS was recommended by the independent Secretarial Panel for the Evaluation of Epidemiological Research Activities (SPEERA, 1990). The 1990 MOU between DOE and HHS was renewed every 5 years. Although the MOU expired in 2005, DOE continued to fund research for some years afterward.

related to radiation exposures needs to be communicated to whom and how best to communicate it by doing message testing with focus groups, hosting roundtables with professionals and subject-matter experts, and conducting individual interviews and surveys. The representative who briefed the committee noted that CDC scientists from the Radiation Studies Section did not have formal interactions with DOE during the previous low-dose radiation program.[13]

4.1.5 Department of Defense

Two entities that are assets of the Department of Defense (DoD) conduct or support low-dose radiation research or have relevant expertise: AFRRI and the Defense Threat Reduction Agency (DTRA).

Armed Forces Radiobiology Research Institute

AFRRI is responsible for preserving and protecting the health and performance of U.S. military personnel operating in potential radiologically contaminated multidomain conventional or hybrid battle spaces and urban environments. AFRRI is the primary DoD entity dedicated to radiation health effects research, education, and operational training. Research areas include biodosimetry, internal contamination, radiation combined injury, radiation countermeasures, and prophylaxis and treatment. In 2014, AFRRI asked the National Academies to identify opportunities to advance its mission for understanding human health risks from exposure to low-dose radiation with special emphasis on DoD military operations and personnel. A report from the Institute of Medicine and the National Research Council concluded that performing substantive work in this area will first require changes in institutional culture and a reorienting of staff expertise, but it identified several opportunities for additional or expanded roles for AFRRI including in preparedness and response to nuclear or radiological emergencies, management of psychological effects associated with a nuclear or radiological emergency, development and management of DoD radiation protection instrumentation, workforce education for radiation professionals, and support of radiation epidemiology and risk research (IOM and NRC, 2014). Since the release of this report, AFRRI has initiated a low-dose radiation program, defining "low dose" as doses below 1 Gy. The expert who briefed the committee did not provide details on specific projects supported under this new program.[14]

---

[13] Armin Ansari, CDC, presentation to the committee on September 24, 2021.
[14] Alexandra Miller, AFRRI, presentation to the committee on September 24, 2021.

Defense Threat Reduction Agency

DTRA is a combat support agency for countering weapons of mass destruction (WMDs). Established in 1998 as part of the 1997 Defense Reform Initiative, it has focused its basic research efforts in areas to reduce, eliminate, and counter the threat and mitigate the effects of WMDs, including those that are radiological in nature. Although the focus encompasses higher doses and dose rates of radiation, DTRA conducts research on single high-energy particle strikes and has provided limited funding for space radiation research (see Appendix D).

4.1.6 National Science and Technology Council

The American Innovation and Competitiveness Act of 2017 (Public Law 114-329) tasked the National Science and Technology Council (NSTC) with coordinating federal efforts related to radiation biology research and with formulating scientific goals for the future of low-dose radiation research in the United States. The report from this effort was publicly released in 2022 (NSTC, 2022). It recommends establishment of an interagency coordination mechanism within the federal government and with international partners for low-dose radiobiology research, with the overall goal to promote communication and a course of research that reduces uncertainty in risk estimates for adverse health outcomes and establishes the shape of the dose-response curve for adverse health outcomes at low doses and low dose rates of radiation (NSTC, 2022). The expert who briefed the committee noted that "defining the threshold of impact for low-dose and low-dose-rate" radiation is a priority for the NSTC committee.[15]

The NSTC report uses the Committee on Interagency Radiation Research and Policy Coordination (CIRRPC) as an example of coordinating mechanism for radiation research and policy among federal agencies. CIRRPC was established in 1984 by the Office of Science and Technology Policy, with the mandate to coordinate radiation matters between agencies, evaluate research, and provide recommendations on the formulation of radiation policy. In 1994, CIRRPC became a subcommittee of the Committee on Health, Safety and Food, under the NSTC (Young, 2020). CIRRPC consisted of two components, a policy committee and a science panel of senior radiation scientists from member agencies. Technical and administrative support for the CIRRPC program was provided through a DOE contract with Oak Ridge Associated Universities. CIRRPC published 20 reports that addressed radiation research

---

[15] Kartik Sheth, White House Office of Science and Technology Policy, presentation to the committee on January 24, 2022.

and policy issues such as radiation compensation, measurements, records, and controls; radiation exposure, dose, and risk assessment; and health effects of low levels of radiation (Young, 2020). It was dismantled in 1995 after 11 years of operation because of challenges with establishing consensus and coordinating agencies' policies. According to a 1994 GAO report, CIRRPC's interagency coordination of radiation protection policy was ineffective.

The expert who briefed the committee[16] did not provide details on how a CIRRPC-type committee would operate to coordinate low-dose radiation research across the federal government. Specifically, details on membership of the committee, funding, and authority remain to be determined.

4.1.7 Intelligence Advanced Research Projects Activity

The Intelligence Advanced Research Projects Activity within the Office of the Director of National Intelligence invests in high-risk/high-reward projects. An unlikely radiation research agency, it recently launched the Targeted Evaluation of Ionizing Radiation Exposure (TEI-REX) program to establish novel minimally invasive biodosimetry methods for low doses of radiation (defined as doses below 0.75 Gy). The TEI-REX program asks research teams in several entities including the Los Alamos National Laboratory (LANL) and LBNL to develop novel approaches to detect radiation-induced changes in noninvasive samples such as skin, hair, nails, and saliva.[17]

4.2 LOW-DOSE RADIATION RESEARCH IN NATIONAL LABORATORIES

National laboratories have traditionally been a vital component of DOE's research capabilities, including radiation research, enabling teams of scientists spanning biology, chemistry, physics, and computation to tackle scientific questions and develop technologies deployed nationally and internationally. For example, national laboratories supported DOE's large radiobiology life-span studies of more than 200,000 mice, 40,000 rats, and 30,000 dogs that were exposed to varying doses, dose rates, and qualities of ionizing radiation. These animals were followed throughout their life span with incredible amounts of recorded experimental detail, pathologies, and reports of disease state (see Zander et al., 2019, for review). The life-span studies involved extensive coordination among the Inhalation Toxicology Research Institute for inhaled radionuclides in dogs and rats,

---

[16] Kartik Sheth, White House Office of Science and Technology Policy, presentation to the committee on January 24, 2022.
[17] See https://discover.lanl.gov/news/stories/010522-biodosimetry.

Pacific Northwest National Laboratory (PNNL) for injected and inhaled radionuclides in dogs, ORNL for mouse genetics studies, ANL for external beam exposures in dogs and mice, and two universities (University of Utah for inhaled radionuclides and University of California, Davis, for a variety of internal exposures). In addition to these studies, technology development in the national laboratories led to tools including flow cytometry, mass spectrometry, molecular cytogenetic methods, electron microscopy, and aspects of systems biology that can be applied worldwide to detect radiation-induced damage and define precise disease phenotypes. PNNL focused on the development of modern proteomic and systems biology, LANL and Lawrence Livermore National Laboratory (LLNL) focused on flow cytometry and sorting, and LBNL contributed to the development of electron microscopes for assessment of cellular ultrastructures.

During the previous low-dose program, national laboratories (primarily LBNL, ORNL, and PNNL) received about 60 percent of the total low-dose radiation program funding from DOE to conduct research in three scientific focus areas:[18]

1. PNNL on linear and nonlinear tissue-signaling mechanisms in response to low-dose and low-dose-rate radiation,
2. LBNL on a systems biology approach to assessment of responses to low-dose and low-dose-rate ionizing radiation, and
3. ORNL on systems genetics approach to low-dose radiation.

In addition to the above-mentioned capabilities, DOE national laboratories supported radiation facilities suitable for inhalation studies, low-dose and low-dose-rate gamma-ray rooms, neutron exposure facilities, and other facilities relevant to low-dose radiation research that were at one time exceptional and recognized worldwide. However, these facilities are no longer operational due to lack of maintenance and eventual decommissioning.

To understand the current role of the national laboratories in low-dose radiation research supported by the federal government, if any, the committee requested from DOE a list of low-dose projects supported by national laboratories, including their scope and funding level. DOE provided to the committee a list of 49 projects carried out in 7 DOE national laboratories (ANL, BNL, LANL, LBNL, LLNL, ORNL, and PNNL) between 2015 and 2021 (see Appendix D). Upon the committee's review, only a few of the projects, primarily those funded in 2016 (the final year of the previous low-dose program), were low-dose radiation projects as would be defined by the committee. The remaining projects aim to answer scientific questions

---

[18] See https://web.archive.org/web/20150906124306/http://lowdose.energy.gov/national_labs.aspx for additional information.

not directly relevant to a mechanistic understanding of low-dose exposure. According to DOE, total funding for these projects was approximately $60 million for the 6-year period, and support for the projects came from DOE, NIH, NASA, Laboratory Directed Research and Development funds, or other sources. NASA was the largest funding source both in terms of number of projects supported and funding amount.

In addition to the information on projects carried out at national laboratories, DOE also provided to the committee some information on current national laboratory capabilities that are relevant to low-dose radiation research.

ORNL has capabilities to study the effects of radiation on two-dimensional cell culture models, three-dimensional spheroid cultures, and tissues-on-a-chip. In addition, ORNL has developed high-throughput DNA damage assays to evaluate the response to radiation with greater sensitivity using a dissociation-enhanced fluorescence immunoassay for detecting -H2AX formation in cell nuclei.

The NASA Space Radiation Laboratory at BNL develops computational models, methodologies, and biological models to support NASA's missions, but these tools also have some applications at low doses. BNL also supports testing of electronic equipment (often the components of satellites) and of radiation detectors and charged-particle radiation beams as cancer treatment options.

LANL has developed transcriptomics, proteomics, and bioinformatics capabilities. LANL also has numerous platforms for single-cell studies (isolation and flow cytometry).

ANL generates radioisotopes at its Low-Energy Accelerator Facility for medical, national security, basic science, and industrial applications and uses the Argonne Tandem Linac Accelerator System facility for cell experimentation.

PNNL's Radiology Exposure and Metrology laboratory supports radiation dosimetry for radiation worker protection and other applications, as well as microdosimetry and shielding effectiveness studies. The Radiation Dosimetry Lab supports male and female anthropomorphic phantoms for external-beam dose studies, including radiation protection garments. PNNL's Environmental Testing Lab provides for concurrent combinations of temperature, humidity, and radiation exposures.

Although important, these capabilities highlight the refocus of the national laboratories on research areas other than low-dose radiation mechanisms and effects.

4.3 LOW-DOSE RADIATION RESEARCH IN UNIVERSITIES

The late William F. Morgan, laboratory fellow at PNNL, presented at a 2014 National Academies meeting a slide (see Figure 1.2) indicating research support by the low-dose radiation program to about 30 universities in the United States and more internationally. Today, much of the funding support for radiation research is provided by NASA for individual investigator-driven projects or collaborative projects on a focused research goal. NASA provides integration for the different projects it funds at annual meetings. NASA also provides physics support for programs that require it, particularly with regard to using the NASA Space Radiation Laboratory at BNL.

Additional radiation research at universities is supported through funding by NIH, DoD, and other agencies, although the vast majority of this work is on high radiation doses and effects relevant to radiation therapy.

4.4 SUPPORT FOR LOW-DOSE RADIATION RESEARCH BY OTHER U.S. ENTITIES

This section summarizes several entities that have an interest in low-dose radiation research and support it in different ways through their activities.

4.4.1 National Council on Radiation Protection and Measurements

The mission of the National Council on Radiation Protection and Measurements (NCRP) is to support radiation protection by providing independent scientific analysis, information, and consensus recommendations. NCRP has not directly addressed low-dose radiation research priorities, but a number of recent NCRP publications address low-dose radiation issues. These include the following:

- A commentary on the implications of recent epidemiological studies for the linear no-threshold (LNT) model and radiation protection (NCRP, 2018a).
- A report on medical doses to patients in the United States (NCRP, 2019), which provides an update regarding medical doses in a previous report on the broader topic on radiation doses to the U.S. population (NCRP, 2009a).
- A report on approaches for integrating radiation biology and epidemiology for enhancing low-dose risk assessment (NCRP, 2020b). The report includes a discussion of the appropriateness of the

adverse outcome pathway (AOP) methodology[19] for the assessment of radiation effects.
- A commentary on naturally occurring radioactive material (NORM) and technologically enhanced NORM from the oil and gas industry (NCRP, 2020a).

NCRP remains interested in assessing the current status of the radiation professionals' workforce and is updating its 2015 statement titled *Where Are the Radiation Professionals?* (NCRP, 2015b).

4.4.2 Electric Power Research Institute

The Electric Power Research Institute (EPRI) is an international member organization that conducts research and development related to the generation and use of electricity. EPRI has published several documents related to low-dose radiation (EPRI, 2011, 2014, 2020) and has been involved in activities such as the appropriateness of the AOP methodology used to evaluate the biological and toxicological effects of chemicals to provide a framework for the assessment of radiation effects. In 2016, it established the International Dose Effect Alliance to organize workshops with participation from national and international researchers to discuss research agendas, programs, and priorities in low-dose radiation research.

4.4.3 Health Physics Society

The Health Physics Society (HPS) supports radiation protection professionals in the practice of their profession and promotes excellence in the science and practice of radiation safety. In 2017, Oak Ridge Associated Universities and DOE's ORNL in partnership with HPS hosted a workshop to address radiation protection research needs. The research needs were summarized in a recent report authored by an HPS Task Force (HPS, 2021) and were broken down into nine broad areas as follows: nuclear fuel cycle and nuclear power production, radiation protection through improved estimates of radiation effects and risk at low doses, use of radiation for medical care, improved measurement of radiation through instrument development, decontamination and decommissioning of nuclear facilities, exploration of

---

[19] AOP is a conceptual framework developed by the Organisation for Economic Co-operation and Development (OECD) to describe a sequence of causally linked events that occur in response to a stressor and lead to an adverse health outcome relevant to risk-based evaluations and management, and regulatory decision-making. The AOP framework is widely used in chemical toxicity testing and there is a growing interest in applying it for radiation effects.

space, national defense, emergency response to nuclear events, and prediction of the fate and effects of radionuclides in the environment.

The HPS Task Force report did not attempt to prioritize the research needs but instead recommended that several factors be integrated in the prioritization process, including the magnitude of risk reduction, potential resource savings, and operational and medical impacts.

4.4.4 American Nuclear Society

The American Nuclear Society (ANS) is an international member organization that promotes the field of nuclear engineering and related disciplines. In 2017, ANS participated in a membership-wide effort to identify "the technical nuclear challenges that need to be resolved by 2030 in order to help solve some of the economic, sociological, or political issues that we face as a society" (ANS, 2017). In this initiative, the ANS membership identified that establishing a modern scientific basis and guidelines for health effects of low-dose radiation regulation is a top-most priority. In 2020, ANS released an updated position statement and recently supplemented it with technical background (ANS, 2022). In this statement, ANS notes that the LNT model used in radiation protection may not adequately describe the relationship between harm and exposure and that long-term research in low-level radiation exposure is needed to improve risk-informed decision-making.

4.5 SUPPORT FOR LOW-DOSE RADIATION RESEARCH INTERNATIONALLY

Several international entities support low-dose radiation research. The committee had the opportunity to learn about some of these programs or initiatives and summarizes them in the following sections. The entities described here are the Multidisciplinary European Low-Dose Initiative (MELODI); the International Commission on Radiological Protection (ICRP); the United Nations Scientific Committee on the Effects of Atomic Radiation (UNSCEAR); the Nuclear Energy Agency/Organisation for Economic Co-operation and Development (NEA/OECD); and programs in Canada and Japan. This list is not exhaustive, and other international entities and countries not described in this section may support low-dose radiation research.[20] The committee discusses the possibility of joint efforts

---

[20] For example, in India, the Bhabha Atomic Research Centre carries out work on high natural background radiation, and in Russia, the Southern Ural Biophysics Institute and the Urals Research Centre Radiation Medicine carry out some low-dose radiation research.

with these and other international programs and possible cost sharing for low-dose radiation projects in Section 6.8.

4.5.1 Multidisciplinary European Low-Dose Initiative

MELODI[21] is a European research platform dedicated to low-dose radiation health risk research, and is one of six such platforms covering the range of disciplines relevant to radiation protection that operate under the European umbrella organization MEENAS (MELODI, EURADOS, EURAMED, NERIS, ALLIANCE, SHARE).[22] MELODI was established in 2010 following the recommendations of the High Level Expert Group on European Low-Dose Risk Research. Currently, MELODI has more than 40 members from 18 countries who represent national bodies, universities, and research institutes committed to low-dose radiation research. While neither MELODI nor MEENAS provides funding for research, support is provided to the research community to ensure that it is able to respond to funding opportunities, especially those issued by the European Commission's Euratom program. For example, the CONCERT European Joint Programme was a large-scale program that supported nine specific research projects, three of which specifically relate to low-dose health risk.

MELODI has made major contributions to focusing European research efforts through the development and regular updating of a strategic research agenda. The latest agenda (MELODI, 2021) proposes research in four main areas: Dose- and dose-rate dependence of cancer risk, risk for non-cancer effects, individual variation in risk, and effects of spatial- and temporal-variation in dose delivery. MELODI supports annual workshops from which several publications have been produced (see, e.g., Averbeck et al., 2020; Gomolka et al., 2020; Kreuzer and Bouffler, 2021; Pasqual et al., 2021; Seibold et al., 2020; Tapio et al., 2021) and has working groups to address research infrastructure needs as well as education and training.

From 2015 to 2020, CONCERT was operating as an umbrella structure for the research initiatives of several European radiation protection research platforms including MELODI. CONCERT supported 3 emergency preparedness and response projects (total of 50 partners funded at the level of €11.2 million over 3 years); 3 radiobiology projects (total of 16 partners funded at the level of €5.5 million over 3 years); 2 dosimetry projects (total of 17 partners funded at the level of €2.1 million over 2 years); and 1 stakeholder engagement project (13 partners funded at the level of €0.8 million over 2 years).[23] Pianoforte, the follow-on project from CONCERT,

---

[21] See https://melodi-online.eu.
[22] See https://eu-meenas.net/doku.php.
[23] See https://www.concert-h2020.eu/concert-info/about-concert.

is currently in contract negotiations and is expected to fund radiation protection projects at a level estimated to be on the order of €4.1 million per year over 5 years.

4.5.2 International Commission on Radiological Protection

ICRP is an independent, nongovernmental organization tasked with radiation protection; its recommendations form the basis of standards, regulations, and practice of radiological protection worldwide. ICRP initiated a review of the system of radiological protection to address changes in scientific knowledge as well as the use of ionizing radiation in different applications including in medicine, industry, and research (Clement et al., 2021). This review is expected to take a decade to complete and could result in revisions to the system and general recommendations to supersede ICRP Publication 103 (ICRP, 2007). ICRP includes in its strategic plan a priority to identify areas of research to support the system of radiological protection. The latest priorities list was published in 2021 (Laurier et al., 2021) and is summarized in Table 4.2.

4.5.3 United Nations Scientific Committee on the Effects of Atomic Radiation

UNSCEAR has been involved in examination of radiation effects for more than 60 years and has provided reports on a variety of radiation-related topics including effects and risks from ionizing radiation, epidemiological evaluation of radiation-induced cancers, biological effects at low radiation doses, combined effects of radiation and other agents, and **levels and effects of radiation exposure following the Chernobyl and Fukushima accidents.** In 2021, UNSCEAR published a report that examined biological mechanisms relevant to the inference of cancer risks following low-dose and low-dose-rate exposures, dose-response relationships, integration of data at different levels of organization, and modeling of cancer mechanisms, and offered directions for future research. The report was limited to mechanisms relating to cancers and did not consider those relating to non-cancer outcomes (UNSCEAR, 2021).

In the context of this report, the most notable conclusions of the UNSCEAR report are as follows (UNSCEAR, 2021):

- There are limited robust data that can be identified at this time that would prompt the need to change the current approach taken for low-dose radiation cancer risk inference as used for radiation protection purposes.

TABLE 4.2 International Commission on Radiological Protection's Research Priorities to Support the Radiation Protection System

	Short Term/Midterm (up to 10 years)	Longer Term (beyond 10 years)
Research to support radiation risk assessment	Appropriateness of the classification of radiation health effects to tissue reactions and stochastic effects.	Basic research, for example, on mechanisms of low-dose effects at molecular, cellular, and tissue levels including non-targeted effects; identification of radiation signatures for cancer; integration of approaches such as considering adverse outcome pathways.
	Characterization of tissue reactions.	Effects of combined exposures.
	Characterization of stochastic effects and radiation detriment, specifically cancer risk models and tissue weighting factors; dose-rate effects and cancer; impact of non-radiation factors in detriment calculations; potential impact of the circulatory system; effects of radiation from in utero exposure; heritable effects of radiation on offspring and next generations; uncertainty analysis.	
	Individual response of humans to radiation.	
	Radiation effects on non-human biota.	
Research to support dosimetry	Relative biological effectiveness, quality factor, and radiation weighting.	Definition of dosimetric targets in organs and tissues.
	Appropriate dosimetric quantities for medicine and other applications.	Strengthening dosimetric targets and methodology for the protection of the environment.
	Dosimetry in emergency situations.	Biokinetic models of radionuclides and radioactive substances in human tissues.
Research to support the application/ implementation of radiation protection system	Development and use of radiation technologies. Ecosystem protection. Research needs for the application of the system of radiological protection.	

- There remains good justification for the use of a non-threshold model for risk inference for radiation protection purposes, given the present knowledge of the role of mutation and chromosomal aberrations in carcinogenesis.
- The implications of the studies on the induction of transmissible genomic instability, bystander effects, abscopal effects, and adaptive responses are still not clear. Adaptive response studies remain without a confirmed mechanistic basis and are of mixed outcome.
- The recommended approach for combining a mechanistic understanding of low-dose radiation carcinogenesis with epidemiological studies is to use mathematical modeling integrating data from experimental systems (e.g., dose-response data for induction of key mutations or epimutations). The use of AOP approaches can help define and formalize key mechanistic steps in carcinogenesis following low-dose exposures.
- Experimental investigations may identify cancer risk indicators that, when validated, could be integrated into epidemiological investigations to improve statistical power or be used for population screening.

4.5.4 Nuclear Energy Agency/Organisation for Economic Co-operation and Development

NEA is an intergovernmental agency that operates within the framework of OECD with the mission to provide assistance to member countries in maintaining and further developing the scientific, technological, and legal bases required for safe, environmentally friendly, and economical use of nuclear energy for peaceful purposes. Coordination and cooperation among member countries is central to the agency's mission. In 2018, participants of an NEA/OECD scoping meeting concluded that global coordination in low-dose radiation research has the potential to improve cost-effectiveness and efficiency, increase international awareness of research, and facilitate data sharing and access to unique facilities. To address these and other issues, participants of the NEA/OECD scoping meeting recommended the establishment of a high-level group by NEA/OECD to support the development of a global coordination initiative in low-dose research. The high-level group in low-dose research (HLG-LDR) was put in place in 2021 and formed three topical groups to carry out its work tasked with (1) the creation of an online register of ongoing or planned low-dose research projects, (2) the development and use of the AOP framework in radiation research and regulation, and (3) the implementation of a communication strategy. Representatives of the HLG-LDR who briefed the committee provided information on the status of these three efforts.[24]

The low-dose research register (named the Global Register of Low Dose Radiation Research Projects) will include current and in-planning research projects in radiation biology, epidemiology, dosimetry, social sciences, and ecotoxicology and a simple description of research projects and contact information for the principal investigators. Collection of data will begin in 2022. Access to the register will be free and is expected to provide researchers with an efficient tool to identify possible collaboration opportunities, avoid unnecessary duplication of efforts, encourage international cooperation in low-dose research, and assist funding agencies in the selection of projects.

The HLG-LDR is undertaking an international effort to evolve the development and use of the AOP framework in radiation research and regulation. As part of these efforts, the group conducted a survey to gather insights on the challenges related to low-dose radiation research, risk assessment, and regulatory decision-making, and then plans to rank the priority questions. More than 250 questions or challenges were received and their categorization and ranking by a steering committee helped to prioritize the set of questions to the top 25 (unpublished).

HLG-LDR aims to improve communication on low-dose risks and uncertainties and adapt it to a targeted audience. To achieve that, the group will identify the available data and tools that can help in making communication more efficient, exercise how to translate technical results into policy-oriented messages, and create a fast track between research results and science-based policies and regulations.

4.5.5 Support for Low-Dose Radiation Research in Canada

The Canadian government and nuclear industry have increasingly directed resources toward low-dose radiation research. The committee describes a joint effort from Health Canada and the Canadian Nuclear Safety Commission (CNSC) and another effort from the CANDU Owners Group (COG).

Canadian Organization on Health Effects from Radiation Exposure

In 2020, Health Canada in partnership with CNSC established CO-HERE (Canadian Organization on Health Effects from Radiation Exposure)

---

[24] Jacqueline Garnier-Laplace, NEA/OECD, and Dominique Laurier, French Institute for Radiological Protection and Nuclear Safety, presentation to the committee on September 24, 2021.

with four primary goals: improve alignment of the two organizations' research priorities to focus and leverage resources; maintain and enhance expertise in dosimetry, radiobiology, and epidemiology; provide informed and consistent messages to the public and stakeholders on matters involving low-dose and low-dose-rate ionizing radiation; and strengthen Canada's contributions toward international efforts.

COHERE published its strategic research agenda in 2020 and identified five research themes (see Table 4.3). The strategic research agenda will be reviewed every 3 years or at a frequency determined by the participating organizations. Following this review, COHERE will revise the research themes with input from stakeholders and based on available resources and national and international developments of interest to the program. COHERE does not currently have dedicated funding.

TABLE 4.3 Research Themes Under the COHERE Strategic Research Agenda

Themes	Cancer Effects	Non-Cancer Effects	Globalized Data Sharing/ Consolidation	Capacity Building	Epidemiological Studies
Research lines	Conduct mechanistic-based studies to examine dose-response relationships and links to adverse outcomes		Develop expertise in the area of data management and interpretation	Test new technologies/ approaches for identifying low-dose-response effects	Link occupational data to cancer/ mortality data
Priority areas	Lung cancer (radon), kidney cancer (uranium), organ-level cancers (tritium)	Cataracts (high and low linear energy transfer), kidney toxicity (uranium)	Adverse outcome pathway, systematic reviews, benchmark dose modeling	Optical spectroscopy, 3D organoid models, stem cell regeneration, phenotypic assays, dosimetry, -omics technology	International pooled studies, uranium miners, other radon cohorts

SOURCE: Canadian Nuclear Safety Commission, https://www.cnsc-ccsn.gc.ca/eng/resources/research/cohere/strategic-research-agenda-cohere.cfm.

CANDU Owners Group

A second effort within Canada to understand risks at low doses of radiation was initiated in 2017 by COG, a private, not-for-profit corporation funded voluntarily by international CANDU operating utilities, Canadian Nuclear Laboratories, and supplier participants. Motivation for this program was the decreasing political support for nuclear power, negative public attitude toward the future deployment of small modular reactors in Canada, cuts in investment and development in nuclear power, and increased industry operating and life-cycle costs. The scientific questions to be addressed by the program are driven by public concerns regarding low doses of radiation as identified by a social science project undertaken by the Centre for the Study of Science and Innovation Policy within the University of Saskatchewan. The representative who briefed the committee noted that the program is expected to generate information that can be used by those responsible for radiation protection and industry.

The operations of the program are facilitated by an advisory committee of academics and representatives of several Canadian government agencies. Tasks of the advisory committee include review of project progress, recommendations for project changes or initiation of new projects, and approval of manuscripts for journal submission. Project progress is summarized in an annual report to the program funders that is not made publicly available.

The budget for the program is approximately $1.5 million per year and currently supports 16 projects conducted primarily by Canadian universities. Embedded within the projects are training opportunities for masters- and doctoral-level research fellows.

4.5.6 Support for Low-Dose Radiation Research in Japan

The committee received briefings from three institutions in Japan that conduct radiation research: RERF, the National Institutes for Quantum Science and Technology (QST), and the Institute for Environmental Sciences (IES). Although RERF does not exclusively conduct low-dose radiation research, the other two organizations focus on low-dose radiation research questions. Japan is investing in a new project called PLANET, which aims to establish an all-Japan network among regulators, academia, research institutes, industrial partners, and other stakeholders with the objective to propose strategies to improve current understanding of low-dose and low-dose-rate risk.

Radiation Effects Research Foundation

Studies of the atomic bombing survivors of Hiroshima and Nagasaki began in 1947 with the founding of the Atomic Bomb Casualty Commission

(ABCC) by the National Academy of Sciences. In 1975 the ABCC was reorganized into RERF, a joint U.S.–Japan research organization supported with funding from the Japanese Ministry of Health, Labour and Welfare and DOE's Office of Health and Safety; the National Academies continue to support RERF research activities through a cooperative agreement with DOE.

The Life Span Study (LSS) is the major epidemiological study conducted at RERF that was initiated in 1950 and continues today. It follows approximately 120,000 men and women of all ages who were atomic bombing survivors and residents of Hiroshima and Nagasaki (exposed individuals) or were not in either city at the time of the bombings (unexposed individuals). Demographically, the cohort consists of about 82,000 individuals from Hiroshima and 38,000 from Nagasaki; about 50,000 are males and 70,000 are females (Ozasa et al., 2018). As of 2017, 25 percent of the LSS was alive, and the average age was 81. The Adult Health Study is a clinical examination program of about 20,000 members of the LSS who were invited to participate in biennial health examinations beginning in 1958. RERF also conducts in utero studies and follow-up studies of the children of the survivors (F1 and F1 clinical studies) conceived after the bombings (Ozasa et al., 2019).

The atomic bombing survivor studies have made extensive efforts to estimate individual doses, based on data obtained from interviews with survivors or their surrogates regarding their exposure conditions and a detailed dosimetry system known as Dosimetry System 2002 (DS02, Cullings et al., 2006, 2017). These individual-level doses have made it possible to quantify risk (primarily cancer) as a function of dose and to investigate the dependency of the dose response on factors such as age and sex. Since 1950, RERF and its predecessor organization have published 14 reports on mortality among the atomic bombing survivors, 3 reports on cancer incidence, and several papers on cancer risks for individual sites (see Table 4.4 for the most recent publications on cancer incidence). For in utero exposures, the latest update found that atomic bomb radiation was associated with mortality from solid cancer for females but not males (Sugiyama et al., 2021). However, only a small portion (14 percent) of the survivors exposed in utero had died at the end of follow-up, so this cohort is expected to continue to provide valuable information on the effects of in utero exposure and cancer mortality later in life. Excess occurrences of leukemia have not been observed. Findings on untoward pregnancies are summarized in Section 2.2.6. Non-cancer effects such as cardiovascular disease, stroke, diabetes, chronic kidney disease, and cataracts are also under study.

Analyses of the atomic bombing survivor cohorts have identified radiation health effects, primarily for cancer mortality and cancer incidence, at higher doses with relative confidence (Grant et al., 2017; Ozasa et al.,

2012). However, estimating the health effects of low-dose or low-dose-rate radiation exposures using this cohort have been challenging. First, statistical uncertainties in health effects at low doses must account for errors that arise due to uncertainty in dosimetry parameters and measurement error in radiation exposure data. Currently, dose estimates for atomic bombing survivors do not fully account for all these sources of uncertainty. Second, while lifetime follow-up allows for a detailed ascertainment of health outcomes, competing risks between outcomes and how those outcomes might be differentially associated with radiation dose can impact the shape of the estimated dose-response association. Third, the LSS has only a limited collection of potential confounders and other risk factors to which small effects at low doses could be particularly sensitive. Therefore, identification of radiation-induced health effects at low doses cannot be based on the LSS alone.

A unique asset of RERF is the longitudinally collected biosamples donated by study participants. Close to 2 million biosample tubes have been collected today and stored at RERF. These samples provide important opportunities to identify potential biomarkers and study in detail the pathogenesis of both cancer and non-cancer effects using a range of -omics approaches. The biosample collection includes 1,000 parent–child trios, in which parents will have varied levels of exposure, suitable for the investigation of heritable genetic effects of parental radiation exposure. Today, biosamples at RERF remain largely underutilized. The foundation is taking steps to assess the ethical, legal, and social implications of human genome studies using these biosamples (Noda et al., 2021) and aims to initiate large-scale genomic and epigenomic analyses to identify differences in exposed and unexposed individuals in 2023.

National Institutes for Quantum Science and Technology

QST's Department of Radiation Effects Research conducts research on the risk of carcinogenesis from low-dose radiation exposure using several animal models on identification of radiation signatures (Ishida et al., 2010; Tsuruoka et al., 2021). These studies have been driven by increasing anxiety regarding the impacts of long-term exposure to low doses of radiation in the context of nuclear accidents as well as medical radiation use. QST also collaborates in dosimetry for the epidemiological study of health effects in Fukushima nuclear emergency workers (Kitamura et al., 2018). The economic and practical limitations of conducting large-scale experiments as well as the ethical considerations led QST to the decision to store and share the pathological data and samples of the animal experiments for future use by constructing an archive called the Japan-Storehouse of Animal Radiobiology Experiments.

TABLE 4.4 Summary of Cancer Incidence in the Life Span Study

Site	Total Incidence of Cases (m; f)	Sex-Averaged ERR at 1 Gy (95% CI)	Effect Modification by ATB, AA	Adjusted Life Style and Other Factors	Publication
All solid	10,473; 12,065	0.47 (0.39, 0.55)	30, 70*	Smoking	Grant et al., 2017
Esophagus	394; 92	0.30 (0.06, 0.66)	30, –	Smoking, drinking	Sakata et al., 2019
Stomach	3,090; 2,571	0.33 (0.20, 0.47)	–, 70	Smoking	Sakata et al., 2019
Colon	782; 1,132	0.63 (0.34, 0.98)	30, 70	Smoking, drinking, meat intake, BMI	Sugiyama et al., 2020
Rectum	518; 528	0.025 (−0.087, 0.14)	30, 70	Smoking, drinking, meat intake, BMI	Sugiyama et al., 2020
Liver	1,166; 850	0.58 (0.27, 0.95)	30, 70	Smoking, drinking, BMI	Sadakane et al., 2019
Pancreas	306; 417	0.45 (0.07, 0.92)	30, 70	Smoking, drinking, BMI	Sadakane et al., 2019
Lung	1,445; 1,001	0.81 (0.51, 1.18)	30, 70	Smoking	Cahoon et al., 2017
Female breast	1,470	1.12 (0.73, 1.59)	30, 70	Smoking, BMI, menarche, menopause, pregnancy-delivery	Brenner et al., 2018
Uterine corpus	224	0.73 (0.03, 1.87)	–, –	Smoking, first pregnancy, menopause	Utada et al., 2018
Uterine cervix	982	0.00 (−0.22, 0.31)	–, –	BMI, pregnancy-delivery, menopause	Utada et al., 2018
Urinary tract, bladder	493; 297	1.4 (0.82, 2.1)	30, 70	Smoking	Grant et al., 2020
Ovary	288	0.30 (−0.22, 1.11)	–, –	None of life style or reproductive factors	Utada et al., 2020
Prostate	851	0.57 (0.21, 1.00)	–, –	None	Mabuchi et al., 2020
Central nervous system	99; 186	1.40 (0.61, 2.57)	–, –	None	Brenner et al., 2020

* Risk estimates for ATB of 30 years and AA of 70 years.

NOTE: AA = attained age; ATB = at the time of the bomb; BMI = body mass index; CI = confidence interval; ERR = excess relative risk; Gy = gray.

SOURCE: Robert Ullrich, Radiation Effects Research Foundation, presentation to the committee on January 24, 2022.

Institute for Environmental Sciences

IES was established in 1990 with the mission to monitor radioactive releases and their effect on the environment and human health from the Spent Nuclear Fuel Recycling Plant in Rokkasho Village, Aomori Prefecture. IES accomplishes this mission by carrying out research activities at the Radioecology and Radiation Biology Departments. The institute currently has two mouse facilities conducting experiments on long-term low-dose-rate (0.05, 1, and 20 milligrays per day [mGy/day]) and medium-dose-rate (200 and 400 mGy/day) exposures to gamma rays, which are comparable to the doses accumulated by radiation workers. These facilities are available to outside investigators upon request. Studies conducted at IES include changes in somatic effects, transgenerational effects, and mechanisms following low-dose exposures. Future directions include studies on individual radiosensitivity including the effect of sex, age, diet, environment, and genetic background; epigenetic changes; neurobiological changes; and tritium internal exposures.

4.6 CHAPTER SUMMARY

A few federal agencies within the United States (primarily DOE, NASA, NIH, CDC, and DoD) have programs that support or conduct research on low-dose radiation relevant to the agency's specific missions. Some offices within these agencies have relevant expertise but the research they support is primarily on higher doses and exposures. National laboratories have traditionally been a vital component of DOE's research capabilities, including radiation research, enabling teams of scientists spanning biology, chemistry, physics, and computation to tackle scientific questions and develop technologies deployed nationally and internationally. Since termination of the previous low-dose radiation research program, national laboratory capabilities have been refocused on research areas other than low-dose radiation mechanisms and effects. Radiation research at universities is primarily supported by NASA for individual investigator-driven projects or collaborative projects on a focused research goal relative to NASA's missions. There is currently no explicitly low-dose radiation research program in the United States. Internationally, several countries and regions, including Canada, Europe, and Japan, have focused low-dose radiation programs.

5

Prioritized Research Agenda

This chapter addresses Charges 2 and 4 of the Statement of Task, which call for the identification of the current scientific challenges for understanding low-dose and low-dose-rate radiation-induced health effects and for recommending a long-term strategic and prioritized research agenda to address scientific research goals. The committee's prioritization process is discussed in Section 5.1 and the research priorities in Sections 5.2–5.4. Section 5.5 provides the timeline and cost estimates for implementing the recommended research agenda, and Section 5.6 compares the committee's recommended agenda to those of other entities.

5.1 LOW-DOSE RADIATION RESEARCH CHALLENGES AND OVERVIEW OF RESEARCH PRIORITIES

The committee addressed Charge 2 of its Statement of Task by listing challenges for epidemiological and biological research as well as some that are common to both research approaches (see Box 5.1). These challenges arise because the effects of low-dose and low-dose-rate radiation exposures are assumed to be subtle and difficult to distinguish from those caused by other stressors or "spontaneous" changes that adversely affect the normal functions of cells, tissues, and organs. Moreover, a full understanding of possible effects may be complicated by change in the magnitude of observed effect with dose, dose rate, type of radiation, and duration of exposure.

The committee addressed Charge 4 of its Statement of Task by proposing an agenda for a multidisciplinary research program intended to improve the evidence base used as the foundation for protection of the U.S. population

> **BOX 5.1**
> **Challenges in Low-Dose Radiation Research**
>
> The list of major challenges presented here was informed by the views that were provided to the committee by experts during its public meetings.[a]
>
> **Epidemiological Approaches**
>
> - The adverse health outcomes to be tested for association with radiation exposure are seldom precisely characterized for molecular and other characteristics. As a consequence, nominally similar health outcomes that differ in etiology and/or radiation response may be combined, thereby limiting efforts to define dose-response relationships and/or reducing sensitivity by including health outcomes that can be demonstrated to arise from causes other than radiation.
> - There may be radiation-related competing risks for the health outcome under study that are often ignored in epidemiological analyses (Andersen et al., 2012). In particular, combining competing risk outcomes into a single outcome can affect the shape of the radiation dose response (Brenner et al., 2022).
> - Radiation dose estimates are often uncertain or imprecise, which can introduce bias, potentially resulting in underestimation of risk differences between the exposed and unexposed groups, and reduce statistical power (Daniels et al., 2020).
> - Observational studies may be affected by both measured and unmeasured or residual confounding factors (Schubauer-Berigan et al., 2020).
> - The radiation dose response may vary by individual characteristics including prior exposures, stress, genetic predisposition, epigenetic profile, and immune history.
> - Establishment of cause-effect relationships, although an important goal of low-dose radiation epidemiological studies, is often challenged by study design conditions which could result in a number of possible explanations for the observed associations or lack thereof. In the absence of an integrated mechanistic understanding, epidemiological studies are unable to make strong judgments as to whether an observed association represents a cause-effect relationship between low-dose radiation exposure and the adverse health outcome.
>
> **Biological Approaches**
>
> - Lack of understanding of how systemic interactions contribute to adverse health effects.
> - Insufficient consideration of more recently discovered mechanisms for tissue, cellular, and genetic regulation, including epigenetic modification, immune status, cellular senescence, aging, and systemic interactions.

- Lack of molecular techniques with sufficient sensitivity and specificity to detect the subtle biological and related effects of low-dose and low-dose-rate radiation exposure.
- Limited use of single-cell and tissue imaging technologies to determine subcellular mechanisms or mechanisms that involve only a few cells.
- Lack of appropriate animal and other biological models (e.g., organs-on-a-chip) for direct translatability of research to human risk.
- Lack of infrastructure such as inhalation and chronic exposure facilities to conduct some specific low-dose and low-dose-rate radiation studies.

Common Challenges

- Inadequate statistical power to detect radiation health effects when the outcome is rare and/or when the magnitude of the effect is small.
- Inadequate consideration and characterization of the types of exposure (internal versus external, radiation type, anatomic location), doses, and dose rates, if such characteristics lead to differences in the magnitude of health effect.
- Traditional dose-response analyses are typically based on a single estimate of radiation dose per person or a univariable summary of multiple potential dose realizations estimated from Monte Carlo simulation methods. Dose-response analysis methods that accommodate multiple potential dose estimates per person (Stram et al., 2021) have the potential to provide more reliable radiation risk estimates by acknowledging the shared and unshared uncertainties in radiation doses.
- Limited biomarkers associated with low-dose and lose-dose-rate radiation-induced adverse health effects (tissues, cell types, individuals) that could be studied earlier or are easier than studying the health effect itself.
- Lack of well-established methodologies to integrate and incorporate data from biological and molecular epidemiology studies into models fit to epidemiological data.
- Lack of incorporation of measurement and data science with computer technology with sufficient sensitivity and specificity to detect the subtle biological and related effects of low-dose and low-dose-rate radiation exposure.

---

[a] This list was informed by Dale Preston (Hirosoft International), presentation to the committee on November 16, 2021; Edouard Azzam (Canadian Nuclear Laboratories), David Brenner (Columbia University), Albert Fornace, Jr. (Georgetown University), Amy Kronenberg (Lawrence Berkeley National Laboratory), and Zhi-Min Yuan (Harvard T.H. Chan School of Public Health), panel discussion on August 26, 2021; and Francesca Dominici (Harvard T.H. Chan School of Public Health), Daniel Krewski (University of Ottawa), and Jonathan Samet (Colorado School of Public Health), presentations to the committee on December 9, 2021.

against the adverse health effects that result from exposures to low-dose and low-dose-rate radiation. Knowledge gaps of the current radiation protection system are summarized in Box 3.1 in Chapter 3. The proposed research agenda aims to fill these gaps by integrating information from epidemiological analyses of the adverse health effects of low-dose radiation with information on cell and molecular responses of humans and laboratory models to exposures to low-dose and low-dose-rate radiation revealed by new-generation analytical tools. Approaches for integrating information from radiation biology and epidemiology to enhance low-dose health risk assessment are described in detail elsewhere (NCRP, 2020a). The greatest benefits and most efficient and rapid progress in the program will be achieved through coordinated multidisciplinary research that harnesses new technologies, methodologies, and biomedical understanding that are being developed by the U.S. scientific enterprise. To achieve this, a sustained and coordinated low-dose and low-dose-rate research community will need to be created and nurtured.

The committee recommended research program leverages advances in modern science and sets ambitious goals for revitalized low-dose radiation research in the United States: to improve understanding of adverse human health effects from exposures at doses and dose rates experienced by the U.S. population, to identify mechanisms for induction of these health effects, to develop improved risk models for doses and dose rates at which direct measurement of risks is not possible or limited, and to develop more individualized risk estimates. As such, it is expected to require multiple decades of investment. These investments are expected to be at the level of $100 million per year over a period of 10–15 years, but periodic reassessments are required as suitable study cohorts and necessary infrastructures are established (see Section 5.4).

The criteria used by the committee to identify priorities for low-dose and low-dose-rate research included (1) existing human, laboratory model, and cellular evidence for adverse health effects resulting from radiation exposure; (2) limitations in the current radiation protection system in the United States; (3) feasibility of improving low-dose and low-dose-rate risk estimation models given newly available technologies and resources as well as increased understanding of human disease mechanisms; and (4) issues of concern for exposed populations and impacted communities. The committee's list of 11 research priorities considered these four criteria, and the proposed approaches for addressing each are summarized in Table 5.1. These research priorities are broadly classified as epidemiological research, biological research, and research infrastructure. The committee strongly emphasizes the need for integration across the research lines and anticipates that the most impactful projects will include work in more than one research line and will be carried out by multidisciplinary teams and that some may require collaboration with international partners.

The epidemiological line of research focuses on directly quantifying the risks of adverse health outcomes following low-dose and low-dose-rate exposures to the types of radiation that are or may be experienced by the U.S. population. The biological line of research focuses on the mechanistic underpinnings of the effects of low-dose and low-dose-rate radiation on molecular pathways including influences from intra- and extracellular interactions and the identification of potential causal relationships to different health outcomes. The infrastructure line of research focuses on developing or deploying new observational and experimental systems, computational technologies, and shared access data systems.

The proposed research will address cancer and non-cancer health outcomes including cardiovascular disease, neurological disorders, immune dysfunction, cataracts, and heritable genetic effects for both internal and external exposures. It also encourages a focus on directly observing health effects from low-dose and low-dose-rate exposures, complemented with biological studies that emphasize exposures below 10 milligray (mGy) representative of the majority of exposures of interest for radiation protection, and/or exposures delivered at dose rates around 5 mGy/h.

The order of the research priorities in Table 5.1 does not imply an order of significance; instead, the priorities are considered to be equally important. Some of these activities can be initiated immediately, and others can only begin after a better foundation is built from current or new research or with additional input from the research and broader stakeholder community, including the impacted communities. The committee's views on the timeline for research activities for the first 10–15 years are discussed in Section 5.5.

In the committee's judgment, the 11 research priorities will enable more accurate estimation of adverse health effects that result from exposure to low-dose and low-dose-rate radiation and will dramatically improve knowledge of the complex cellular and molecular processes that are engaged during transduction of low-dose and low-dose-rate radiation damage into adverse health outcomes. The committee also noted that some of the research priorities can have additional benefits including capacity building, training of the next generation of radiation researchers, and development of tools that could be transferrable to other lines of research. However, the committee recognizes that these research priorities do not represent a complete list of important low-dose and low-dose-rate radiation research questions. For example, studies designed to confirm or strengthen the basis for existing scientific findings, particularly those that are controversial or lack a clear interpretation, are also important. In addition, research in radioecology, in the psychological effects following low-dose radiation exposures, and in radiation risk communication are not included in the recommended strategic agenda but are topics that are worth exploring by the low-dose radiation program in the future.

TABLE 5.1 Committee Recommended Research Priorities for Low-Dose and Low-Dose-Rate Radiation Research

Priority Research Goal	Approach	Integration Across Research Lines
Epidemiological Research		
E1 Develop and deploy analytical tools for radiation epidemiology.	Develop cohorts of sufficient size, with detailed health information and biosample collection and accurate dosimetry, to support epidemiological studies of radiation-induced health effects in medically, occupationally, and environmentally exposed U.S. populations.	B2–B4; I1–I3
E2 Improve estimation of risks for cancer and non-cancer health outcomes from low-dose and low-dose-rate external and internal radiation exposures.	More precisely define health outcomes to enable exclusion of diseases caused by other effects, identifying easily measured signatures that can serve as disease surrogates by improving dosimetry and identifying and compensating for confounding and modifying factors.	B1–B4; I1–I3
E3 Determine factors that modify the low-dose and low-dose-rate radiation-related adverse health effects.	Assess the impact of genetic makeup, epigenomic status, DNA repair efficacy, comorbidities, exposure history to radiation and other agents, lifestyle and psychosocial factors, and immune status on radiation-induced adverse health outcomes.	B1–B4; I1–I3
Biological Research		
B1 Develop appropriate model systems for study of low-dose and low-dose-rate radiation-induced health effects.	Identify laboratory model systems in which molecular, cellular, and pathological features of radiation-induced health effects are similar to humans.	E2–E3; I1–I4
B2 Develop biomarkers for radiation-induced adverse health outcomes.	Identify radiation-induced changes in cellular and molecular features that causally link to adverse health effects in appropriate model systems.	E1–E3; I1–I4
B3 Define health-effect dose-response relationships below 10 mGy and below 5 mGy/h.	Establish radiation dose-response curves for molecular and cellular endpoints and for associated early- and late-stage diseases at doses below 10 mGy and dose rates below 5 mGy/h.	E1–E3; I1–I4

B4 Identify factors that modify or confound estimation of risks for radiation-induced adverse health outcomes.	Assess the impact of genetic makeup, epigenomic status, DNA repair efficacy, comorbidities, exposure history to radiation and other agents, lifestyle factors, and immune status on low-dose and low-dose-rate radiation-induced adverse health effects and associated cellular and molecular response endpoints.	E1–E3; I1–I4
Research Infrastructure		
I1 Tools for sensitive detection and precise characterization of aberrant cell and tissue states.	Identify, develop, and deploy bulk and single-cell -omics[a] and image measurement and computational analysis workflows to quantify disease-linked cellular and molecular signatures that are sufficiently sensitive, reliable, and low cost for wide-scale application.	E1–E3; B1–B4
I2 Harmonized databases to support biological and epidemiological studies.	Develop accessible databases that document exposure levels, rates, types, and durations as well as cell, molecular, and health outcomes for human populations and experimental models.	E1–E3; B1–B4
I3 Dosimetry for low-dose and low-dose-rate exposures.	Elucidate biological localization of internalized radionuclides; directly measure radiation-induced damage and associated response mechanisms; develop high-fidelity anatomically and physiologically based dosimetry; develop and apply modern statistical and computational methods for dose reconstruction.	E1–E3; B1–B4
I4 Facilities for low-dose and low-dose-rate exposures.	Ensure access to low-dose and low-dose-rate exposure facilities, including those allowing internal exposure in model systems by a variety of routes (e.g., inhalation, ingestion) or invest in new facilities.	B1–B4

[a] The broader field of "-omics" includes genomics, transcriptomics, proteomics, metabolomics, and radiomics.

NOTE: mGy = milligray.

The research priorities are discussed in Sections 5.2–5.4 with emphasis on significance, current status, and promising research directions. The committee expects that the specific tactics for addressing these priorities will be developed with input from the extended research community and other stakeholders, including the impacted communities. Importantly, the committee recognizes that the list of priorities will likely evolve as biological understanding and research tools advance and as the research community and other stakeholders are engaged with the program (see Chapter 6).

5.2 EPIDEMIOLOGICAL RESEARCH PRIORITIES

Epidemiological studies of radiation-exposed human populations have provided the information that is used worldwide to estimate risks of adverse health outcomes from these exposures and to guide regulatory decision-making. However, past studies have been limited in their ability to inform on risks from low-dose and low-dose-rate radiation exposures that are of most relevance to U.S. populations because of the challenges described in Box 5.1. The following sections suggest several ways to help overcome some of these challenges and therefore increase understanding of the adverse health effects that result from exposure to low-dose and low-dose-rate radiation. These include development and deployment of analytical tools for radiation epidemiology (see Section 5.2.1), improved estimation of risks for cancer and non-cancer health outcomes (see Section 5.2.2), and identification of factors that modify the low-dose and low-dose-rate radiation-related adverse health effects (see Section 5.2.3).

5.2.1 Develop and Deploy Analytical Tools for Radiation Epidemiology (Priority E1)

Scientific and Decision-Making Value

Powerful analytical tools are now available or are being developed that allow more accurate measurement of radiation exposures and exposure rates and more precise definition of the adverse health effects that may arise due to radiation exposures. Application of these tools in epidemiological studies of human populations will improve investigations of adverse health effects that may be caused by low-dose and low-dose-rate exposures. Selection of the most appropriate study populations and study designs can best be done by the low-dose and low-dose-rate research community with input from the broader research community and other stakeholders, including the impacted communities. These might include populations exposed during childhood, those exposed during medical procedures or occupationally, and those who are environmentally exposed, for example, those living near nuclear waste sites who may ingest or inhale radioactive materials from contaminated environments, or those exposed to background radiation including residential radon (see Table 2.1).

Current Status and Promising Research Directions

Epidemiological studies aiming to directly quantify the adverse health effects that result from low-dose and low-dose-rate radiation exposures, either internal or external, will require careful selection and detailed characterization of study populations that allow examination of lifetime risks of radiation exposures. These study cohorts may be assembled in several ways, for example, by

1. Building on existing historic cohorts. These cohorts may have been assembled to address a different scientific question but might be repurposed to assess risks at low doses of radiation. In this case, investigators would take advantage of data already collected and collect additional information through medical records, Medicare and Medicaid claims, death records, or other means to support studies of radiation risks. In some cases, this may require data harmonization in order to enable combination of multiple cohorts. An example of that approach is the Million Person Study that consists of more than 30 historic cohorts (Boice et al., 2022a). Historic cohorts for which biological samples exist may be of great value as they could allow more precise definition of disease phenotypes or assessment of molecular response endpoints—assuming that sample collection and preservation methods are compatible with the assays to be performed. In some cases, active follow-up of a subgroup of cohort members may be possible to collect additional information and biosamples or passive follow-up at regular intervals, to update the incidence or mortality data and to conduct new dose-response evaluations.
2. Initiating new retrospective cohorts. These cohorts might be assembled by reconstructing exposures to the populations of interest over time and examining how these exposures affected health endpoints over the years by looking for disease occurrence or death from disease through cancer registries, medical records, Medicare and Medicaid claims, death records, or other means. The EPI-CT cohort of medically exposed individuals (see Section 2.1.2) is an example of an international retrospective cohort that was facilitated by electronic record linkage, and uses an improved and standardized dosimetric approach.
3. Initiating studies that have both retrospective and prospective phases. These cohorts might be assembled using a retrospective

approach to recruit participants who already have substantial follow-up and obtaining more detailed information for a subsample of the cohort, for example, socioeconomic and lifestyle factors during lifetime via interviews or other means and biosamples for molecular and other analyses.

4. Developing prospective cohorts. Assembly of the very large numbers of individuals (likely millions) and the long follow-up (several decades depending on the population) for disease occurrence needed for low-dose and low-dose-rate epidemiological studies requires significant effort and resources. However, assembly of informative, new cohorts may become feasible in the future by employing more efficient sampling methods and by taking advantage of more precise information about radiation exposures and disease phenotypes that inform on etiology that is expected to be captured in future, computationally accessible electronic medical records (EMRs). Work on development of a "Learning Health System" (Kuntz et al., 2019) and on sharing and aggregation of data for COVID-19-related research (Dron et al., 2021; Park et al., 2021) suggest strategies that might be adopted to move radiation epidemiology in this direction.

Irrespective of the study design, desired characteristics recorded for each cohort member include (1) information on radiation types and exposure routes and precise estimates of dose and dose rates; (2) detailed health status including incidence[1] of precisely defined adverse health outcomes; and (3) information on physical, chemical, and social environmental factors that may confound or modify radiation dose-adverse health-effect associations. When such information is difficult or expensive to collect for all cohort members, principled study designs based on sampling (e.g., case-cohort design, nested case-control design, validation sampling design) can be used, together with modern statistical analysis methods (Kim, 2015; Langholz and Thomas, 1990). In addition, two-phase study designs offer

---

[1] To understand the etiology of cause-and-effect associations following low-dose radiation exposures, there is a need to conduct incidence-based follow-up studies. It is broadly recognized that the absence of a nationwide cancer incidence registry in the United States has detrimental effects on epidemiological research. The Virtual Pooled Registry Cancer Linkage System, coordinated by the North American Association of Central Cancer Registries with funding from the National Cancer Institute, is an ongoing effort to connect researchers performing minimal risk linkage studies with multiple U.S. population-based cancer registries. Acquiring incidence information for endpoints other than cancer will require electronic medical record linkages because there are no registries for these other disease endpoints.

cost-effective sampling strategies for the collection of additional information (which may be expensive) on a subset of the overall cohort (Tao et al., 2020).

Relevant to issue (3), above, is the issue of confounding. Without the benefit of random assignment, comparison groups in epidemiological studies may differ with respect to factors other than radiation exposure. If these factors are also related to the adverse health outcome of interest, then the observed effect of radiation on adverse health outcome risk may be indistinguishable from the effects of these other risk factors (Schubauer-Berigan et al., 2020), that is, be confounders. Inadequately accounting for confounding can lead to bias in an estimate of the association between radiation exposure and adverse health outcome.[2]

Strategies to increase the accuracy of radiation exposure estimates may include accessing records of medical exposure types and levels; using individual and in-home radiation monitors that report continuously on occupational and environmental exposures; generating accessible geospatial databases of environmental radiation and other contaminants; and utilizing computational algorithms that accurately estimate organ- and cell-specific dose and dose rates from external and/or internal sources and that account for source radiation type, internal versus external exposure, and body size and composition, anatomic location, and sex. These algorithms may be further improved by incorporating information from biological studies using new-generation nanoscale analysis tools that reveal how individual photons or ions alter DNA, individual proteins, and organelles in individual cells and how these alterations are subsequently processed biologically. Relevant analytical technologies are described in more detail in Section 5.4.1 (Priority I1). In addition, it is crucial to understand the random and systematic errors in this information, which could lead to dose estimation errors.

Resources that may be exploited to improve individual cohort members' health status assessments may include

- EMRs made accessible for purposes authorized by law or by the patient while maintaining individual privacy. Concepts and tools developed to support research in COVID-19 testing, treatments, and vaccines and/or the development of a "Learning Health System" (Kuntz et al., 2019) may be particularly important guides.[3] The utility of EMRs for low-dose and low-dose-rate radiation research can be increased by developing and promoting nationwide use of health outcomes data standards that will guide collection of

---

[2] Not all risk factors are confounders. In addition, confounding is more likely to impact exposed-unexposed comparisons than dose-response analyses.

[3] Mike Snyder, Stanford University, presentation to the committee on November 17, 2021.

the information needed for low-dose and low-dose-rate radiation epidemiology (e.g., precisely defined disease states and accurate, anatomically precise measures of radiation exposure). Information on individual medical exposures to radiation will be especially important.

- Information from cellular and molecular analyses of tissues including associated microbiomes in which low-dose and low-dose-rate radiation-induced diseases may originate and biofluids[4] that interact with these tissues. Technologies for precise disease phenotyping are described in detail in Section 5.4.1 (Priority I1). These analyses may include assessment of the presence of signatures that have been associated with low-dose and low-dose-rate radiation-induced disease in laboratory model systems. They may quantify individual characteristics (e.g., genetic, epigenetic, and immune status) that may influence risk of developing adverse health outcomes from low-dose and low-dose-rate radiation exposures. Studies of cells and biomolecules in biofluids that interact with radiation-induced disease sites may be particularly important because not all anatomical sites are easily accessible (Bhawal et al., 2020; Hampel et al., 2021; C. Huang et al., 2021; Quigley et al., 2017). Indeed, recent genomic studies demonstrate the existence of clonal subpopulations within individuals including those irradiated in utero (Applegate et al., 2021) that originate and are propagated during development (Li et al., 2021; Moore et al., 2020). These clonal subpopulations may carry genomic or epigenomic changes that put the cells carrying them at increased risk of radiation-induced disease. New-generation single-cell analysis tools may identify and characterize these at-risk cells (Adhikari et al., 2020; HuBMAP Consortium, 2019; Rozenblatt-Rosen et al., 2020; Stuart et al., 2019) but biofluid sampling will likely be needed to enable their practical detection in humans.

- Information on health status from Internet of Medical Things (IoMT) devices (Popov et al., 2022). These devices may include wearable and in-home sensors and smart phones that can provide information on health endpoints such as weight, gait and balance, voice pathology, heart function, temperature, glucose and other aspects of blood chemistry, cognitive function, and eye movement, which may be adversely affected by exposure to low-dose and low-dose-rate radiation. These devices may also reveal information about food and drug consumption that may alter or mimic

---

[4] Biofluids may include blood, oral swabs, urine, and fecal material and would be collected at appropriate time points based on the hypotheses to be tested.

radiation-induced health effects. This type of data can be collected on a sample of the cohort population over a long time span. Selected technologies available for characterization of human health endpoints are summarized in Section 5.4.1 (Priority I1).

- Information from geospatial databases that can be accessed to provide information about physical, chemical, and social environmental factors that may influence aspects of human physiology that may directly or indirectly influence or confound the identification of low-dose and low-dose-rate radiation-induced adverse health effects (Olney, 2021). Examples of geospatially defined features that might be associated with individuals in study cohorts include aspects of health[5] climate,[6] environmental pollutants,[7] and levels and types of environmental radiation (Dindaroğlu, 2014). The information from geospatial databases could complement the individual-level factors obtained by the IoMT devices or be the source of information when individual-level monitoring is not available. Harmonized databases to support biological and epidemiological studies are discussed in Section 5.4.2 (Priority I2).

5.2.2 Improve Estimation of Risks for Cancer and Non-Cancer Health Outcomes from Low-Dose External and Internal Radiation Exposures, Including Suitable Surrogate Biomarkers of Health Risk Where Appropriate (Priority E2)

Scientific and Decision-Making Value

The quantitative relationship between exposure to radiation and cancer risk at the low doses (<100 mGy) most commonly encountered by the U.S. population and low dose rates (below 5 mGy/h) is assumed to be linear, but linearity is not well established experimentally or epidemiologically at these low doses. Even less is known about the levels of risk for health outcomes other than cancer, including cardiovascular disease, neurological disorders, immune dysfunction, cataracts, and heritable genetic effects. However, if such risks exist at low doses and dose rates, they could lead to substantial changes in risk-benefit analyses for activities that involve low-dose radiation exposures. Also, the health impacts of internal exposures to low-dose and low-dose-rate radiation are not well studied, although both routes of exposure are relevant to the U.S. population. Advances in dosimetry, biology, geospatial epidemiology, and disease phenotyping are now sufficient

---
[5] See https://www.cdc.gov/dhdsp/maps/gisx/resources/geo-spatial-data.html.
[6] See https://www.climate.gov/maps-data.
[7] See https://www.epa.gov/geospatial.

to encourage the design of epidemiological studies that can identify and quantify adverse health outcomes resulting from low-dose and low-dose-rate radiation exposures, while identifying and excluding factors other than radiation that may affect the same adverse health outcomes (i.e., confounding and modifying effects).

Current Status and Promising Research Directions

Cancer is the most well-established adverse health outcome resulting from radiation exposure (Berrington de González et al., 2017; Hauptmann et al., 2020; Kitahara et al., 2015; Little et al., 2022a; UNSCEAR, 2006a). Evidence from a range of exposure scenarios at higher doses consistently demonstrates elevated cancer risks for nearly all tissues based on data from the atomic bombing survivors (Grant et al., 2017) and other exposed populations (UNSCEAR, 2008), with highest risks for leukemia (excluding chronic lymphocytic leukemia) and tumors of the brain, bladder, skin, and thyroid. Evidence accumulated during the past decade has shown that these patterns persist even in populations exposed to low-dose and low-dose-rate radiation (mean doses <100 mGy; see, e.g., Berrington de Gonzalez et al., 2020; Kitahara et al., 2015), although direct evidence at doses around 10 mGy remains limited, and uncertainties remain as to how these endpoints are influenced by radiation type and route of exposure.

Even greater uncertainty exists regarding low-dose radiation-associated health effects for outcomes other than cancer (cardiovascular, neurological, heritable genetic, and other effects; see Section 2.2), but, generally, associations have been observed over the past decade at doses lower than previously considered important for these effects. For example, although the International Commission on Radiological Protection (ICRP) considers cardiovascular effects to fall under the category of tissue reactions and assumes a threshold for induction of 500 mGy, some epidemiological analyses and meta-analyses indicate an elevation of risk at doses less than 500 mGy (e.g., Little et al., 2012; Tran et al., 2017) and indicate that risk of circulatory disease may follow a linear dose-risk relationship at doses below 500 mGy (Little et al., 2012). Association of cardiovascular disease with low doses of radiation remains controversial due to the possibility of uncontrolled confounding by lifestyle factors.

The future availability of detailed and precise information on cancer and non-cancer health outcomes (see Section 5.3.2 for Priority B2), coupled with accurate information on levels and rates of radiation exposure (see Section 5.4.3 for Priority I3), offers the opportunity to explore dose-response relationships at doses relevant to exposed U.S. populations more precisely. This will require appropriate study designs and deployment of new association discovery methodologies to ensure that these associations are statistically significant and false discovery is minimized in these high-dimensionality datasets. During study design, consideration needs to be given to focusing on health outcomes that are precisely defined (e.g., using molecular, cellular, and/or physiological assessment tools), ideally with respect to factors relevant to etiology and that are not influenced by treatment strategies that may change over time or with economic status. Quantitative health outcomes and molecular surrogates thereof that are suggested by epidemiological studies at higher doses or that have been shown in laboratory model studies to be related to low-dose and low-dose-rate radiation exposure might be given special attention. Association discovery may be based on traditional statistical methods or may take advantage of the recent development of computational methods (e.g., machine learning algorithms and artificial intelligence). The ultimate goal is to identify adverse health outcomes that are caused by exposure to low-dose and low-dose-rate radiation.

Statistical and computational methods for association discovery need to address statistical power and bias. Bias can be ameliorated by applying Bradford Hill's considerations for assessing causality, together with modern statistical methods for making causal inference from epidemiological data (Marshall and Galea, 2015). In addition, statistical methods have recently been introduced to estimate causal dose-response curves, based on generalized propensity score models to account for confounding, together with parametric, semi-parametric, or non-parametric dose-response models.[8] Non-parametric models do not rely on an assumed functional form for the association between radiation dose and outcomes (e.g., linear no-threshold). These methods have been applied to low-level air pollution research and could be applied to low-dose radiation epidemiology but require extension to accommodate measurement error in radiation doses. Additional methodological research is needed to establish and compare the statistical properties of new analysis methods, in order to understand their appropriate application in different scientific contexts.

Analyses of low-dose radiation effects do not need to be overly reliant on arbitrary levels of statistical significance (Wasserstein and Lazar, 2016). In fact, within individual studies, the type I error rate (i.e., the false-positive rate) can be inflated due to conducting multiple statistical hypothesis tests for several outcomes, both overall and among subgroups. Instead, inference can be focused on confidence intervals, which provide the range of (excess) risks over which the data are consistent. In addition, it is essential to recognize that a single study is unlikely to provide definitive evidence of radiation effects at low doses and whether those effects differ according to biological

---

[8] Francesca Dominici, Harvard T.H. Chan School of Public Health, presentation to the committee on December 9, 2021.

factors, lifestyle factors, or other environmental exposures. Instead, evidence needs to be combined from multiple studies. Meta-analyses of study-level data can be useful to estimate average effects across studies but require that similar statistical models are fitted to the underlying individual-level data. Alternatively, pooled analyses of harmonized individual-level data can be used, if they are available, together with mixed-effects models that allow for unobserved heterogeneity across studies. To this end, Bayesian methods (full or empirical) need to be developed and applied (Smith et al., 1995). Dose-response shapes and patterns of effect modification can be informed by, but not explicitly depend on, a model for effects at higher doses. They may also be informed by the dose-response curve shape observed in exposed laboratory models as described in Section 5.3.3 for Priority B3.

Classical machine learning and newer artificial intelligence algorithms implemented on increasingly powerful computational platforms are now being used to integrate large-scale -omics, image, biological, and clinical datasets (Goecks et al., 2020) in ways that identify regulatory mechanisms that may control biological and clinical phenotypes and/or that predict biological or medical behavior. Artificial intelligence has an increasing impact in biological (Jumper et al., 2021) and medical areas (Topol, 2019). Application of classical machine learning and newer artificial intelligence algorithms to identify adverse health endpoints that are associated with low-dose and low-dose-rate exposures and the operative response mechanisms will become increasingly productive as robust and accessible datasets are developed for carefully designed study retrospective or prospective cohorts. These tools are summarized in Section 5.4.1 for Priority I1.

5.2.3 Determine Factors That Alter the Low-Dose and Low-Dose-Rate Radiation-Related Adverse Health Effects (Priority E3)

Scientific and Decision-Making Value

Several factors may influence an individual's sensitivity to radiation and therefore need to be considered in risk assessment and risk management. Age at exposure has been shown to modify the radiation dose-response relationship for some cancer types. Higher risks have generally been reported for individuals exposed at younger ages (Grant et al., 2017), and for breast and uterine cancers, reported risks were higher for women exposed around the age of menarche (Brenner et al., 2018; Utada et al., 2018). Animal studies have provided some insights on the biological mechanisms underlying the influence of age at exposure to individual response to radiation (see Applegate et al., 2020, for review). Radiation dose-response relationships may also vary between sexes with some studies suggesting higher risks for women compared to men (ICRP, 2007). One notable example of radiation sensitivity of women versus men comes from analyses of the Life Span Study cohort of atomic bombing survivors which showed a three times higher excess risk of incident lung cancer due to radiation exposure among women compared to men (Cahoon et al., 2017; Hu et al., 2021). However, recent analyses of occupational cohorts within the Million Person Study did not provide evidence of significant differences in the lung cancer risks between men and women (Boice et al., 2022c). The National Council on Radiation Protection and Measurements (NCRP) is currently evaluating sex-specific differences in lung cancer radiation risks and assesses their use in transfer models and lifetime risk projections. Little is known about the effects of other factors and on other health outcomes. Plausible modifiers may involve the host (e.g., inherited genetic susceptibility, existence of clonal subpopulations, immune constitution, comorbid medical conditions) and/or lifestyle (e.g., smoking, obesity, physiological stress, diet). Knowledge of the effects of these other factors on low-dose and low-dose-rate radiation-induced health outcomes may allow for more individualized risk assessments and risk management. Variation in individual response to radiation is a topic of growing importance for radiological protection (Rajaraman et al., 2018; Wojcik et al., 2018) and of an ongoing ICRP task group.[9]

Current Status and Promising Research Directions

Evidence for inherited genetic susceptibility to radiation response derives largely from rare genetic syndromes in which individuals demonstrate hypersensitivity to the killing effects of radiation and frequently have increased risk for developing cancer, such as ataxia-telangiectasia, Nijmegen breakage syndrome, and others (Pollard and Gatti, 2009). Much of the research on radiation-related health impacts in individuals who are autosomal recessive for these deleterious mutations in genes has been used to understand pathways related to high- and low-dose radiation responses, particularly DNA damage responses. Evidence from both in vitro and animal studies suggests that at least some radiation responses differ when comparing low- to high-dose exposures. Nevertheless, the research on genetic modifiers of high-dose radiation effects on health provides important proof of principle that such studies are important. To date, because of small sample sizes and lack of replication in independent populations, these studies have not robustly identified germline genetic variants that modify radiation-related health risks. Future studies that assess potential germline variation in radiation-related health risks need to follow best practices

---

[9] See Task Group 111 Factors Governing the Individual Response of Humans to Ionising Radiation, https://www.icrp.org/icrp_group.asp?id=169.

established over the last decade, including sufficient sample size and replication of results in independent populations.

Immune constitution is thought to modify the effects of radiation either by altering the efficacy with which damaged cells are removed or by altering cytokine levels that alter cell phenotypes including differentiation state, proliferation, and motility. Advances in immunology over the past three decades led to the extension of the original self/non-self-theory, adding common alarm signals, so-called damage-associated molecular patterns, or danger signals as chief drivers for immune engagement (Matzinger, 1994). More recently, recognition systems for RNA and DNA have been added to the list of biomolecules that signal danger to the immune system. This is important because radiation exposures, like many stresses and injuries, get relayed in vivo through shared pathways, especially along the danger sensing and inflammatory/immune signaling cascades, that are open to amplification and exacerbation over time (McBride et al., 2004). Permanent damage may be localized, such as the stem cell compartments or their niches, whose function can be directly or indirectly affected along with their resilience to other stresses (Rodrigues-Moreira et al., 2017). Such permanent radiation damage has been shown largely in studies utilizing higher radiation doses and in infectious, inflammatory, and autoimmune diseases, for example through epigenetic modifications or through persistent senescence that disturbs tissue dynamics causing inflammation (Campisi et al., 2011).

Low-dose radiation scenarios are less studied, but one example that might be relevant is inflammatory recall where open chromatin memory domains become readily accessible to homeostatic transcription factors and in essence change the threshold for activation (Larsen et al., 2021). It is possible that low-dose and low-dose-rate radiation also alter the homeostatic intracellular redox rheostat to affect responses to other challenges, just as much as other challenges might affect the redox rheostat and therefore the response to radiation. It is currently also unclear if the immunological changes following low-dose radiation exposures actually link to the same long-term and late clinical disease outcomes as high-dose radiation exposures or if other outcomes are more relevant (Boerma et al., 2022). It is also still unclear whether there is memory of low-dose radiation exposures or what the importance in the context of other stressors such as obesity, infection, or trauma might be. Feasibility and cost have limited most of these studies primarily to detecting imbalances in peripheral immune cell subsets with immune function. However, this is changing as more powerful tools (see Section 5.4.1 for Priority I1) for assessment of immune phenotypes are developed. These can now be deployed to determine whether immunological changes seen post-exposure are associated with adverse health impacts and how these are modified by other stressors. The latter is of interest because an expert who briefed the committee on aspects of brain function and human physiology[10] noted that the brain operates as a strong signal amplifier to help the body respond to stress, infection, and other evolutionarily important survival endpoints. The brain, and particularly the hypothalamus, receives and sends chemical signals that modify cellular behavior throughout the body, especially aspects of immune function. Depending on context, these interactions can be either beneficial (e.g., by enhancing immune response to invading pathogens) or deleterious (e.g., by stimulating cancer cell growth or contributing to cachexia). Overall, these mechanisms raise the possibility that stress, immune function, and neural signaling interact to influence how cells, tissues, and organs respond to radiation.

Regarding lifestyle factors, perhaps the best studied factor to date is tobacco exposure and its impact on estimates of radiation-related lung cancer risks, with most evidence supporting a sub-multiplicative effect (Cahoon et al., 2017; Tomasek, 2013). Whether these findings are consistent for tobacco and radiation exposures on other outcomes also associated with tobacco exposure (e.g., bladder cancer and cardiovascular disease) or for combined effects of radiation and other lifestyle factors such as obesity and diet is unknown. Understanding these combined effects is important because both obesity and diet contribute to disparities in many diseases, including cancer and cardiovascular disease.

There is also limited evidence relating to the health risks associated with combined exposure to radiation and other agents to which people are exposed and which may modify the effect of radiation. However, this is of great importance in different occupational and environmental exposure settings where populations are exposed to radiation and chemicals or other harmful agents. The last comprehensive review of co-exposure effects (UNSCEAR, 2000) concluded that, in general, genotoxic agents with similar biological and mechanistic behavior when acting at the same time will interact in a concentration-additive manner. This conclusion was supported by more recent studies (Nuta et al., 2014), but other reports demonstrated greater-than-additive effects of radiation and arsenic compounds on some cellular endpoints (Hornhardt et al., 2006).

Epidemiological studies with high-quality data on host and lifestyle factors (e.g., from increasingly powerful geospatial databases) as well as biospecimens that can be used for germline genomics or other biomarker studies (e.g., epigenomic, protein, and transcriptional signatures that regulate cell and tissue behavior; see Section 5.3.2), together with statistical and

---

[10] Daniel Marks, Oregon Health & Science University, presentation to the committee on November 16, 2021.

computational methods discussed in Section 5.2.1 (Priority E1), can provide evidence on how these factors modify low-dose and low-dose-rate radiation health effects. Major advances in genomic technologies that now allow for large-scale genotyping and sequencing to assess both common and rare genetic variants hold promise for the development of studies aimed toward understanding heritable genetic contributions to radiation-related health impacts (see Section 5.4.1 for Priority I1).

5.3 BIOLOGICAL RESEARCH PRIORITIES

Elucidation of the mechanisms that are involved in the conversion of low-dose and low-dose-rate radiation-induced damage into adverse health effects provides important support to epidemiological studies of radiation risk. Mechanistic understanding also may suggest strategies to mitigate adverse health effects that result from low-dose and low-dose-rate exposures. Mechanistic studies can focus on adverse effects in humans and/or on laboratory models thereof. Laboratory model-based studies tend to be better controlled, adequately statistically powered, and less prone to confounding, therefore substantially strengthening the evidence for disease causation and the underlying dose-response relationships, provided they accurately model the disease pathogenesis following irradiation. The following sections suggest several aspects of mechanism-based biological research that may increase understanding of how low-dose and low-dose-rate radiation exposures lead to adverse health effects, including development of improved laboratory models (see Section 5.3.1), identification of biomarkers for radiation-induced health effects (see Section 5.3.2), defining health effect-dose relationships below 10 mGy and below 5 mGy/h (see Section 5.3.3), and identification of factors that modulate or mimic radiation health effects (see Section 5.3.4).

5.3.1 Develop More Accurate Model Systems for Study of Low-Dose and Low-Dose-Rate Radiation-Induced Health Effects (Priority B1)

Scientific and Decision-Making Value

Biological studies of low-dose and low-dose-rate radiation health effects in humans will rely on the use of laboratory model systems. Informative models may be engineered cells and tissues grown in the laboratory (Suckert et al., 2021; Tognon et al., 2021) and/or engineered animal models (Collaborative Cross Consortium, 2012; Paunesku and Woloschak, 2018). The utility of information from the study of these models depends on the extent to which they accurately mirror the aspects of human biology targeted for study. The development of these models can be guided by the increasing information about the molecular, cellular, and physiological characteristics of normal and aberrant human tissues and human diseases revealed using new-generation analytical tools. Multiple models may be used to cover different aspects of radiation-induced adverse health outcomes, and multiple models of the same outcome can be employed to guard against artifacts that may be specific to a single model. Extrapolation from experimental data to possible effects in humans is considered more reliable when similar molecular responses and/or outcomes are observed in a variety of model systems. Integration of the information gained from laboratory models and from epidemiological studies will improve understanding of the mechanisms underlying low-dose and low-dose-rate radiation-induced adverse health outcomes, improve risk estimates for the low-dose and low-dose-rate exposures experienced by the U.S. population, and suggest strategies to mitigate risks.

Current Status and Promising Research Directions

Laboratory models have strengths and weaknesses for low-dose radiation studies. In general, models comprising engineered cells, organoids (collections of cells grown in three-dimensional [3D] cultures), and tissues grown in the laboratory are more convenient and lower cost than engineered animal models but are limited to studies of specific cellular and molecular processes and mechanisms. However, animal models are better suited to studies of disease outcomes. Several characteristics and uses of engineered cells and tissues and animal models are discussed in the following sections.

For decades, studies of the biological effects of radiation have focused on cells isolated from humans and laboratory animals. These studies have revealed much of what is currently known about cellular mechanisms to respond to radiation-induced damage. In general, the cell types most studied have been those that can be easily grown in the laboratory. However, these cell types typically have been grown in two-dimensional cultures, and often they are not the cell types in which radiation-induced diseases arise. Moreover, they typically have not included the diversity of cells (e.g., epithelial, endothelial, and immune) that may interact in tissues to alter responses to radiation. These limitations can be reduced by employing new bioengineering technologies that generate 3D, multicellular biological systems, either organoids (Nagle and Coppes, 2020) or "organs-on-a-chip" (also known as tissue chips) (Low and Tagle, 2017). Tissue chips are now routinely used and have even been launched into space (Low and Giulianotti, 2019). Tissue chips coupled with microfluidics are becoming increasingly sophisticated to allow for interaction of tissue-specific cells with immune cell subsets and the microbiome, more closely modeling aspects of human and animal physiology. Artificially engineered scaffolding that supports

3D organ development in the laboratory environment is another example of designing advanced functional biomimetic structures (Nikolova and Chavali, 2019). Collectively, these systems provide exciting new tools for the investigation of molecular, cellular, and tissue responses to low-dose and low-dose-rate radiation. Processes that appear important can then be promoted for assessment in animal models and eventually for association with radiation exposure in epidemiological studies.

Mice are the animal species most commonly used for studies of physiology and disease formation, and several strains have been exceedingly well characterized biologically and genetically. Transgenic mouse strains are readily available for study of the influence of specific genes on radiation-induced adverse outcomes. Development of crosses between mouse strains that vary substantially in many aspects of disease formation also provides tools to discover the genes, molecular processes, and disease processes that may be influenced by exposure to low-dose and low-dose-rate radiation. The Collaborative Cross (Complex Trait Consortium, 2004), which combines the genomes of eight genetically and phenotypically diverse founder strains, has been created as a community resource to facilitate the genetic analysis of complex traits and may be particularly useful in dissecting the biology and genetics of low-dose and low-dose-rate radiation-induced adverse outcomes (Collaborative Cross Consortium, 2012).[11] Genetic engineering tools such as CRISPR gene replacement (Doudna, 2020; see Section 5.4.1 for Priority I1) also will be useful in studies of the impact of defined human gene sequences. However, commonly used mouse strains are limited since they were derived from relatively few original sources, mostly at the beginning of the 20th century, so they do not represent the genetic diversity found in humans or even in wild-type mice. In addition, they may acquire new genetic variations over time that alter key aspects of radiation responses that are not typically found in mice or humans. A case in point is the C3H/HeJ mouse strain that derived from the C3H/HeN mice and developed a mutation in Toll-like receptor 4 (TLR-4); as a result, it only poorly responds to lipopolysaccharide challenge with suboptimal tumor necrosis factor-alpha production and as such might not be the preferred model to study radiation-induced danger signaling and inflammation. Similarly, using BALB/c mice for radiation mutagenesis might be misleading considering the DNA-dependent protein kinase catalytic subunit (DNA PKcs) deficiency and hence abnormal DNA repair efficacy of these mice. Comparisons of genotypes between mice and humans can reveal such phenomena.

The use of mice to study cancer endpoints is particularly well established. These studies can be conducted in the context of a well-developed

---

[11] Andrew Wyrobek and Antoine Snijders, Lawrence Berkeley National Laboratory, presentation to the committee on January 24, 2022.

and expanding framework of the key biological processes that contribute to disease pathogenesis known as the Hallmarks of Cancer (Hanahan, 2022; Hanahan and Weinberg, 2011; Paunesku et al., 2021). This framework includes aspects of tumor cell survival and dissemination, vascularization, immune surveillance, and tumor-stromal interactions that are important in cancer genesis and progression. In addition, the National Cancer Institute's (NCI's) Mouse Models of Cancer Consortium and follow-on efforts have developed a wealth of genetically engineered mice for the study of processes leading to cancer. Many are available through the NCI Mouse Repository at the Frederick National Laboratory.[12] NCI is currently developing a community resource of well-characterized patient-derived xenografts (Sun et al., 2021). Studies of low-dose and low-dose-rate radiation-induced cancers will benefit from these concepts and resources.

The above-mentioned and other developments in cell and animal models have led to a good but incomplete understanding of the mechanisms underlying radiation-induced cancer (see, e.g., UNSCEAR, 2021). In addition, most investigations so far have focused on the early stages of carcinogenesis, initiation in particular, and relatively little is known about the effects of radiation exposures on later stages of carcinogenesis. New experimental models including new model organisms apart from the mouse may be needed for these studies, possibly including pigs, dogs, and nonhuman primates—in compliance with legislation and guidelines governing biomedical research—because of the greater resemblance to human anatomy, immunology, and lifespan compared to small laboratory animals (Maynard et al., 2021). A full appreciation of radiation-induced disease formation, and therefore the experimental system to model that, will need to take into account both the genomic and epigenomic abnormality carried by the target cells (e.g., the breast epithelial cells that may develop to breast cancers) as well as the proximal and distal environments in which these cells exist.

Animal models also are being developed for the study of adverse health outcomes other than cancer that might be caused by low-dose and low-dose-rate radiation exposures. Specific disease models exist for cardiovascular disease progression (Jia et al., 2020; Liao et al., 2015) and neurocognitive deficits (Dawson et al., 2018) as examples. Humanized mouse models with bone marrow reconstitution using human hematopoietic stem cells (Ando et al., 2008) permit detailed investigation into lineage development in the context of external or internal exposures, but might not be an appropriate model for long-term studies. Finally, patient-derived single-cell models and construction of tissue array models can provide personalized determination of treatment options and responses to radiation, including risk assessment.

---

[12] See https://frederick.cancer.gov/resources/repositories/nci-mouse-repository.

Mouse strains modeling these endpoints exist but have not been fully exploited. The adverse outcome pathway (AOP) framework (see, e.g., NCRP, 2020b; Svingen et al., 2021) is likely going to provide a means to integrate knowledge on the pathogenesis of radiation-associated non-cancer health effects. These and future models will facilitate studies of possible radiation-induced pathologies that so far have been only lightly explored.

It is increasingly recognized that cells function within a specific biological context and that they are strongly controlled by the signals they receive, as illustrated in Figure 5.1. The fact that these signals can come from cells that are in close proximity to the irradiated cell or from distal organs such as the brain only adds further complexity and underscores the need to study radiation responses in vivo as much as possible. Proximal interactions are often referred to as "bystander responses" and are well recognized by radiation biologists (Tomita and Maeda, 2015; UNSCEAR, 2021). Not only do these interactions determine how individual cells respond to radiation but they are also ultimately critical for the maintenance of tissue and organ viability. In other words, indirect effects of radiation on cells surrounding the cells of origin for radiation-associated cancers and non-cancerous pathologies could be as important as the direct radiation effects noted above in determining the outcomes of exposures and therefore need to be modeled accordingly. This is clearly demonstrated by pioneering studies that have shown that the incidence of cancers and by extension other diseases can be strongly influenced by the microenvironment(s) in which abnormal cells

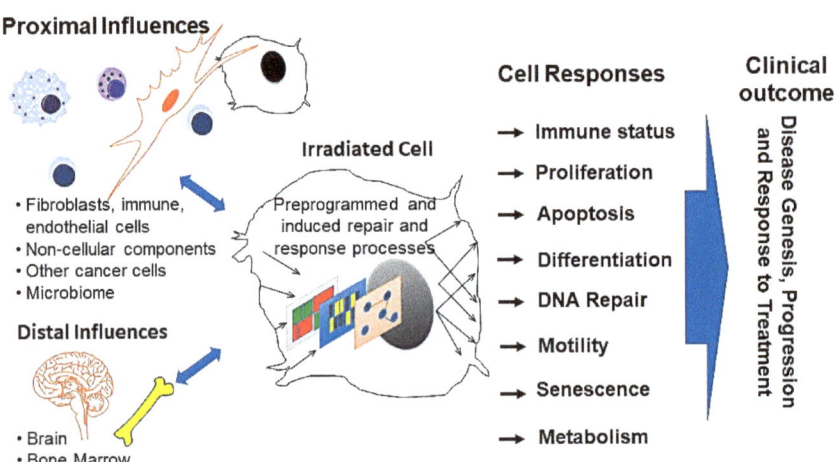

FIGURE 5.1 Schematic representation of proximal and distal influences on the irradiated cell and cellular response. SOURCE: Courtesy of committee chair, Joe Gray, Oregon Health & Science University (emeritus).

exist (see Bissell and Hines, 2011; Mintz and Illmensee, 1975; Nelson and Bissell, 2006; Radisky and Bissell, 2004). Indeed, cells that form cancers in one environment can behave normally in another (Mintz and Illmensee, 1975). Models genetically engineered to enable study of cellular interactions (e.g., by genetically labeling or functionally modifying cells of interest) will facilitate study of cellular interactions on low-dose and low-dose-rate radiation-induced adverse outcomes.

5.3.2 Develop Biomarkers for Radiation-Induced Adverse Health Outcomes (Priority B2)

Scientific and Decision-Making Value

The Food and Drug Administration's *Biomarkers, Endpoints, and other Tools (BEST) Resource* glossary defines a biomarker as a "characteristic that is measured as an indicator of normal biological processes, pathogenic processes, or responses to an exposure or intervention, including therapeutic interventions."[13] The BEST glossary further defines biomarkers for susceptibility or risk, diagnosis, monitoring, prognosis, prediction of behavior, response to perturbation, and safety. Biomarkers for risk, diagnosis, and response will be particularly important for low-dose and low-dose-rate radiation research. Biomarkers of risk may identify individuals who are susceptible to radiation-induced adverse outcomes. Diagnostic biomarkers may identify adverse outcomes that are preferentially induced by low-dose and low-dose-rate radiation such that these can be assessed in epidemiological studies or that are associated with other etiologies so that cases with these biomarkers can be excluded. Biomarkers of response may identify cellular and molecular features or biological processes that change in response to low-dose and low-dose-rate radiation exposures. Importantly, all biomarkers can be measured with increasing precision, sensitivity, and reproducibility using new-generation analytical tools. The integration of biomarkers of radiation-induced and non-radiation-induced risk and response discovered in biological studies into epidemiological studies promises to increase the power to identify subtle effects and enable the exploration of factors that influence individual susceptibility. Measurement of response biomarkers will provide important insights about the mechanisms that are engaged as humans respond to low-dose and low-dose-rate radiation exposures.

---

[13] See https://www.fda.gov/drugs/biomarker-qualification-program/about-biomarkers-and-qualification.

Current Status and Promising Research Directions

New and powerful analytical tools (see Section 5.4.1 for Priority I1) now enable precise and sensitive measurement of the cellular and molecular components and the organizations thereof (i.e., biomarkers) for normal, irradiated, and diseased tissues. This section provides examples of how biomarker analyses are already being deployed by the radiobiology research community and suggests areas where additional research is needed to inform on low-dose and low-dose-rate radiation effects with emphasis on response and diagnostic biomarkers. Risk biomarkers are discussed in Section 5.3.4 (Priority B4).

Regarding response biomarkers, measurements of changes in large-scale gene expression biomarkers after many different perturbations of biological systems have resulted in the definition of thousands of regulatory and functional networks and signaling pathways that enable cell and tissue function. The National Institutes of Health's (NIH's) Library of Integrated Network-Based Cellular Signatures has made important recent contributions in this area (Keenan et al., 2018). Many pathways and networks are now curated and publicly available. For example, the Molecular Signatures Database[14] includes 50 "Hallmark Gene Sets" that represent well-defined biological states or processes.

Recent work has identified some of the major signaling pathways that are activated by different, mostly high doses of radiation (Brackmann et al., 2020; Mukherjee et al., 2019; Paul et al., 2019) and low-dose radiation-induced persistent transcriptome changes in genes associated with immune function (Snijders et al., 2012), but expansion of such studies and replication of results is essential for establishing robust biomarkers. Indeed, it remains to be determined whether activation of each response biomarker is associated with an increase or decrease in adverse health effects. In addition, it is already known that circulating small molecules such as miRNA can act as radiation-damage signaling molecules and that they tie in with health outcomes (Chakraborty et al., 2020; Soares et al., 2021). These and follow-on studies to elucidate the mechanisms engaged as cells and tissues respond to low-dose and low-dose-rate radiation are promising but will benefit from cohesive approaches similar to those deployed by The Cancer Genome Atlas (TCGA; Collins and Barker, 2007), Human BioMolecular Atlas Program (HuBMAP Consortium, 2019), and Human Tumor Atlas Network (HTAN; Rozenblatt-Rosen et al., 2020). The multidisciplinary low-dose and low-dose-rate radiation research program envisioned by this committee might directly engage with these programs. Importantly, these

---

[14] See https://www.gsea-msigdb.org/gsea/msigdb/index.jsp.

studies will require increased access to low-dose and low-dose-rate exposure facilities as described in Section 5.4.4 (Priority I4).

In the context of cancer or non-cancer health outcomes, advanced-omics technologies include those with single-cell resolution capabilities, promise to reveal the relevant biomolecules, the pathways involved (including both DNA damage signaling and other signaling pathways), and the dose dependence of low-dose effects. Analytical technologies that efficiently assay multiple endpoints in single cells (see Section 5.4.1 for Priority I1) allow simultaneous assessment of genomic, epigenomic, and transcriptomic events in individual cells. This is especially useful at the low-dose radiation range because these technologies can identify the response of the small number of cells that stochastically incur damage as a result of exposures to low doses of radiation. These studies on individual cells could lead to development of an "atlas" of mechanistic changes that may enable more precise definition of disease subtypes that are more strongly associated with low-dose radiation exposure. Such approaches will also aid the identification of biomarkers that could be applied in population studies and for the development of AOPs.

The development of low-dose and low-dose-rate response biomarkers will benefit from analysis of biospecimens collected longitudinally. It is expected that the majority of studies that allow for longitudinal sample collection will be carried out using laboratory models (see Section 5.3.1 for Priority B1) exposed in facilities designed for low-dose and low-dose-rate exposures (see Section 5.4.4 for Priority I4); however, longitudinal studies in humans are also possible (Johnson et al., 2022). Both engineered tissues and animal models will be informative; however, animal models will enable studies of irradiated tissues as well as biosamples including blood (whole blood, serum, and plasma), urine, saliva, buccal cells, skin swabs, hair follicles, fecal material, and cerebrospinal fluid. All biomaterials can be preserved in appropriate materials (e.g., for stabilization of RNA or phosphoproteins) and can be analyzed for biomarker identification of disease progression in a retroactive manner or with targeted approaches for quantitation of biomarkers and changes associated with known disease progression. As an example, changes in circulating lipid composition are often associated with cardiovascular disease, and lipidomics could offer an informative collective profile of lipid classes in addition to particular species with high correlation to this outcome.

Diagnostic biomarkers are increasingly being identified and can subdivide anatomically defined diseases into subgroups that differ according to prognosis, etiology, anatomic origin, pathway usage, and response to therapy. Breast cancer, for example, can now be subdivided into at least five subgroups depending on the diagnostic biomarkers used (Ellis and Perou, 2013). The TCGA PanCancer effort has identified biomarkers that define four cell-of-origin biomarker patterns that persist across 33 different types of cancer (Hoadley et al., 2018). Finally, genome sequencing studies have identified genomic signatures in cancers that suggest specific, non-radiation causative agents for individual tumors (Alexandrov et al., 2020). The observed differences in etiology between the subtypes raise the possibility that some cancer subtypes (and by extension other disease subtypes) could be more susceptible to induction by low-dose and low-dose-rate radiation than others. The observation by Ahadi et al. (2020) of cell-of-origin subtypes suggests that some will be more affected by internal radiation than others. Biomarkers are also being developed for other health endpoints that may be important in low-dose and low-dose-rate radiation research including cardiovascular diseases (Dhingra and Vasan, 2017), neurodegenerative diseases (Hansson, 2021), and aging (Ahadi et al., 2020).

The concept that disease subtypes are differentially susceptible to induction by low-dose and low-dose-rate radiation and mode of delivery can be tested for biological plausibility in laboratory models that accurately represent specific disease subtypes. Subtypes that appear most strongly influenced by aspects of low-dose and low-dose-rate radiation exposure can then be tested in humans in epidemiological studies (see Section 5.2.2 for Priority E2).

5.3.3 Define Health-Effect Dose-Response Relationships Around 10 mGy or 5 mGy/h (Priority B3)

Scientific and Decision-Making Value

Experimental studies at the molecular, cellular, tissue, and whole-organism levels can be used to examine the shape of the dose-response relationships for each of the relevant endpoints and inform the biological and physical factors that influence the response at doses nearing 10 mGy and 5 mGy/h (i.e., at the range where epidemiological studies may not be able to provide firm conclusions). Studies that integrate this information with that from epidemiological studies will increase understanding of the mechanisms involved and reduce the uncertainties of current risk estimates for low-dose and low-dose-rate exposures experienced by the U.S. population.

Current Status and Promising Research Directions

Radiation exposures around 10 mGy lead to molecular, cellular, and health outcomes that are not as well defined as those at higher doses, in particular cytotoxic doses. Advancements in assay technologies and in the ability to accurately measure these outcomes increase the ability to establish radiation dose-response curves for molecular and cellular endpoints and for associated early- and late-stage diseases at different dose rates. Because these endpoints may differ from those related to radiation cytotoxicity, new models will have to be developed rather than relying for guidance on cytotoxic outcomes (see Section 5.3.1 for Priority B1) and will require increased access to low-dose and low-dose-rate exposure facilities (see Section 5.4.4 for Priority I4).

Direct induction of DNA damage and subsequent mutations by radiation are well studied, particularly in the case of DNA double strand breakage and the cellular response to it, sensing and repairing that damage. However, double strand breakage is rare at low doses and at low-dose rates for low linear energy transfer (LET) radiation[15] but the repair may be not as efficient as at higher doses, and the responses in most cells will ultimately be determined by other forms of damage. While the importance of DNA damage and misrepair resulting in mutations in driving carcinogenesis is recognized, there remains little consensus on the existence of a distinct mutational signature of radiation exposure that would allow more confident attribution of an individual case to the exposure. However, there is growing evidence that genetic signatures can be defined that identify risk factors other than radiation as causative for individual cancers (Alexandrov et al., 2020), so these can be excluded from radiation epidemiological studies.

Similarly, there is an incomplete catalogue of the target genes for radiation carcinogenesis, the target cell populations for specific cancer types, and their radiation dose dependence. The impact of low-dose radiation exposures, and exposures to differing radiation qualities, on mutational loads in individuals is unknown but can now be assessed by modern high-throughput sequencing methods in human and animal model studies.[16]

Also relevant to low-dose radiation exposures is the role of transmissible genomic instability (i.e., the phenomenon of persistent elevation of mutation frequency in the descendants of irradiated cells). However, there are some indications that a threshold of exposure, around 100 mGy low-LET radiation, needs to be exceeded to trigger such instability (see UNSCEAR, 2021). The relevance and importance of "adaptive response," whereby a low "priming" dose of radiation can induce DNA repair or immune response mechanisms that reduce quantitatively the outcome of a second higher-dose exposure, are equally undefined (see UNSCEAR, 2021). New tools for comprehensive analysis of DNA, modified DNA, RNA, and proteins in single-cell analysis tools (see Section 5.4.1 for Priority I1) will provide information about the mechanisms that operate following low-dose and low-dose-rate radiation exposures. Importantly, the damage caused by

---

[15] Damage produced by high-LET radiation including from alpha particles from ingested radionuclides typically does cause double strand breaks (Stap et al., 2008).

[16] Phil Jones, Sanger Institute, presentation to the committee on November 17, 2021.

radiation or other exposures is not necessarily immediately proximate in time to the disease-causing alteration, as illustrated by the human genetics of chromosomal or gene-specific diseases. Often the molecular incident cause is present long before the chromosomal damage, which poses an immense challenge for studies of disease etiology and pathogenesis, one that AOP approaches maybe be helpful in addressing.

The role of DNA damage and repair in the context of non-cancer health outcomes and the radiation doses at which this damage occurs is little understood. In cataract formation, for example, genes such as *ATM*, *RAD9*, and *PTCH1* are known to modify the induction of lens opacities following radiation exposures, but these genes are generally not considered to be significant contributors to atherosclerotic disease.

There are alternatives to direct mutation as causative mechanisms for health effects, namely epigenetic modifications, which include DNA methylation which is generally associated with gene silencing; post-translational modifications (PTMs) of chromatin, and more than 200 known covalent modifications of the histone octamer by methylation, acetylation, phosphorylation, or ubiquitination, all associated with gene activation or silencing; chromatin remodeling that affects transcription factor accessibility and thereby gene expression; and structural changes including nucleosome replacement or higher-order nuclear topology controlling tissue-specific and tissue-appropriate gene expression (Feinberg et al., 2016; Jenuwein and Allis, 2001).

Epigenomic changes can be induced at a distance from radiation-damaged cells via chemical signaling from the damaged cells (Sprung et al., 2015). Epigenetic changes occur in many epithelial tissues including skin after aging and sun exposure in precisely those genomic regions with mutational errors in invasive squamous cell carcinoma (Vandiver et al., 2015), a concept likely extending to ionizing radiation exposure. Epigenetic changes also cause various other human diseases in addition to cancer such as protein aggregation diseases, metabolic diseases, neurological and psychiatric diseases, and imprinting disorders (Kungulovski and Jeltsch, 2016). Several recent studies support a direct link between low-dose radiation and epigenetic changes (reviewed in Lei et al., 2020; Leung et al., 2021; Miousse et al., 2019; Tharmalingam et al., 2017), and a comprehensive analysis in terms of the full range of epigenetic modifications and alterations to chromatin structure after low-dose exposures is clearly warranted. Understanding these genomic dynamics and their low-dose-response relationships as they relate to cancer and non-cancer disease pathologies will have a bearing on risk assessment. How much of low-dose effects are in fact mediated through reactive oxygen damage forms an intricate part of this equation and needs to be explored in detail. The modulation of reactive oxygen species is likely directly or indirectly related to changes in mitochondrial function that have been observed after low-dose exposures (Shimura et al., 2016). Some studies suggest that reactive oxygen damage from low-dose and repeated low-dose exposures may even contribute to the proliferation of pre-cancerous cells in tissues (Fernandez-Antoran et al., 2019). Furthermore, the role of radiation damage to other organelles (excluding the cell nucleus) has received little attention, but this too may have an impact on health outcomes and follow different dose-response relationships (Paunesku et al., 2021). These biological endpoints are increasingly accessible for study using the analytical tools described in Section 5.4.1 (Priority I1).

5.3.4 Identify Factors That Modify or Confound Estimation of Risks for Radiation-Induced Adverse Health Outcomes (Priority B4)

Scientific and Decision-Making Value

Estimates of the risks of adverse health outcomes from low-dose and low-dose-rate radiation exposures may be modulated by events unique to an individual or confounded by exposure to factors other than low-dose and low-dose-rate radiation that produce the same adverse health outcomes. Modifiers that are identified in studies of laboratory model systems can be tested in epidemiological studies for their impact on risk estimation in human populations.

Current Status and Promising Research Directions

Studies of the responses of genetically and biologically diverse laboratory model systems (see Section 5.3.1 for Priority B1) to low-dose and low-dose-rate radiation and/or to chemical and environmental perturbagens will facilitate identification of risk modifiers and confounders. Numerous factors might be considered as risk modifiers by altering aspects of the processes by which radiation-induced DNA damage is translated into adverse health outcomes (e.g., DNA damage repair, damage surveillance, immune competence, stress response). These may vary between individuals or populations and may include functional genetic polymorphisms; epigenomic modifications that vary with age, sex, dietary intake, and environmental exposure and lifestyle; immune function including past "education"; and overall health status. Risk biomarkers for these events can be defined in laboratory model systems (see Section 5.3.1 for Priority B1) and then evaluated in epidemiological studies of U.S. populations (see Section 5.2.1 for Priority E1).

The immune system is the conduit where intracellular and intercellular responses merge and where local responses have systemic reach. Immune system alterations following exposure to high doses of radiation are well established in that radiation damage gets sensed and interpreted through common pattern recognition receptors that signal danger from damaged "self" (Harding et al., 2017; Härtlova et al., 2015; Mackenzie et al., 2016). This response feeds into evolutionary conserved innate immune cell activation/inflammatory pathways (e.g., NFϰB and type-I interferons) that potentially bridge to the adaptive arm of the immune system through dendritic cell cross-priming and T-cell activation. Redox reactions play a significant role in this, derived in part from these inflammatory cascades involving reactive oxygen species (ROS)-generating reactions (e.g., inducible nitric oxide synthase or nicotinamide adenine dinucleotide phosphate oxidase) which are very similar to the initial radiation-induced ROS. Traditionally, this relationship has been thought to be dose dependent with low doses being considered anti-inflammatory in certain disease states but not others. This concept needs to be reexamined under well-defined conditions and over a wide range of doses using modern technologies.

Because defects in danger signaling are known to contribute to a host of human diseases including cardiovascular, autoimmune, and cancerous, it is conceivable that low-dose radiation-induced danger signals could affect disease initiation and/or progression and therefore health outcomes, especially if poorly controlled. In fact, there is already evidence from high-dose exposures linking persistent and/or unrepaired DNA damage to tissue senescence and sustained inflammatory infiltration in vivo (Rodier et al., 2009). Focused studies could determine the low-dose radiation response to danger signaling and the sensitivity of the different mechanisms for immune sensing of danger and tissue damage and how these affect immune balance and outcome in the short and long terms. For instance, redox status sensing through Nrf-2 reportedly acts at doses as low as 20 mGy while micronuclei (i.e., DNA damage) remain unrepaired, highlighting the possibility of different dose responses for different mechanisms (Rodrigues-Moreira et al., 2017; Rothkamm and Löbrich, 2003). Similarly, the engagement of central-systemic feedback loops, especially hematopoietic imbalances or amplification of signals in the hypothalamus, which are known in the context of higher radiation doses, can be evaluated; this will be highly relevant for organ interaction, amplification, morbidity, and mortality. Evaluating the effect of low-dose radiation on tumor incidence and the immune reactions that are generated in susceptible and resistant animal models will be important as will be the role of immunogenetics, including major histocompatibility pathways, and how they factor into radiation sensitivity and immune activation post-exposure.

There is still much to understand about the mechanistic basis for the differences in radiosensitivity in various tissues, though differences in DNA damage response are likely to contribute given their importance to cancer induction. Differences between tissues are primarily due to epigenomic changes that occur during development. However, they also may be influenced by lifestyle and other factors. Additionally, the number of cells at risk for transformation into cancer cells is likely to be important. The target cells and tissues for radiation-associated non-cancer outcomes are not well characterized, and information on these and their responses to radiation insult will be important in making judgments on low-dose risk extrapolation. For circulatory diseases and cognitive dysfunction, inflammation is likely going to play a key role. Hence, identifying and characterizing the target cells and tissues involved will be crucial in developing appropriate risk models. Overall, a better understanding of the pathogenesis of radiation diseases, especially non-cancer outcomes, at all organizational levels is required.

These processes can now be studied in laboratory models using the suite of -omics and multiscale molecular imaging tools that are described in Section 5.4.1 (Priority I1). Moreover, these tools can be integrated with similar data on normal and diseased tissues that are available in public databases emerging from NIH and international programs such as TCGA, the International Cancer Genome Consortium, HuBMAP, and NCI's HTAN to facilitate identification of precise disease signatures that can be tested for association with low-dose radiation exposure. The application of these and other methods to further characterize mechanisms of low-dose and low-dose-rate health effects combined with the AOP approach to integrate knowledge provides a route to develop a framework on the critical steps in the pathogenesis of radiation health outcomes that can inform risk assessment for all health outcomes. Even for radiation carcinogenesis where the mechanisms are relatively well studied, many questions remain as to the modifiers of risk such as comorbidities, underlying genetic variants, and exposures to other agents. Collectively, these efforts can be geared toward assessing the impact of genetic makeup, epigenomic status, DNA repair efficacy, comorbidities, history of exposure to radiation and other agents, lifestyle factors, and immune status on radiation response outcomes and biomarkers for ensuing health effects.

If unique biomarkers for low-dose and low-dose-rate radiation-induced adverse health effects are defined, they can be compared to unique biomarkers for adverse health effects produced by causes other than radiation. These can be identified by treating laboratory models with agents known from the literature or public-domain genetic or chemical perturbation databases to produce adverse health outcomes or biomarker responses similar to those produced by low-dose and low-dose-rate radiation. If a biomarker is not unique to radiation, then agents that induce the same diagnostic biomarkers as low-dose and low-dose-rate radiation are potential confounders of the radiation-biomarker association in observational epidemiological studies (see Section 5.2.2 for Priority E2). However, potential confounders may be eliminated if they manifest cellular or molecular biomarkers that identify adverse health effects that are associated with etiologies other than radiation (e.g., genomic signatures in cancers that suggest tobacco use, defective DNA mismatch repair, ultraviolet light exposure, or aflatoxin exposure as causative events; see Alexandrov et al., 2020).

5.4 RESEARCH INFRASTRUCTURE PRIORITIES

The low-dose radiation research program can take advantage of the remarkable advances that have been made in the past two decades in understanding the behavior of complex biological systems and disease phenotyping that may improve the sensitivity of future epidemiological and experimental studies. These advances have been powered by the health research programs supported by NIH and by advances in measurement, data science, and computer technology supported by the Department of Energy (DOE), NIH, and the National Science Foundation.

5.4.1 Tools for Sensitive Detection and Precise Characterization of Aberrant Cell and Tissue States (Priority I1)

Scientific and Decision-Making Value

Major advances in measurement, data science, and computer technology over the past 20 years have resulted in a wealth of tools that can be deployed to report on the molecular compositions and multiscale molecular and physical structures that comprise normal and diseased cells and tissues. These tools can be readily applied to reveal the responses to perturbations including those induced by low-dose and low-dose-rate radiation. These revolutionary tools, in aggregate, allow quantification of subtle cellular and molecular processes important in radiation research that have previously not been possible, including changes in single cells as a result of the interactions of those cells with radiation.

Current Status and Promising Research Directions

-Omics analysis tools enable assessment of the molecular components that comprise cells and tissues. Work in this area was initiated by the development of robust, fast, and low-cost nucleic acid sequencing tools to support the Human Genome Program co-led by DOE and NIH. Development of these tools was further stimulated by TCGA (Collins and Barker, 2007) in the United States and by the International Cancer Genome Consortium (ICGC, 2010) worldwide. As a result, robust tools are available in many research and clinical laboratories in the United States that can quickly generate sequences for entire genomes and transcriptomes for less than $1,000.[17] Work in this area continues today, driven by NIH and DOE programs and substantial U.S. industry investments. Long-read-length sequencing technologies are emerging that may enable identification of genomic abnormalities in otherwise difficult-to-sequence regions of the genome (Nurk et al., 2022) and make it possible to assess alternative splicing solutions. These tools have been enhanced by the development of experimental and computational workflows that allow analysis of DNA and RNA in archived tissues and by the development of easily accessible reference databases, against which test sequences can be compared in efforts to identify differences between normal and diseased cell populations and between individuals and to identify contaminating microbial species and/or changes that result from external perturbations including exposure to ionizing radiation.

Nucleic acid sequencing tools have been further enhanced by the development of experimental and computational workflows that enable assessment of aspects of the spatial organization of chromatin within cells and/or epigenomic DNA modifications that influence gene expression and cellular function. The epigenome comprises several types of chemical or conformational modifications to DNA and the associated proteins. These include DNA methylation (i.e., the addition of a methyl group to cytosine, generally at CpG dinucleotides); PTM of nucleosomes, including methylation, acetylation, phosphorylation, and ubiquitinylation; chromatin compaction; and higher-order chromosomal folding. In addition, long-read sequencing can allow indirect measurement of chromatin compaction and even higher-order folding.[18] The NIH Roadmap Epigenomics Mapping Consortium has been instrumental in advancing this area (Bernstein et al., 2010).

The successful development of genome analysis tools inspired the development of tools to study other cellular components including new and more efficient mass spectrometry–based approaches for analysis of proteins, metabolites, cellular carbohydrates, and lipids (Aardema and MacGregor, 2002). Protein analysis has progressed to include protein modifications beyond phosphorylation, with fine mapping of glycans (Y. Huang et al., 2021). Metabolites are now considered an integral part of human physiological status and progression of disease, with many acting as signaling

---

[17] See https://www.genome.gov/about-genomics/fact-sheets/Sequencing-Human-Genome-cost.

[18] A recent multi-investigator study examined the three most popular protocols for whole-genome methylation sequencing analysis, all of which involve bisulfite conversion, which is selective for unmethylated cytosine, as well as enzymatic deamination, targeted methylation capture, long-read sequencing, and array-based methods. This study showed high concordance between assays and specific advantages and disadvantages of the individual methods that can be used to select assay designs for a given study (Foox et al., 2021).

molecules and contributing to a pro-inflammatory status. Lipids, an integral part of metabolism, are shown to have a high degree of structural complexity, particularly in the context of increased oxidative stress, with contribution to progression of adverse health effects (Natesan and Kim, 2021). Many aspects of mass spectrometry–based analysis are being accelerated by NIH's Clinical Proteomic Tumor Analysis Consortium (Ellis et al., 2013).

Early-generation -omics analysis tools enabled analysis of materials isolated from collections of cells or tissues. However, tools for analyses of single cells or parts thereof are also increasingly available. These began with the development of flow cytometry and sorting for high-speed cell analysis and purification (Herzenberg et al., 1976), including at Los Alamos National Laboratory (Fulwyler, 1965; Van Dilla et al., 1969) and Lawrence Livermore National Laboratory (Gray et al., 1987). However, recent developments based on nucleic acid barcoding allow efficient analysis of DNA, DNA modifications, and RNA in isolated single cells (Quake, 2022) and in situ (Moses and Pachter, 2022). Others enable single-cell mass spectrometry (Lanekoff et al., 2022).

These techniques, when applied to tissues exposed to low-dose radiation or to diseased tissues from individuals in exposed populations, will provide fine phenotyping of cell populations (e.g., immune system); tissue-specific responses and microenvironment interactions including with microbiomes; and identification of small molecules (e.g., metabolites, lipids) that have the potential to act as signaling molecules and transcription factors or induce epigenetic changes. New methods such as Repair-seq can map the genetic dependencies of DNA repair outcomes (Hussmann et al., 2021).[19]

Applications of -omics technologies are already being employed in space biology research, cancer research, and neuroscience, to name a few. Given that perturbations with low-dose exposures may not be quantifiable at a whole-tissue level with multiple cell populations due to a low signal, current knowledge is lacking in understanding how single changes may lead to long-term health effects. Such technological advances can provide important information on initiation and advancement in a range of low-dose radiation-associated health effects other than cancer.

Imaging analyses complement -omics analyses by providing information about the hierarchical organizations of the molecules, organelles, cells, and tissues; the functional consequences of interactions between these entities; and how these organized entities respond to perturbations including radiation. Work in imaging and -omics is currently being accelerated by the HuBMAP Consortium (2019) and HTAN (Rozenblatt-Rosen et al., 2020), which aim to develop comprehensive -omics and image-based atlases of

---

[19] Dale Ramsden, University of North Carolina at Chapel Hill, presentation to the committee on November 16, 2021.

normal and cancerous tissues. Similarly, NIH's Brain Research Through Advancing Innovative Neurotechnologies® (BRAIN)[20] initiative, which aims to revolutionize understanding of the human brain, also contributes to accelerating work in imaging and -omics. In medicine, radiomics use data-characterization algorithms to extract features from medical images beyond what can be observed by radiologists and can improve disease classification and predict clinical outcome among other benefits (Mukherjee et al., 2020).

Recent progress in noninvasive, anatomic imaging now enables more precise definition of the extent of disease as well as assessment of the molecular state of disease and quantification of variations therein. This capability comes from advances in imaging technology, reporter chemistries, and image visualization and analysis tools. Areas of advance include (a) easy-to-use 3D ultrasound imaging for quantification of flow, fibrosis/stiffness, and other molecular features revealed by injected microbubbles coupled to affinity ligands (Ajmal, 2021); (b) improved computed tomography (CT) and micro CT imaging at lower radiation dose based on photon counting and spectral analysis for assessment of tissue composition, and precise mapping of contrast reagents (Garnett, 2020); (c) faster magnetic resonance imaging (MRI) resulting from high-density receivers, highly undersampled acquisitions and faster scan times, and improved image reconstruction and visualization (Kataoka et al., 2022); (d) faster positron emission tomography (PET) imaging informed by radiotracers engineered to report on molecular or cellular status (e.g., metabolic activity, fibrosis, DNA synthesis, apoptosis, drug concentration, and inflammation; see Choudhury and Gupta, 2017); and (e) optical coherence tomography and diffuse optical spectroscopy for imaging of eyes, skin, bone, brain, breast, and other accessible tissues (Wilson et al., 2016). Integration of images acquired from different imaging modalities (e.g., ultrasound/CT, PET/CT, and PET/MRI) further increases the information that can be obtained. Reconstruction and characterization of image features from all modalities have benefited substantially from recent developments in artificial intelligence and machine learning that are made possible by new-generation computational technologies.

More precise disease phenotypes (e.g., in cancer, cardiovascular disease, cataracts, and dementias) revealed by these technologies may increase the precision of epidemiological studies of the effects the low-dose and low-dose-rate radiation. Their increasing availability in medical centers throughout the United States, increasing safety, and decreasing cost make it reasonable to consider deploying them in future radiation health effects studies. These technologies are being applied to improve disease detection and treatment so that overall mortality resulting from radiation exposures may be decreased.

---

[20] See https://braininitiative.nih.gov.

Multi-omics image analyses of disease biopsies (and normal tissue) can provide information on cellular and subcellular proteins, cell distributions, and interactions between them (Lun and Bodenmiller, 2020; Schapiro et al., 2022). Multi-round immunostaining and imaging technologies allow expression of many different proteins to be measured in the same tissue section, thereby allowing assessment of cellular composition, interactions between cells, assessment of signal transduction cascades, and detailed immunophenotyping (Black et al., 2021; Lin et al., 2015). Similar multi-protein analysis can be accomplished using multiplexed ion beam imaging (Coskun et al., 2021) and spatially defined mass spectrometry–based techniques (Gessel et al., 2014), with applications in spatial distribution of lipids and metabolites. Metabolic imaging can also be achieved with methods such as fluorescence lifetime imaging microscopy (Datta et al., 2020) to characterize metabolic states and involvement of specific processes such as in mitochondria (glycolysis or oxidative phosphorylation). Spatial genomics and transcriptomics technologies and interactions are particularly well suited to study clonal heterogeneity in tissues (Marx, 2021; Zhao et al., 2022).

The information these tools provide on the cellular compositions of normal and diseased tissues, on functional states, and on the functional consequences of interactions between cells may be used to define more precise disease phenotypes in epidemiological studies and to elucidate the cellular and molecular mechanisms that are influenced by low-dose and low-dose-rate radiation. The single-cell capabilities seem particularly well suited to study the stochastic interactions of low-dose radiation with the cells and components that comprise tissues.

Advances in fluorescence, X-ray, and electron microscopy, chemistry, and computation have been combined to allow imaging of the organization and dynamics of single molecules, protein complexes, and organelles (Liu et al., 2015). Innovations in fluorescence microscopy and fluorescence labeling chemistries include super-resolution fluorescence microscopy for single-molecule localization and tracking and fluorescence correlation spectroscopy and single-molecule fluorescence resonance energy transfer for assessment of molecular movements and interactions (Nickerson et al., 2014). In addition, novel sample preparation techniques, such as tissue clearing, and preparation techniques that expand the biospecimen itself coupled with large-format imaging tools, such as light sheet microscopies, facilitate rapid 3D imaging of extended cellular volumes (Zhang et al., 2017). New X-ray microscopes allow 3D imaging of structures as small as 20 nanometers (nm), while scanning electron microscopes coupled with serial block-face sectioning or focused ion beam sectioning allow 3D imaging of structures as small as 4 nm (Riesterer et al., 2020). The development of cryoelectron tomography offers the possibility of subnanometer imaging of molecular complexes in single cells (Chua et al., 2022). Additional innovations in microscopy, chemistry, and image integration allow specimens to be moved between imaging platforms, thereby enabling multimodal imaging (e.g., correlative light and electron microscopy; López et al., 2017).

These tools, when applied in radiation biology, will allow direct study of the structures and organizations of the proteins, protein complexes, and organelles that are directly and indirectly affected by ionizing radiation. These include DNA repair complexes in nuclei and nucleoli; organelles such as mitochondria, macropinosomes, and lamellipodia that may be involved in cell death responses; and filopodia-like protrusions that mediate intercellular interactions and motility (Johnson et al., 2022).

Revolutionary advances in single-particle cryogenic electron microscopy (cryo-EM) are now being made through NIH-supported cryo-EM centers that enable atomic resolution measurements of single-molecule and protein-complex structures that do not readily form crystals.[21] In addition, DOE supports next-generation synchrotrons (e.g., bright, storage ring, and X-ray free-electron lasers),[22] which can enhance studies of the dynamics of protein interaction and responses to perturbations as well as intracellular structures. Development of these technologies will support fundamental studies of the molecular responses to radiation. These technologies could be deployed in future research into the biophysical effects of cell interactions with single photons or ions and direct measurements of the damage to specific cellular components including DNA, associated repair complexes, mitochondria, membranes, and other features of cells that may be influenced by the passage of ionizing radiation. Such information may be useful in the development of more precise multiscale dosimetry models.

The Internet of Things refers to devices equipped with sensors that connect and exchange data over the internet or other communications networks. IoMT refers to devices that inform all aspects of human health or performance or exposure (Dwivedi et al., 2022). IoMT devices may include smart phones, in-home monitors, implantable devices, and wearable devices that allow continuous assessment and reporting of a wide range of physiological and psychological endpoints or exposures in humans (Greco et al., 2020). The growing list of accessible endpoints includes weight, gait and balance, voice pathology, heart function, temperature, glucose and other aspects of blood chemistry, cognitive function, eye movement, food and drug consumption, disease detection, geographic location, and exposure to environmental agents.

Deployment of IoMT devices for low-dose and low-dose-rate radiation studies offers the possibility of accurate assessments of individual exposures to radiation and physiological changes that may be associated with such exposures. Wearable dosimeters may continuously report exposures of radiation from environmental or medical procedures. In-home and geographically

---

[21] See https://www.cryoemcenters.org/cryoem-centers.
[22] See https://science.osti.gov/User-Facilities/User-Facilities-at-a-Glance/BES/X-Ray-Light-Sources.

dispersed environmental sensors may also improve estimates of exposures to radioactive materials. Wearable monitors of aspects of human physiology and cognitive function that report continuously may allow more accurate assessment of changes in health status that may be associated with radiation exposures. Deployment of IoMT devices already exists in some occupational settings (where personal electronic dosimeters are used) and can be considered for future-generation epidemiological studies aimed at improving estimates for risk of exposure to low-dose and low-dose-rate radiation.

Advances in -omics, image analysis, and distributed sensor technologies can now provide measurements of the molecular and cellular compositions, organizations, and static and dynamic interactions between them in normal and diseased tissues both prior to and as they respond to more precisely known levels of radiation and other perturbagens. Computational tools are now being developed with support from NIH and DOE that interpret these data to reveal how biological systems function and make the data and analytical tools available to the scientific community. Machine learning tools reveal networks that regulate behavior and discover differences between normal and diseased tissues that may be causally related to disease genesis and progression. Dynamic modeling tools describe how complex systems respond in the short and long terms to perturbations and, more importantly, predict how they will respond to perturbations including radiation.

Several computational concepts implemented on increasingly powerful computational platforms are used to integrate -omics, images, and biological phenotypes and clinical data (Goecks et al., 2020) in ways that identify regulatory mechanisms that may control biological and clinical phenotypes and/or identify molecular signatures and phenotypes that are associated with perturbations. These concepts include (1) dimensionality reduction to select the most important features in integrated datasets, (2) Bayesian learning methods that include prior knowledge during learning, (3) supervised and unsupervised classification and regression methods that organize health effects into discrete categories (e.g., disease subtypes, genomic or epigenomic[23] states, and/or functional molecular networks) and that identify associations

---

[23] One of the most exciting developments in both epigenome analysis methods and their computational interpretation is the development of single-cell -omics methods that can measure, most typically, pairwise combinations of DNA methylation, chromatin modifications, and gene expression but have been extended to chromatin structure as well. These measurements are more limited in the genome-scale comprehensiveness of a given analysis, compared to bulk (non-single-cell measures), but they open the door to advanced methods from statistical mechanics, including entropy, stochastic processes, and critical phenomena, which allow for time-dependent modeling, epigenomic landscape analysis, and, most importantly, bottom-up modeling—namely, the ability to predict and model the underlying molecular network state using measurements taken only from within that cell (Teschendorff and Feinberg, 2021). Such approaches are particularly important in the study of low-dose radiation effects since their cellular effects are comparatively low frequency and stochastic but will impact multiple molecules within the radiation-impacted cells.

of these with response to perturbations, (4) deep learning methods that use multilayer neural networks to identify complex relationships in complex datasets (typically without providing information about the mechanisms that drive the relationships), and (5) ensemble learning wherein many models of associations are developed and averaged to produce predictions. These machine learning tools applied to measurements of cells and tissues following exposure to low-dose and low-dose-rate radiation will allow identification of the features and regulatory mechanisms that are influenced by radiation as well as precise health effects that result from exposures. Tools that link features and mechanisms to health effect phenotypes will suggest potentially causal relationships that can be tested in experimental systems.

Dynamic models are central to understanding the behavior of complex biological systems including responses to perturbation. Elucidation of the emergent properties of the system is an important goal of many such models. Models have been developed that describe chemical reactions, protein folding, cell phenotypes, immune function, interactions of cells that comprise complex tissues, and interactions between organs and between individual organisms and their environments. The model used depends on scale and complexity of the system and on the level of understanding of the processes that influence the behavior of the system. Commonly used model types include agent-based models (ABMs; Metzcar et al., 2019), differential equations (Chaves and de Jong, 2021), and molecular dynamic (MD) models (Ingólfsson et al., 2022).

ABMs typically consist of computational objects situated in space and time, called agents, that represent biological objects of interest (e.g., the diverse organelles, cell types, mechanical structures, and/or organs that comprise irradiated systems). Rules are defined that describe how each agent sends and receives signals and how it acts based on received signals (e.g., change in state, movement, growth, death). These rules are based on biological understanding or hypotheses, can be as simple or complex as biological understanding allows, and can be different in scale and type (e.g., cell phenotype, molecular activity, and organs) as long as rules can be defined that link them. Such models are well suited for the exploration of how cells and tissues respond to radiation-induced changes in the signals encoded in the rules. The number of agents and complexity of rules can be as large as computational capability allows. ABMs are already used to describe the responses of complex biological systems to ionizing radiation.[24]

Partial differential equation (PDE) models calculate the concentrations and/or the velocities of the components comprising a system. In general, the components in PDE models are similarly scaled (e.g., describing interacting

---

[24] Sylvain Costes, National Aeronautics and Space Administration, presentation to the committee on September 24, 2021.

chemicals or components of the immune system). The number of components of PDE models can become large, but modern computers make managing millions of equations tractable. However, development of models that integrate across biological and molecular systems is difficult. PDE models may be useful in understanding the behavior of regulatory networks that are influenced by radiation.

MD models predict how every atom in a protein or other molecular system will move over time, based on physical laws governing interatomic interactions. The utility of MD simulations is increasing as better structures of proteins and protein complexes are determined (e.g., using single-particle cryo-EM or next-generation synchrotrons) and as computing power increases to allow simulation of biological processes at relevant timescales. MD models may be particularly useful in exploring radiation–matter interactions but are computationally demanding. The high-performance computers available in DOE's national laboratories are well suited to MD simulations; the exoscale systems now being deployed at Argonne National Laboratory and Oak Ridge National Laboratory and the powerful cloud computing platforms that are now available from public domain providers are particularly noteworthy.

Major advances in computing technologies and architectures have powered many advances in biomedical analysis technologies—for example, by providing the computational power for massively parallel sequencing, multiplex imaging, MD simulations, artificial intelligence, cryo-EM, secure federated computing, and more.

5.4.2 Harmonized Databases to Support Biological and Epidemiological Studies (Priority I2)

Scientific or Decision-Making Value

Funding agencies and publishers of scientific articles increasingly require plans for data management and data sharing for research they support or publish. Several frameworks for data management and stewardship have been published; for health sciences, the most cited are the FAIR (findable, accessible, interoperable, and reusable) principles (Wilkinson et al., 2016). Despite major advances in open and free exchange of data in many fields of science, transparency and application of the FAIR principles in human studies of environmental health issues remain highly controversial.

Current Status and Promising Research Directions

The Human Genome Project and follow-on cancer analysis programs stimulated the development of databases of healthy individuals against which new populations could be conveniently compared. A key feature of these reference databases is their public accessibility and convenience of use. Examples of commonly used resources include GenBank, an NIH genetic sequence database of annotated collections of publicly available DNA sequences;[25] NCI's Genomic Data Commons, a unified repository and cancer knowledge base that enables data sharing across cancer genomic studies in support of precision medicine;[26] the University of California, Santa Cruz's Genome Browser, which describes the sequences, genes, and other components of the normal genome;[27] CBioPortal for Cancer Genomics, which provides visualization, analysis, and download of large-scale cancer genomic datasets;[28] the ENCODE portal, which informs on functional elements in the human genomes;[29] the Genome Aggregation Database (gnomAD), which aggregates exome and genome sequencing data from various large-scale sequencing projects;[30] the Catalog of Somatic Mutations in Cancer, which helps explore the impact of somatic mutations in human cancer;[31] and the Trans-Omics for Precision Medicine (TOPMed) program, which provides disease treatments tailored to an individual's unique genes and environment.[32] Recently, work during the COVID-19 pandemic demonstrated the feasibility of making EMRs computationally accessible to identify higher-risk populations and for other purposes, while maintaining the required confidentiality. In addition, a growing number of geospatial databases are becoming available that inform on aspects of the environment, health care, economic status, social status, transportation, and other factors, which may reveal confounding events when included in next-generation epidemiological studies. Importantly, NIH, the National Aeronautics and Space Administration, and other federal agencies are increasingly committed to the development of databases in which information is available under FAIR principles (Wilkinson et al., 2016). The availability of data under FAIR principles already has stimulated the development of thousands of computational tools that access these reference databases. These tools can be aggregated, as in done in Galaxy, to support accessible, reproducible, and transparent computational research.[33] These and similar reference databases will be valuable in low-dose radiation research—for example, by serving as references against which radiation-perturbed normal

---

[25] See https://www.ncbi.nlm.nih.gov/genbank.
[26] See https://gdc.cancer.gov.
[27] See https://genome.ucsc.edu.
[28] See https://www.cbioportal.org.
[29] See https://www.encodeproject.org.
[30] See https://gnomad.broadinstitute.org.
[31] See https://cancer.sanger.ac.uk/cosmic.
[32] See https://topmed.nhlbi.nih.gov.
[33] See https://elixir-europe.org/communities/galaxy.

and diseased tissues can be compared in order to more accurately define aspects of biology that are influenced by exposure to radiation, documenting the levels of environmental exposures experienced by individuals in U.S. populations, and improving understanding of the phenotypes of diseases that may be caused by radiation exposures.

5.4.3 Dosimetry for Low-Dose and Low-Dose-Rate Exposures (Priority I3)

Scientific or Decision-Making Value

Understanding the effects of exposures to low-dose and low-dose-rate radiation depends on accurate information about the levels of such exposures and consideration of radiation type, mode of exposure, and individual characteristics. Recent developments in several aspects of radiation dosimetry suggest that future low-dose and low-dose-rate radiation studies can benefit from improved personal dosimeters, computational phantoms, biokinetic and source-term models, and tools for environmental radiation exposure. In parallel with these developments for radiation dosimetry, modern statistical and computational methods for dose reconstruction are needed to fully integrate detailed dosimetry data into modern analyses of epidemiological studies.

Current Status and Promising Research Directions

Accurate measurements of cell-, tissue-, and organ-specific radiation exposures experienced by medically and occupationally exposed individuals will improve understanding of the health effects that result from those exposures. Recent work in harmonization efforts demonstrates high variability in reported monitoring results (Fantuzzi et al., 2014; Mayer et al., 2021; Stadtmann et al., 2018), thereby necessitating investigation of the effects of calibration bias in dosimetry monitoring systems and periodic harmonization intercomparison studies. Further harmonization regarding reconstruction from reported exposure quantities spanning generational application of ICRP Publications 26, 60, and 103 in reconstruction of fundamental organ dosimetry further mobilizes existing data sources.[34] Use of IoMT wearable dosimeters may facilitate harmonization for occupationally exposed individuals. Inclusion of detailed information in EMRs of lifetime organ-specific radiation doses from medical diagnostic procedures will enable more accurate assessment of such exposures and support epidemiological studies of the adverse health effects that result from such exposures.

---

[34] See https://oriseapps.orau.gov/cedr/default.aspx.

This will be an important undertaking given that exposure from medical diagnostic procedures is the biggest human-made radiation source but will require substantial changes in medical practice and recordkeeping and good records of the doses delivered and the reasons for exposure.

In the case of neutron dosimetry, recent international harmonization intercomparisons demonstrated greater variability compared to photon-based systems (Fantuzzi et al., 2014; Mayer et al., 2021; Stadtmann et al., 2018). This variability was attributed to the breadth of energies from source neutron fields and the high variability in the neutron dose coefficients at low energies (10 kilo-electronvolts [keV] to 100 keV). Neutron dosimeters (e.g., thermoluminescence albedo dosimeters, etched-track detectors, superheated emulsions, and direct ion storage chambers) have inherent limitations, with ongoing challenges in determination of directional response, making dose estimation and reconstruction a continuing challenge (Stricklin et al., 2021). Improving characterization of source radiation fields with directional dependence will improve occupational neutron dosimetry and enable more accurate assessment of organ-specific doses. Furthermore, knowledge of worker activities (source exposure based on radiation work permit, posture, and duration) informed by IoMT wearable detectors coupled with innovation in rapid Monte Carlo radiation transport modeling can provide near-real-time organ dose estimation to accompany typical reported values of effective dose (lacking organ-specific information). The quantitative information from these health and exposure monitoring devices, coupled with health information from EMRs, can provide increasingly accurate health and exposure metrics for next-generation studies of the health effects of low-dose and low-dose-rate radiation, assuming that personal privacy issues can be properly managed.

Improved computational tools and Monte Carlo radiation transport modeling capabilities are now emerging that can be leveraged and further developed to allow integrated, multiscale dosimetry from the track structure to the organ and organ-system levels. Anthropomorphic phantom models were originally rooted in the "Reference Man" paradigm, which evolved to an age-specific stylized (mathematical) model employed in the MIRD Schema[35] and CT-based voxel phantoms adopted by ICRP (2009, 2016a,b), which corrects for sex- and age-specific (newborn, 1-year-old, 5-year-old, 10-year-old, 15-year-old, and 20- to 25-year-old) differences. Currently, ICRP has improved upon limitations of organ contouring and has improved resolution (e.g., thin-walled organs, expanded definition of organ targets) of adult male and female hybrid mesh-type phantoms (ICRP, 2020). The mesh phantoms have the added functionality of being deformable, permitting

---

[35] Developed by the Medical Internal Radiation Dose (MIRD) Committee of the Society of Nuclear Medicine.

the creation of expanded morphometry (beyond reference), in addition to articulated postures (ICRP, 2020; Yeom et al., 2019, 2021).

These phantoms can be further developed for use in estimation of organ doses for prospective and retrospective studies of low-dose and low-dose-rate radiation effects beyond reference models based on 50th percentile Western European Caucasian anatomical parameters (ICRP, 1975). This includes development of phantoms representative of non-reference ages beyond the six reference ages described above, as well as representative of cohort demographics, as has been conducted with the Japanese phantom-based models of the J45 phantoms (Sato et al., 2020). Underrepresented cohorts currently not adopted by ICRP models, notably pregnant women of various gestational periods, need to be adopted to accurately assess organ doses for specific populations (Makkia et al., 2019; Maynard et al., 2011, 2014, 2015a,b; Petoussi-Henss, 2021). Improved computational capabilities permit the implementation of these enhanced mesh-type phantom models. Although the mesh-type phantoms represent anatomic fidelity in reference models, expansion to include realistic distribution of anatomical parameters, for example, adipose tissue in addition to subcutaneous, will more accurately model individuals in non-reference populations.

Phantom models can be further improved by taking advantage of innovations in targeted radionuclide therapies in nuclear medicine such as targeted alpha therapies. These include development of 3D models of tissue microstructure (e.g., definition of kidney model at the nephron level) to model internal radionuclide deposition and archived samples to determine 3D spatial distribution of deposition.[36] At the whole-organ level, models of both intraorgan and interorgan blood vasculature used to differentiate radionuclide decays in organ parenchyma from radionuclide decays in organ blood content can further inform the dose distribution in the human body using phantom models to estimate radiation dose, bridging organ-level with organ microstructure dosimetry for low-dose radiation exposures and uptakes.

Computational dosimetry based on anatomically enhanced phantom models to permit individual or subcohort dose assessment now appears feasible. However, widespread use will require enhancements in commonly used Monte Carlo radiation transport codes to accommodate mesh-type phantoms and proposed multiscale anatomical enhancements without degraded computational performance. Radiation transport, especially at low energies, must be enhanced through appropriate variance reduction techniques or establishment of justified low-energy cutoffs for particle transport to maintain reasonable computational processing times, with challenges

---

[36] See http://janus.northwestern.edu/janus2/index.php.

mostly lying with radiation transport of changed particles, whether secondary from indirectly ionizing radiation or primary.

While dosimetric models for internal emitters depend primarily on the emission properties of radionuclides, biokinetic models depend on radionuclide inventory (and progeny), chemical form (e.g., solubility, transformed states in the body), physical form (e.g., particle size), route of intake, and age of intake. Existing models are well described in national and international consensus-based reports (ICRP, 1995, 2016b; NCRP, 2009b). However, current biokinetic models of occupational cohorts have largely reflected healthy Caucasian working adult males, resulting in deterministic (i.e., "reference") biokinetic models (NCRP, 2009b, 2018b) with few recent exceptions (Martinez et al., 2022). Expansion of biokinetic models representative of the broader public or cohort (age- and sex-specific) can lead to internal dose assessment models that include expanded morphometry and other associated factors (diet, smoker dosimetry, radon background). Current innovations in nuclear medicine have adopted patient-specific radionuclide biodistribution (Fisher, 2021), whose principles can be expanded to cohort-specific (e.g., age, sex, pregnant women) factors of radionuclide metabolism for both prospective epidemiological study design and retrospective dose reconstruction to improve identification of dose-response relationships for internalized radionuclides.

Applications of variability of internal dose coefficients have been preliminarily explored in the field of consequence management in the establishment of dose-based public protection–derived response levels (Cochran et al., 2020). Current tools permit consideration of population-specific cohorts[37] whose dose estimation must be expanded to reflect impacts from internalized radionuclides. Where dose reconstruction for internal radiation uptakes is often limited by available data, integration of high-fidelity source-term modeling, such as from reactor models (Bixler and Nosek 2021; Wieselquist et al. 2020) or consequence management or fallout tools (Auxier et al., 2017), may supplement both prospective and reconstructive efforts correlating internal dosimetry quantities with high-fidelity source-term modeling of radionuclide inventory and validating with in-field experimental data (environmental monitors, personnel monitors, nuclear forensics tools).

Despite advances in dosimetric modeling, errors in estimated radiation doses can arise from uncertainty in dosimetry parameters, as well as from measurement error in the underlying radiation exposure data (see Section 5.2.1) that are supplied to dosimetry systems. These dose errors can introduce bias in estimation of the dose-response shape and reduce statistical power. Modern statistical and computational methods for dose

---

[37] See https://maccs.sandia.gov/secpop.aspx.

reconstruction and risk estimation can be applied to account for dose errors that are classical or Berkson in form and that are independent or shared across individuals. These include flexible (i.e., semiparametric or nonparametric) statistical models and simulation-based approaches. In particular, recent research has focused on two-dimensional Monte Carlo approaches that simulate alternative sets of doses for an entire cohort rather than a single set that emerges when each individual's dose is estimated independently from other individuals; these sets of doses are then integrated into dose-response analyses (Kwon et al., 2016; Simon et al., 2015; Stram et al., 2015, 2021). At the same time, a growing body of statistical research has developed methods for measurement error in epidemiological data, particularly in nutritional epidemiology, including methods that correct for correlated errors in exposures (e.g., dose error) and outcomes (e.g., errors to outcome misclassification; Bennett et al., 2017; Keogh et al., 2020; Shaw et al., 2020, 2021; Wu et al., 2019).[38] Failure to further develop and apply these methods in epidemiological studies, particularly the large studies that will be required to detect radiation health effects at low doses with sufficient statistical power, will continue to limit the statistical analysis and interpretation of large and complex dose reconstructions for quantifying radiation risk.

5.4.4 Facilities for Low-Dose and Low-Dose-Rate Exposures (Priority I4)

Scientific and Decision-Making Value

The potential gains from a new low-dose radiation research program are highly dependent on available facilities that are tailored to the specific needs of this line of research. These facilities significantly differ from facilities that are used primarily for higher-dose experiments or applications that tend to involve a high-dose-rate delivery, making it very difficult to "turn the source down" to deliver low-dose and low-dose-rate exposures. In other words, a higher-dose activity facility cannot be adjusted easily for use in low-dose radiation research.

Current Status and Promising Research Directions

The committee reached out to several radiation facilities that have capabilities to support low-dose research to understand and document those capabilities. The committee selected "larger" facilities, but it recognizes that other smaller facilities including several cesium-137 irradiators or X-ray sources are routinely used for low-dose research in universities, hospitals,

---

[38] See Supplementary Appendix B of Gilbert et al., 2020, for a full discussion on dose-error methodology for radiation epidemiology studies.

and other settings. Responses from the facilities, except the response from the Argonne Tandem Linac Accelerator System (ATLAS) facility at Argonne National Laboratory, are shown (unedited) in Appendix E. These responses contain information useful to the research community other than what is summarized in Table 5.2 for the purposes of this committee's task. In addition to the facilities listed in the table, the committee also reached out to the National Institute of Standards and Technology (NIST) and the University of North Carolina (UNC) at Chapel Hill. NIST did not respond to the committee's request and a UNC representative told the committee that facilities that house nanobeams for irradiation of cells and animals at UNC are still in the research stage.

An assessment of multiple large radiation facilities that have capabilities to carry out low-dose research revealed that diminished support for radiation research in the United States has left the radiation research community with inadequate exposure facilities to support low-dose and low-dose-rate radiation research and address high-priority issues:

- There are no facilities available to facilitate inhalation studies to understand the effects of internal emitters on the lungs; in the past, the United States had a facility at the Inhalation Toxicology Research Institute in New Mexico, but this facility was terminated. The construction of instrumentation that delivers doses to animals via inhalation and dosimetry support for inhalation studies is complex.
- Facilities for low-dose-rate exposures (similar to those at the Institute for Environmental Sciences in Japan and several in Europe including FIGARO in Norway, and others in the United Kingdom, France, and Italy)[39] are not available in the United States. These facilities permit animal exposures and can tune the dose down to be delivered over long exposure times, unlike facilities in the United States.
- Facilities similar to the deep underground facilities in Europe and Canada designed to eliminate the effects of background radiation are of restricted access or of limited capabilities. The committee is aware of the underground radiation biology laboratory at the radioactive waste disposal site Waste Isolation Pilot Plant in New Mexico (Castillo et al., 2021; Van Voorhies et al., 2020).
- High-LET sources such as carbon ion and others can be found in Japan and Germany; several are under construction in Russia, but none are currently available in the United States.

---

[39] See https://www.concert-h2020.eu/en/Concert_info/Access_Infrastructures/Bulletins.

TABLE 5.2 Available Facilities for Low-Dose and Low-Dose-Rate Research in the United States

Facility	Radiation Type or Description of Facility	Location	Start; End Year	Main Purpose	Dose Range (max; min)
AFRRI	Triga reactor (mixed field gamma/neutron)	AFRRI complex	1969; no plan	Materials, cells, animals; equipment	Information not provided
AFRRI	High-level cobalt (mono-energetic)	AFRRI complex	1968; no plan	Materials, cells, animals	Information not provided
AFRRI	Low-level cobalt (mono-energetic)	AFRRI complex	1974; no plan	Materials, cells, animals	Information not provided
AFRRI	Linac (mono-energetic, 4, 10, 15 MeV)	AFRRI complex	2013; no plan	Materials, cells, animals	Information not provided
ATLAS	Ion beams	Argonne National Laboratory, Physics Division	Not provided	Basic research in nuclear physics; production of radioisotopes; currently no radiobiology	Information not provided
CSU	Low-dose-rate γ ray (137Cs) tissue culture facility	Main CSU campus (MRB 08)	Not provided; not planned	Radiobiology experiments	Information not provided
CSU	Low-dose-rate γ ray (12 individual 137Cs) tissue culture facility	Main CSU campus (MRB 12)	1997; no plan	Radiobiology experiments	Information not provided
CSU	Low-dose-rate neutron tissue culture facility (14.1 MeV)	Main CSU campus (MRB 02)	Expected to be operational in 2022; no plan	Engineered human tissues ("tissues on a chip")	Information not provided

Dose Rate (standard setup)	Inhalation Experiments	Available to Outside Users; Available Adjacent Infrastructure	References Demonstrating Capabilities
From less than 10 R/h to more than 100 kR/h	No	Yes; Yes	Bene et al., 2021
From less than 1 R/h to more than 100 kR/h	No	Yes; Yes	Bene et al., 2021
From less than 1 R/h to more than 100 kR/h	No	Yes; Yes	Bene et al., 2021
From 0.05 to 6 Gy/min	No	Yes; Yes	Bene et al., 2021
Low dose rate not standard but possible	No	Yes but not for radiobiology; Not available	Information not provided
Currently 9.3 mGy/h but can increase to 500 mGy/h or decrease to background	No	Yes; Yes	Kato et al., 2006
1 mGy/h to 100 mGy/h	No	Yes; Yes	Amdur and Bedford, 1994; Bedford, 2001; Huang et al., 2011; Kato et al., 2006, 2007; Ochola et al., 2019; Peng et al., 2012; Ulsh et al., 2001; Wilson et al., 2008
3.6 mGy/h to a factor of 20 lower	No	Intended; Yes	Information not provided

continued

TABLE 5.2 Continued

Facility	Radiation Type or Description of Facility	Location	Start; End Year	Main Purpose	Dose Range (max; min)
CSU	Low-dose-rate γ ray (137Cs) vivarium	Main CSU campus (MRB 06)	—; No plan	Mice and medaka fish	Information not provided
CSU	Low-dose-rate neutron (252Cf) vivarium	CSU Foothills Campus	2017; not planned (new source planned for 2022)	Small animals	Information not provided
LLUMC	Synchrotron-based proton facility (50–250 MeV)	G2	1990; not planned	Patient treatment; clinical research; radiobiology (cells and tissues)	Information not provided
LLUMC	Synchrotron-based proton facility (50–250 MeV)	HBL	1990; not planned	Physics and radiobiology (cells, tissues, and animals)	Information not provided
LLUMC	Linear accelerator (2–22 MeV)	TrueBeam	2019; not planned	Patient treatment; clinical research; radiobiology (cells and tissues)	Information not provided
NSRL	Protons (linac or tandem Van de Graaff)	Brookhaven National Laboratory	~2003; >2030	Radiobiology research (cells, tissues, or animals) and electronics testing	>>1 Gy; as low as 0.1 to 0.2 mGy
NSRL	Ions (electron-beam ion source, tandem Van de Graaf)	Brookhaven National Laboratory	~2003; >2030	Radiobiology research (cells, tissues, or animals) and electronics testing	>>1 Gy; as low as 0.1 to 0.2 mGy
RARAF	Neutrons	RARAF, Irvington, NY	2015; not planned	Radiobiology (mice, tissue, and cells)	Up to 10 Gy; no lower limit

Dose Rate (standard setup)	Inhalation Experiments	Available to Outside Users; Available Adjacent Infrastructure	References Demonstrating Capabilities
10 cGy/day to 0.41 cGy/min	No	Yes; Yes	Ochola et al., 2019; Shakhov et al., 2012
1 mGy/day	No	Yes; Yes	Acharya et al., 2019; Borak et al., 2021; Perez et al., 2020
Standard setup is 100–200 cGy/min but can range from 1 to 300 cGy/min	No	Yes but limited; Yes	Unternaehrer-Hamm et al., 2020
Standard setup is 100–200 cGy/min but can range from 1 to 300 cGy/min	No	Yes but limited to outside clinical care hours; Yes	Information not provided
5–600 cGy/min	No	Yes but limited; Yes	Information not provided
Between 0.01 and 1 Gy/min	No	Yes; Yes	La Tessa et al., 2016; Simonsen et al., 2020
Between 0.01 and 1 Gy/min	No	Yes; Yes	La Tessa et al., 2016; Simonsen et al., 2020
Up to 3 Gy/h	No	Yes; Yes	Marino, 2017; Xu et al., 2015

continued

TABLE 5.2 Continued

Facility	Radiation Type or Description of Facility	Location	Start; End Year	Main Purpose	Dose Range (max; min)
RARAF	Ion beams (LET = 8–1,000 keV/ μm)	RARAF, Irvington, NY	1980; not planned	Radiobiology (cells and thin tissues; microbeam available)	Up to 100 Gy; single particle
RARAF	FLASH (6 or 9 MeV electrons)	RARAF, Irvington, NY	2020; not planned	Radiobiology (mice, tissues, and cells)	Up to 100 Gy; 0.1 Gy
RARAF	FLASH (4.5 MeV protons)	RARAF, Irvington, NY	2018; not planned	Radiobiology (cells and thin tissues)	Up to 100 Gy; 1 msec at selected dose rate
RARAF	VADER ^{137}Cs gamma	CUIMC, New York	2017; not planned	Radiobiology (mice and cells)	1 month; 5 min at selected dose rate

NOTE: AFRRI = Armed Forces Radiobiology Research Institute; ATLAS = Argonne Tandem Linac Accelerator System; CSU = Colorado State University; CUIMC = Columbia University Irving Medical Center; HBL = horizontal beam lateral; LET = linear energy transfer; LLUMC = Loma Linda University Medical Center; NSRL = NASA Space Radiation Laboratory; RARAF = Radiological Research Accelerator Facility.

Overall, a substantial investment in facilities specifically designed for internal and external exposures to low-dose and low-dose-rate radiation of types relevant to exposed or potentially exposed U.S. populations will be needed to support a revitalized low-dose radiation research program in the United States.

5.5 ESTIMATED TIMELINE AND COSTS

The development of a robust research program that can provide information about the risks to humans that may result from exposures to low-dose and low-dose-rate radiation and about the involved mechanisms will require significant investments in biological research, dosimetry, epidemiology, facilities, data curation and coordination, education and outreach, and communication. This might be accomplished by establishing and nurturing an interactive multidisciplinary program as illustrated conceptually in Figure 5.2 comprising interacting hubs focusing on basic and translational biology, analytical and computational technologies, and epidemiology. The

Dose Rate (standard setup)	Inhalation Experiments	Available to Outside Users; Available Adjacent Infrastructure	References Demonstrating Capabilities
Adjustable	No	Yes; Yes	Miller et al., 1999; Randers-Pehrson et al., 2009
16 mGy/sec to 600 Gy/sec	No	Yes; Yes	Garty et al., 2022
Up to 4 kGy/sec	No	Yes; Yes	Grilj et al., 2020
0.1–1 Gy/day (time-variable)	No	Yes; Yes	Garty et al., 2020

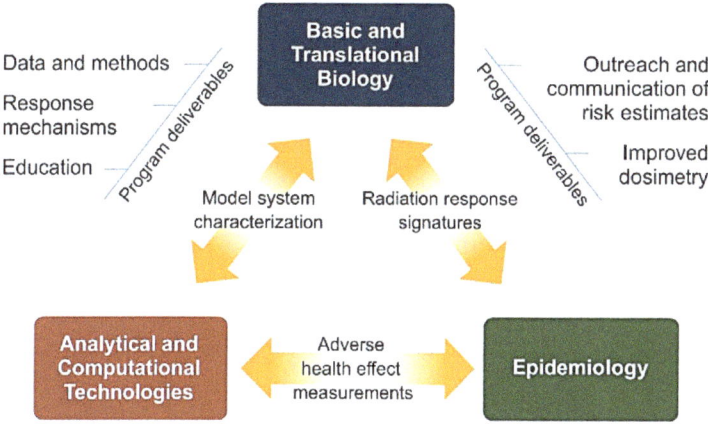

FIGURE 5.2 Illustration of the interacting hubs of the low-dose radiation multidisciplinary program.

analytical and computational technology hub would provide tools for model system characterization to the biology hub and for assessment of adverse health effects to the epidemiology hub. The biology hub would elucidate mechanisms of response and provide radiation response signatures for assessment in the epidemiology hub. The epidemiology hub would explore associations between radiation and adverse health events and refer strong associations to the biology hub for assessment of mechanism and causality. Program output might include data and methods, radiation response mechanisms, risk estimates, and improved dosimetry

The committee's research agenda extends for 15 years, to 2037. By that time, several of the biological research priorities (e.g., development of model systems [Priority B1] and development of biomarkers for radiation-induced adverse health outcomes [Priority B2]) and research infrastructure priorities (e.g., tools for detection and precise characterization of aberrant cell and tissue states [Priority I1] and dosimetry for low-dose and low-dose-rate exposures [Priority I3]) are expected to be completed or to be approaching completion and providing critical information. However, it is likely that the epidemiological research priorities will extend further into the future based on progress with improving dosimetry for epidemiological studies (Priority I3), further establishment of database infrastructure (Priority I2), and advances on the most biologically important components of low-dose and low-dose-rate radiation (e.g., through research on Priorities B2 and B4). That said, certain aspects of the epidemiological research priorities can begin immediately to complement planning for future epidemiological studies. Notably, these efforts should include engagement with the research and other stakeholder communities to examine to what extent some of the committee-recommended research can be conducted by adding to existing population studies and to identify the appropriate study populations for next-generation radiation epidemiology studies. Certain epidemiological studies could require substantial time for completion, possibly three decades or more. This means that long-term commitment for the program (see Section 6.1) is essential for its success.

The committee estimates that funding needed to set up the program is on par with the congressionally authorized funds for 2023 and 2024 (see Appendix A), that is, at the level of $30 million and $40 million annually, respectively, but needs to rise to the level of $100 million annually thereafter and remain at that level through about 2037. Periodic reassessments are required as large epidemiological studies and necessary research infrastructures are established. Although the committee recognizes that the exact form of the program will be determined by the funding agency after consultation with stakeholders, the following prototypical program is intended to justify the $100 million annual funding level. Specifically the program might include

- A basic and translational biology hub comprising approximately 20 individual laboratories, 6 multidisciplinary centers, 3 technology development and deployment centers, and a basic science data coordinating center (cost ~$50 million annually). This effort would be similar in scale and composition to other targeted basic and translational biomedical research programs now operated by NIH (e.g., NIH HuBMAP; the NCI HTAN program, the NCI Cancer Systems Biology program).
- An epidemiology hub comprising three epidemiology centers, an epidemiology data coordinating center, and a dosimetry center (cost ~$30 million annually) dedicated to quantification of risks to U.S. populations exposed to low-dose and low-dose-rate radiation. This program is similar in size to the one carried out at the Radiation Effects Research Foundation (see Section 4.5.6).
- An education, outreach, and policy hub comprising an education center that develops training curricula and administers a training grant program, a science policy center, and an outreach and communication center (cost ~$10 million annually).
- A facilities development program for low-dose and low-dose-rate exposures (cost ~$5 million annually).
- Program administration, internal and external coordination, grants management, and operation of an external advisory committee (cost ~$5 million annually). A key aspect of program administration will be to ensure coordination between low-dose basic research, epidemiological research, technological research, education, and outreach efforts within the U.S. program and with non-U.S. low-dose radiation research programs.

Congressionally authorized funds for the program were at the level of $20 million in 2021 but much lower amounts ($5 million) were appropriated. Congressional staff who briefed the committee noted that additional funds could become available, with the appropriate justification and with evidence of research progress.[40] The committee recognizes that the research priorities it identified need to be achievable within reasonable budgets. Although it did not make a detailed assessment of the costs associated with the proposed research agenda, the committee used its informed collective judgment to provide a rough estimate of the research costs. Overall, it found that for the period 2023–2024, the currently authorized funds (if fully appropriated, which is rarely the case) may be sufficient to initiate

---

[40] Alyse Huffman and Adam Rosenberg, Committee on Science, Space, and Technology, Energy Subcommittee, U.S. House of Representatives, presentations to the committee on August 26, 2021.

the low-dose radiation program, but significant investments, at the level of $100 million annually, will be required for the period 2025–2037.

The estimate of $100 million annually provided by the committee is larger than the amount authorized so far for the low-dose radiation program. However, the large number of individuals within the U.S. population that are exposed to low-dose and low-dose-rate radiation annually as a result of medical, occupational, and environmental exposures (see Table 2.1 for examples) and the substantial costs for complying with radiation protection standards and guidelines make it critical that the risk management and mitigation efforts for the U.S. population be guided by complete information about possible risks for cancer, cardiovascular disease, neurological disease, and other disease risks that may exist. This will require the $100 million annual program scale recommended by the committee. Appropriations at the level of $5 million per year are not adequate to even initiate a meaningful low-dose radiation research program—as seen in 2021 when funds for the program were at that level and the program was not initiated. The committee cautions that inadequate funding for the program will lead to continued scientific and policy debates about risks of low doses of radiation and the possible inadequate protection of patients, workers, and members of the public from the adverse effects of radiation.

5.6 COMPARISON OF THE COMMITTEE-RECOMMENDED RESEARCH AGENDA TO THOSE OF OTHER ENTITIES

The committee reviewed the research agendas proposed by other entities, in particular, the Multidisciplinary European Low-dose Initiative (MELODI; see Section 4.5.1), ICRP (see Section 4.5.2), and the Canadian Organization on Health Effects from Radiation Exposure (COHERE; see Section 4.5.5), and compared those with its recommended agenda. Overall, it found consistency in the main scientific issues recognized to be of highest priority by the different entities. These include improving cancer risk assessments for different radiation types and modes of exposure, understanding risks of health outcomes other than cancer, and improving dosimetry. Similar to this committee's research agenda, ICRP and MELODI prioritize the need for a more individualized risk assessment. ICRP is also concerned with the effects of radiation on non-human biota, a topic not addressed by the research agendas proposed by MELODI, COHERE, and this committee. The overall concordance in these research agendas indicates that collaboration and cooperation at the international level will be important to avoid unnecessary duplication of efforts, to share costs for projects, and to identify the most promising synergies among the different research programs.

In addition to the general consistency in the main scientific topics recognized to be of highest priority by the different entities, there is also consistency in the approach of phrasing these priorities. Specifically, this committee, similar to MELODI, ICRP, and COHERE, is neutral regarding the possible outcomes of the research and does not favor or appear to favor a certain possible outcome. A notable exception to this approach is that of the National Science and Technology Council (see Section 4.1.6), which phrased its priority as "defining the threshold of impact for low-dose and low-dose rate," implying that such a threshold does exist.

Despite the general similarities in the research topics and approach, this committee's approach to defining the research agenda differs in four important ways:

1. It emphasizes the need for integration between the epidemiological and biological research lines it identified and true partnerships between the two research lines to achieve the program's goals.
2. It provides equal emphasis on understanding the risks of cancer and non-cancer health outcomes.
3. It proposes the establishment of new epidemiological studies that can address questions about risks at low doses and dose rates and proposes that the appropriate populations are selected with input from the research community and other stakeholders, including the impacted communities.
4. It is based on leveraging advances in biotechnology and research infrastructure to help address the research priorities.

5.7 CHAPTER SUMMARY, FINDINGS, AND RECOMMENDATION

Epidemiological and biological research on low-dose and low-dose-rate radiation faces several challenges (see Box 5.1). These challenges are most often ascribed to the fact that effects of low-dose and low-dose-rate radiation exposures are assumed to be subtle and difficult to distinguish from those caused by other stressors and/or "spontaneous" changes that adversely affect the normal functions of cells, tissues, and organs. Moreover, the magnitude of the effects may change with dose, dose rate, type of radiation, and mode of exposure.

The committee identified 11 research priorities broadly classified in three research lines: epidemiological research, biological research, and research infrastructure (see Table 5.1). These research priorities can help overcome the existing research challenges, will enable more accurate estimation of adverse health effects that result from exposure to low-dose and low-dose-rate radiation, and will improve knowledge of the complex cellular and molecular processes that are engaged during transduction of low-dose and low-dose-rate radiation damage into adverse health outcomes. The committee emphasizes the need for integration across the research lines and anticipates that the most impactful research projects will include work in more than one research line and will be carried out by multidisciplinary teams. These research priorities do not represent a complete list of important low-dose and low-dose-rate radiation research questions. For example, studies designed to confirm or strengthen the basis for existing scientific findings, particularly those that are controversial or lack a clear interpretation, are also important. Some of the research priorities can have additional benefits including capacity building, training of the next generation of radiation researchers, and development of tools that could be transferrable to other lines of research.

The order of the research priorities does not imply an order of significance; instead, the priorities are considered by the committee to be equally important. Some of these activities can be initiated immediately, and others can only begin after a better foundation is built from current or new research or with additional input from the research and broader stakeholder community, including the impacted communities.

The committee expects that the specific tactics for addressing the research priorities and integrating epidemiological and biological components will be developed with input from the extended research community and other stakeholders, including the impacted communities. Importantly, the committee recognizes that the list of priorities will likely evolve as biological understanding and research tools advance and as the research community and other stakeholders are engaged with the program.

The committee estimates that funding needed to set up the program is on par with the congressionally authorized funds for 2023 and 2024, that is, at the level of $30 million and $40 million annually, respectively, but need to rise to the level of $100 million annually thereafter and remain at that level through about 2037. Although the committee recognizes that the exact form of the program will be determined by the funding agency after consultation with stakeholders, it provided a prototypical program comprising interacting hubs focusing on basic and translational biology, analytical and computational technologies, and epidemiology, intended to justify the $100 million annual funding level. The committee also notes that appropriations at the level of $5 million per year are not adequate to even initiate a meaningful low-dose radiation research program—as seen in 2021 when funds for the program were at that level and the program was not initiated. The committee cautions that inadequate funding for the program will lead to continued scientific and policy debates about risks of low doses of radiation and the possible inadequate protection of patients, workers, and members of the public from the adverse effects of radiation.

Finding 4: Epidemiological studies have played a crucial role in identifying risks (primarily for cancer) from medical, occupational, and environmental radiation exposures at low doses. Existing epidemiological studies are unable to address a number of outstanding questions of low-dose and low-dose-rate exposures of concern to the U.S. population including the full range of potential adverse health effects, risks associated with doses around 10 milligray, and the potential impacts of genetic, lifestyle, environmental, and other factors that may also affect radiation-related risk estimates. Epidemiological studies designed to overcome these limitations can better elucidate adverse health effects of radiation exposure at low doses and low dose rates relevant to the U.S. population today.

Finding 5: Radiation biology studies have contributed to the mechanistic understanding of the effects of radiation on molecular pathways and intra- and extracellular processes. The application of novel and developing technologies will enable more precise definition of the cellular and molecular processes that are affected by low-dose and low-dose-rate exposures. Integration of this information with that from epidemiological studies will enable better quantification of the adverse health effects from low-dose and low-dose-rate exposures relevant to the U.S. population, increase understanding of the involved mechanisms, and inform on the most appropriate risk assessment models to be used.

Finding 6: Advances in biotechnology and research infrastructure have been driven by the vast research and development enterprise in the United States. These include new observational and experimental systems, tools for measurement and genetic manipulation, increased computational power, improved interpretative algorithms, and shared data access systems. These advances have enabled innovation and breakthroughs in many scientific areas including cancer research and treatment, environmental health effects research, and vaccine production. A revitalized low-dose radiation research program can likewise leverage and further develop these capabilities to enable scientific innovation and breakthroughs in radiation biology and epidemiology.

Recommendation A: Agencies responsible for the management of the multidisciplinary low-dose radiation program should fund low-dose and low-dose-rate radiation research in the 11 high-priority research topics identified by the committee and can address the scopes outlined in Finding 1. (See Table 5.1 for listing and approach for addressing the recommended priorities.) These research priorities are broadly classified as epidemiological research, biological research, and research infrastructure and are of equal importance.

Finding 7: Significant investments over a sustained period spanning several decades are necessary to develop a multidisciplinary low-dose radiation research program in the United States that leverages existing and developing research infrastructure that will achieve the goals outlined in Finding 1. The committee's best estimate is that the investments required during the first 10–15 years of the program are at the level of $100 million annually and periodic reassessments are required as large epidemiological studies and necessary research infrastructures are established.

6

Essential Components of the Low-Dose Radiation Program

This chapter addresses the fifth charge of the Statement of Task, which calls for defining the essential components of the low-dose radiation research program that would address the prioritized research agenda recommended by the committee in Chapter 5. This chapter also addresses the sixth charge of the Statement of Task regarding coordination between federal agencies and with other national and international efforts to achieve the program's scientific objectives.

The committee identified eight essential elements of a robust, multidisciplinary low-dose radiation program: (1) programmatic commitment, (2) independent advice and evaluation, (3) transparency, (4) prioritized strategic research agenda, (5) appropriate research-sponsorship mechanisms, (6) training, (7) engagement and communications with relevant stakeholder communities, and (8) coordination. A description of these elements and the committee's views on how to incorporate them in the low-dose radiation program are described in Sections 6.1–6.8.

Recognizing that the research agenda proposed by this committee extends beyond the resources of a single federal agency and will require coordination across several agencies, these elements apply to any agency that is involved or will be involved in low-dose and low-dose-rate radiation research. The committee also summarizes its views on a possible model for leadership of the coordination of low-dose radiation research in the United States (see Section 6.8) and discusses whether the Department of Energy (DOE) is the appropriate entity to manage the low-dose radiation program (see Section 6.9).

Relevant to the discussion of the essential elements and effective management of the program is a clear understanding that multidisciplinary researchers will be needed to effectively address the strategic agenda recommended by the committee. Expertise from different disciplines that contribute to understanding low-dose radiation issues includes but is not limited to biology, epidemiology, statistics, -omics and data science, imaging, and physics and dosimetry. Intellectual input from those with broader expertise not directly associated with radiation research is also needed; for example, improved knowledge about the impact of low-dose and low-dose-rate exposures on epigenetic effects may come from those who have not previously studied radiation effects as long as there is access to the required radiation exposure equipment or data. Additionally, immunologists, modelers, social scientists, and specialty clinicians such as cardiologists, neurologists, and ophthalmologists are also expected to contribute to multidisciplinary low-dose radiation research; therefore, the program needs to identify ways to attract them to radiation research and offer appropriate training.

6.1 PROGRAMMATIC COMMITMENT

A long-term commitment—over several decades—to low-dose radiation research is essential to address the research priorities discussed by the committee in this report and to take advantage of the continuing technological and biological advances (see Chapter 5). This will enable the agency or agencies involved in low-dose radiation research to develop a strategic vision for the research, formulate specific plans to meet the vision, implement the plans and fund the research, communicate the findings, evaluate the progress toward achieving the research priorities, and make any midcourse adjustments necessary to meet the goals. Importantly, the programmatic commitment for low-dose research needs to be evident at all levels of the agency that carries out the research. Commitment at the highest level signals a priority for such research within the agency's overall mission and activities, and it is important in the agency's representation at the congressional and interagency levels to advocate for resources, as necessary. Commitment at the highest levels is also necessary for the agency staff to see this research as an important and rewarding aspect of the agency's programs and activities; this, in turn, ensures that adequate resources—both personnel and finances—will be devoted to the program. Commitment at the program management level is needed to develop and nurture the overall research program that must be developed neutral to outcome in terms of the impact of the research on assessment of radiation health risk and consequently its potential impact on radiation protection policy and practice in the United States, and to coordinate program activities with complementary activities underway worldwide.

6.2 INDEPENDENT ADVICE AND EVALUATION

The success and long-term viability and credibility of the low-dose program will require independent expert advice that (1) helps ensure that the program supports research based on modern science, (2) is relevant not only to the managing agency's or leading agencies' interests but also to those of other stakeholders, (3) provides ongoing strategic direction to increase the program's impact, (4) helps navigate difficult challenges of distrust toward some government-led research in radiation and maintain a research program neutral to outcome, (5) enhances overall confidence of all stakeholders in the program and its findings, and (6) ensures that all research results are communicated in appropriate ways to experts, stakeholder communities, and the general public. When government alone cannot provide the solution to the problem, particularly because of issues of distrust and conflicts as well as scientific complexity, independent advice and evaluation from a trusted entity are important to enhance the program's viability and credibility.

Advisory committees are often used to bring in experts to provide nonbinding strategic direction to an agency, which is generally followed, although the agency is not legally bound to do so. The committee recommends that an independent advisory committee should be formed at the beginning of the program and be maintained throughout its operations. Although the advisory committee will not be directly responsible for managing program activities nor will it have any operational responsibilities, it will be a valuable resource and make important contributions to the program, using processes that are transparent and open to the public. For example, material prepared by the independent advisory committee can be made available to the public and its meetings can allow public access.

The committee has identified the following specific functions for the low-dose radiation program independent advisory committee:

- Address recommendations of this committee on the research agenda and develop specific objectives, a strategic plan, and metrics of evaluation including milestones.
- Monitor the implementation of the strategic plan and research progress.
- Propose updates and adjustments to the strategic plan based on research progress and on new circumstances, including scientific advances and policies and stakeholder needs, to improve both the relevance and the timeliness of the program's research activities.
- Provide advice on programmatic processes that are transparent and that include the call for proposals, project selection and funding mechanisms, research oversight and coordination, training, stakeholder engagement, and the reporting of research results.

- Engage with the scientific and other relevant communities nationally and internationally through annual workshops and other meetings of opportunity to receive input on the program's management and strategic plan, and to further promote coordination, partnerships, and awareness.
- Contribute to the periodic evaluation of the program, according to proposed metrics, and its impact and assess adequacy of funding.
- Assist with dissemination of research findings in effective ways for the diverse audiences. Effective ways may include but are not limited to presentations at annual workshops, traditional and social media, and websites.

Membership of an advisory committee is key to its effectiveness and needs to convey to the stakeholders that it can be trusted. The advisory committee needs to include members who are accomplished in diverse disciplines relevant to low-dose radiation health effects research as defined by the research priorities identified in Chapter 5. It also needs other (nontechnical expert) stakeholder representation including members of impacted communities. The independent advisory committee members would be required to meet conditions described under the Federal Advisory Committee Act, including a disclosure of conflicts annually and on an ongoing basis, as potential conflicts may arise. The activities and functions of four previous independent advisory committees might be considered when establishing an advisory committee for the revitalized low-dose radiation research program in the United States:

1. The Advisory Committee for Energy-Related Epidemiological Research (ACERER) was created to provide advice and strategic direction in conducting the program as outlined in the memorandum of understanding (MOU) between DOE and the Department of Health and Human Services (HHS; 1990–2005). The first meeting of ACERER was in 1993, and ACERER continued to meet periodically between 1994 and 2000. Members of ACERER were selected by the Secretary of HHS and included research scientists, public health officials, representatives of public interest groups, and representatives of impacted communities. Both DOE and HHS had nonvoting representatives on the advisory committee (U.S. Congress, Senate, 1998). The ACERER Subcommittee for Community Affairs helped to ensure community engagement and advised ACERER on matters related to community needs.
2. The Santa Susana Field Laboratory Advisory Panel of independent experts was created in response to community calls for independent health studies of the health consequences of radioactive releases

and contamination from the Santa Susana Field Laboratory operations.[1] The panel and its consultants conducted a series of studies about the potential offsite impacts of contamination from accidents at the site. These studies were initiated by the local community, which played an active role in determining priorities among the questions to be explored (SSFL Advisory Panel, 2006).
3. An independent technical steering panel was created to provide technical direction to the Hanford Environmental Dose Reconstruction project, established to estimate radiation doses to the public from operations at the Hanford Site. The steering panel evaluated and approved all technical decisions and reports. Panel members included technical experts and representatives from the states of Washington and Oregon, the Indian tribes, and the public. The panel hosted public meetings and provided access to the data used in reconstructing doses (Haerer et al., 1989).
4. A Committee on Research Priorities for Airborne Particulate Matter was created by the National Research Council to advise the Environmental Protection Agency (EPA) administrator on the development of a research agenda on airborne particulate matter and to monitor implementation and research progress. The committee authored four reports to address its task (NRC, 1998a, 1999b, 2001, 2004) but had no operational responsibilities. After outlining research priorities and approaches in the 1998 report, it met every few years to evaluate progress and to provide additional guidance to EPA.

This National Academies committee envisions that the majority of an advisory committee's members will be technical experts who can advise on scientific and research management issues. Community members selected to serve on the independent advisory committee are unlikely to fully reflect the range of people impacted by radiation exposures, though they would have a broad understanding of these issues or the views of these communities. Research that involves a specified exposed human population or community needs to include additional engagement from members of the exposed populations or communities in designing and implementing these research activities. This additional engagement can be accomplished by the establishment of special advisory subcommittees specific to the research activities. For example, participation of patients, patient advocates, and health care professionals on these special advisory subcommittees would be necessary

---

[1] The Santa Susana Field Laboratory in southern California was a complex of industrial research and development facilities that operated about 10 low-power nuclear reactors with a history of accidents and releases.

to provide advice on research that involves studies of medically exposed populations; similarly, participation of members of impacted communities and technical experts whose work has focused on research on the impacted communities would be necessary to provide advice on research that involves communities impacted by the nuclear weapons program.

In two follow-on written communications, a group of impacted community members and advocates who also briefed the committee during its October 28, 2021, meeting (see Section 6.7) proposed reinstitution of the community Monitoring and Technical Assistance (MTA) Fund[2] and its successor the Community Involvement Fund (CIF).[3] According to this group, both MTA and CIF functioned well and provided grants for important independent studies related to DOE's nuclear weapons complex that advanced efforts to protect impacted communities from the adverse effects of radiation. The committee agrees with the group that MTA and CIF proved useful in the context of studies related to DOE's nuclear weapons complex, which was their specific function. However, the research program described by the committee in this report includes but is not limited to studies related to exposures from the nuclear weapons complex. Instead, the research program described in this report is a comprehensive biology and epidemiology research program, which requires the organizational structure of an advisory committee that is described in this section. The group of impacted community members and advocates also provided recommendations for best practices for working with Indigenous nations and communities.[4] Among these suggestions, the committee found useful ideas that need to be considered when research activities that involve these communities are proposed. The committee received additional input on this issue during its information-gathering meetings.[5]

---

[2] The fund was established in 1998 as part of a national settlement with community groups about cleanup at DOE sites. The fund helps nonprofit nongovernmental organizations and federally recognized tribal governments procure technical and scientific assistance to perform independent reviews and analyses of environmental management activities at DOE sites.

[3] Letters to the committee from impacted community members and members of advocacy groups on January 6, 2022, and February 1, 2022.

[4] For example, the group notes that any research relating to Indigenous communities must undertake government-to-government consultation and comply with the necessary permissions and protocols set up by the Indigenous governments. The group also notes that research relating to Indigenous communities and nations should prioritize trust building and make use of local community expertise. (Letter to the committee from impacted community members and members of advocacy groups on February 1, 2022.)

[5] Johnnye Lewis, University of New Mexico, presentation to the committee on November 16, 2021.

6.3 TRANSPARENCY

Since its start in the 1940s, research on adverse health effects of radiation exposure has been marred by deep mistrust among the public of the government sponsors of that research. Reasons for this mistrust are addressed in Section 2.1.6 and as discussed in Section 6.7, the public's misgiving about the impartiality of government agencies and their sponsored research persists and runs very deep. Based on the input of community representatives to the committee, it is apparent that there is continuing distrust toward the U.S. government and there is a belief that the U.S. government has failed to accept responsibility for past radiation exposures and has failed to develop programs that adequately compensate all impacted communities.

In addition to the impacted communities and the public, the other important audience for radiation research is the scientific community. Although some degree of tension between any research sponsor and the investigator community is understandable, in the case of radiation health research sponsorship by DOE, these tensions have been palpable (see Section 6.9). Without a long-term commitment to low-dose radiation research, the agency's priorities and milestones were not known, creating an atmosphere of uncertainty and doubt. There was also a genuine concern among some investigators that DOE was less interested in the science than in the bottom line of how the results they obtained would impact regulations, particularly at the DOE cleanup facilities. This was inevitably viewed as having an influence on the research activities supported by the program.[6]

The committee offers recommendations for both research priorities (see Chapter 5) and the organizational framework for such research (this chapter). The committee also judges that for the low-dose program to succeed, the establishment of trust among the government agency, the impacted communities, and scientific researchers is critical. This chapter presents the many processes that would play roles in creating trusted relationships; transparency of the entire research enterprise will be essential.

Transparency in this context is not limited to disclosure of conflicts of interest or responses to Freedom of Information Act requests, which are very important and statutorily mandated; it also entails dedication to openness and communication at every step, including processes for public participation and engagement, clear statements and communication of plans and milestones for research, and communication of all findings irrespective of their implications, to name just a few.

---

[6] Experience of some committee members, some of them recipients of awards from the previous low-dose program.

6.4 A PRIORITIZED STRATEGIC RESEARCH AGENDA

A strategic research agenda is an essential element for any large-scope scientific undertaking. The agenda must identify and prioritize research questions, appraise appropriate methodologies and technologies, and lay out budgetary outlays necessary to meet the scientific goals. Moreover, any such plan—especially when it spans a period of time—must make allowances for scientific discoveries, unanticipated results or events, and new questions that may arise during the course of research while maintaining neutrality to the research outcomes.

In this report, the committee has recommended a prioritized strategic research agenda (see Chapter 5) that is a path forward for the scientific understanding of the health effects of low levels of radiation exposure. Unlike some other efforts in radiation health, the committee's recommendations constitute a comprehensive, multidisciplinary program that is likely to span several decades. Importantly, the committee's recommended research priorities are informed by input from over 80 scientific experts and members of the stakeholder and public interest communities (see Appendix C). The committee anticipates that the new low-dose radiation program will use this recommended agenda, along with other recommendations presented in this chapter, to develop the overall framework for a successful multidisciplinary program. As noted in Chapter 5, a number of the recommended research priorities are intentionally nonprescriptive; additional specificity and decisions, for example, on what populations need to be examined (see Section 5.2.1, priority E1) will need to be made in consultation with the stakeholder communities including impacted communities. As the program matures, the committee expects that appropriate revisions and updates to specific aspects of the prioritized research agenda may be needed. Again, these updates will be made in consultation with the stakeholder communities.

6.5 RESEARCH-SPONSORSHIP MECHANISMS

During the past several decades, the practices and policies relevant to the research enterprise—including solicitation, selection and funding of research applications, coordination and oversight of the research, and communication of findings—have matured, and today most government agencies use similarly robust and transparent procedures.[7] Any agency that manages and supports the low-dose radiation program needs to follow these established procedures. The committee leaves the myriad details

---

[7] See https://grants.nih.gov/grants/grants_process.htm; https://www.nsf.gov/publications/pub_summ.jsp?ods_key=pappg.

of processes for research management to the sponsoring agency, but some highlights of the best practices for such management are provided below.

6.5.1 Development of Research Solicitation

The sponsoring agency needs to work with the recommended independent advisory committee to develop a specific strategic plan, using this report as the starting point (see Section 6.2). Such a plan would also include the optimum order in which specific research topics may be pursued as well as milestones for the process. These mechanisms and milestones need to offer flexibility to support projects with a range of scope and duration, from pilot or focused studies that require short-term funding (2–3 years) to projects with longer-term objectives that require long-term funding (5 years or more). After conducting literature reviews or holding workshops for information gathering as needed, agency staff can then take the steps necessary to develop specific research solicitations (or calls for applications) that are aligned to the strategic plan. It is also a common practice to have the draft solicitation reviewed either by advisory committee members or outside experts, being careful to avoid any conflicts that could arise by asking the reviewers in advance to commit to not responding to the solicitation.

6.5.2 Review of Applications

The cornerstone of research funding procedures is external application review, with the objective to evaluate the proposed projects using a process that ensures scientific merit and is also considered fair, equitable, timely, and free of bias.[8] The steps and criteria for the review process need to be transparent to the applicants and other interested parties. External project review, by a group of experts who are outside the funding agencies, helps determine whether the proposed activities and supporting methodologies and technologies represent a technically valid, cost-effective, and realistic means of accomplishing the project's stated objectives within a given budget and time constraint. This external project review may also provide constructive recommendations for improvements to the proposed projects. The review process results in scores or rank-order of all applications, which can then provide the basis for funding of applications.

6.5.3 Funding Mechanisms

The National Institutes of Health (NIH) is a model agency for its well-documented and diverse funding mechanisms that generally fall into

---

[8] See https://grants.nih.gov/grants/peer-review.htm.

three categories: grants, contracts, and cooperative agreements.[9] For NIH grants, investigators are generally responsible for developing the concepts, methods, and approach for a research project and, once funded, are left alone to conduct the research. For contracts, the awarding unit is responsible for establishing the detailed prerequisites for accomplishing certain tasks, and the agency then directs the best-qualified group to perform the specific tasks. For cooperative agreements, both the awarding unit and the recipient have substantial responsibility in developing the concepts, methods, and approaches for a research project, and the research is generally conducted with ongoing interactions and feedback. Within these funding mechanisms, different NIH activity codes identify categories (e.g., research, training, cooperative agreements) to be funded. Other federal agencies, including DOE's Office of Science, also have diverse funding mechanisms to support research but do not differentiate across categories using activity codes. Instead, the solicitation will describe any limitations on eligibility for a specific funding mechanism. DOE also issues program announcements, but these are only available to DOE national laboratories.

As the committee outlined in Chapter 5, the complexity and scope of the scientific problems involved in low-dose radiation research favor funding mechanisms that support well-planned and integrated teams of specialists from different disciplines and institutions, such as NIH's U-type awards, which support a research program of multiple projects directed toward a specific major objective.[10] The current National Institute of Allergy and Infectious Diseases' (NIAID's) Radiation and Nuclear Countermeasures Program (see Section 4.1.3) provides an excellent model that demonstrates the strengths of this approach. A second example is the National Cancer Institute's (NCI's) RAS Initiative which aims to better understand the RAS oncogene and RAS-driven cancer development.[11] The initiative, headquartered at the Frederick National Laboratory, built an open model of research collaborations across government, academia, and industry to reenergize efforts to develop RAS therapeutics.

Funding mechanisms also need to promote the training and development of early-career investigators in radiation research across different disciplines (see below). Promotion of training can be achieved by allowing funding for investigators at graduate and postgraduate levels and ensuring their inclusion in U-type awards. This is a change from the previous low-dose DOE program, which expected projects to include graduate students and postdoctoral trainees to enhance training but did not provide dedicated training grants. In addition, similar to the R25 or T32 awards to support

---

[9] See https://grants.nih.gov/grants/funding/ac_search_results.htm.
[10] See https://grants.nih.gov/grants/funding/ac_search_results.htm.
[11] See https://www.cancer.gov/research/key-initiatives/ras.

research education activities, establishment of predoctoral training programs in radiation epidemiology, biostatistics, and related disciplines would be essential to prepare the necessary workforce for the epidemiological studies supported by this committee (see Section 5.2).

6.5.4 Research Oversight

Cooperative agreements (U-class of grants) typically involve extensive effort on the part of the sponsoring agency staff in terms of research oversight. This ensures that the direction of research is consistent with the goals agreed upon in advance and any midcourse adjustments are made with the agreement of all parties. Also, when research is conducted by multidisciplinary teams, the staff is needed to facilitate the various teams working together. Therefore, the committee envisions that the role of the funding agency staff will continue after the initial funding decisions have been made, and the agency needs to appreciate this as it assigns staff.

6.5.5 Data Management and Sharing

During the past two decades, there has been an evolution in thinking about data management and data sharing policies, resulting in recent policies and recommendations and exemplified by a final NIH policy,[12] the FAIR (findable, accessible, interoperable, and reusable) guidelines (Wilkinson et al., 2016), and a recent National Academies of Sciences, Engineering, and Medicine workshop.[13] The deepening interest in this area comes from the recognition that the interpretation of publicly available large-scale data benefits from analysis and integration by the extended bioinformatics and computational biology communities and from the associated transparency of analysis. Recent reanalyses of data generated by The Cancer Genome Atlas program by the PanCancer initiative[14] illustrates the power of the process. These public processes should also facilitate assessment and reanalyses of data used for policy making. Thus, in epidemiology, the interest in data sharing is rooted in the desire to validate findings (i.e., repeating the original investigator's analyses), to extend the analyses (using alternative methods), and to combine the findings of multiple studies (for meta-analyses or pooled analyses). In view of these developments, investigators applying to NIH for support today are required in their application to outline a plan and budget for data

---

[12] See https://grants.nih.gov/grants/guide/notice-files/NOT-OD-21-013.html.
[13] See https://www.nationalacademies.org/event/04-29-2021/changing-the-culture-of-data-management-and-sharing-a-workshop#sectionWebFriendly.
[14] See https://gdc.cancer.gov/about-data/publications/pancanatlas.

stewardship and management. Several scientific journals also require or strongly recommend that authors of papers reference the data repository where the original data, metadata, and codes may be found. The committee expects that the new low-dose radiation program would conform to contemporary standards for data management and sharing. At the same time, the committee is aware that adhering to such guidelines can be challenging—for example, when working with historical data for which data management and sharing agreements were not in place—and expects that some flexibility would be needed in certain situations. Finally, data sharing is an aspect of transparency, and this will also help the agency build a trusted relationship with various communities.

In addition to data management and sharing, the agency will also need to develop protocols for applications to access biosamples collected by low-dose radiation program–funded projects, processes for reviewing the applications, and biosample use agreements. Support from an external review panel, similar to the process followed by the Chernobyl Tissue Bank, may be appropriate to ensure the scientific merit and appropriate use of resources.[15]

6.5.6 Dissemination of Scientific Results

Dissemination of scientific results comes naturally to scientists who are used to publishing articles in peer-reviewed professional journals when one or more observations can be interpreted to confirm or refute a hypothesis. Such publications are valuable in communicating results and conclusions with other scientists working in the same or adjacent fields. However, by necessity such publications tend to be dense and complex or have other features that make them difficult for the public or scientists working outside of the field to understand. Therefore, it is important that the agency provide opportunities where the results of its sponsored research are presented in a comprehensible fashion to the impacted communities (see also Section 6.7). For improved understanding, it would also be desirable to have independent experts comment on the results and put them in the broader context of knowledge about radiation and health. In this context, since editors often favor publishing positive results because they are more interesting and ultimately more citable (Duyx et al., 2017) and scientists may choose to only publish results that confirm their prior views or hypotheses, it is important that the agency identifies mechanisms for *all* results—whether positive or not—to be published.

---

[15] See https://www.chernobyltissuebank.com/access-to-materials.

6.6 TRAINING

A decline in the number of professionals with expertise in radiation-related research and applications was recognized by the National Council on Radiation Protection and Measurements almost a decade ago (NCRP, 2015b) and the same organization is working toward understanding whether the downward trend continues today.[16] Establishing a low-dose radiation community of scientists including physicists, biologists, and epidemiologists, as well as medical professionals, communicators, and risk management experts by providing the appropriate training in low-dose and low-dose-rate radiation health effects and radiation protection principles will be needed to (1) support the proposed multi-decade research, (2) engage experts who are not already engaged in radiation research, (3) manage exposures to the U.S. population, and (4) communicate and engage with exposed populations. Establishing this low-dose radiation community of scientists and medical professionals will require dedicating considerable resources toward training at all career levels while promoting diversity, equity, and inclusion. Training of individuals in communities that are traditionally underserved or underrepresented will be important because these communities may be more likely to be exposed to radiation in the environment.

Training of students, faculty, and management at all levels will be needed to support the multi-decade research proposed and engage experts who are not already engaged in radiation research. Several funding options directed toward training are discussed in Section 6.5.3. These may include training grants, visiting fellowships similar to those provided by the Radiation Epidemiology Branch,[17] or partnerships such as those between the Radiation Effects Research Foundation and several universities in Japan and the University of Washington.[18] Additionally, training can be in the form of informal collaborations between radiation experts and those outside the field, as well as through courses offered by institutions involved in radiation research. The committee was informed about several such courses (see Table 6.1), and additional courses may exist that were not brought to the committee's attention. Unlike training courses in Europe, those in the United States are geared toward higher doses and not at low doses and low dose rates to be addressed by the revitalized low-dose radiation program described in this report. Also, most available courses are not

---

[16] The committee's observation is that several organizations that engaged in low-dose radiation research in the past, notably the national laboratories, have lost their radiation expertise because work has refocused on other research topics. That said, it is likely that the downward trend of radiation professionals, at least in research settings, continues today.

[17] See https://dceg.cancer.gov/fellowship-training/apply/reb.

[18] See https://www.rerf.or.jp/en/programs/general_research_e/partners_e.

TABLE 6.1 Examples of Radiation Courses Available in the United States and Internationally

Course	Topics Covered
NCI's Radiation Epidemiology and Dosimetry training course	Fundamentals of radiation epidemiology, dosimetry, and risk modeling; radiation health effects and exposure assessment; medical radiation exposure (diagnostic and therapeutic); environmental and occupational exposures; and susceptibility to radiation health effects
CDC's Radiation Studies Section	Radiation emergency response; radiation risk, health effects, and risk communication
AFRRI's Medical Effects of Ionizing Radiation	Biomedical consequences of radiation exposure and management of radiation effects
NIAID scientific meetings	Animal models of radiation injuries, medical countermeasures, biodosimetry, and decorporation following radiation scenarios; regulatory approaches
NIAID's Radiation and Nuclear Group	Medical countermeasures, biodosimetry, and decorporation following radiation scenarios
NASA's STAR Program	Fundamental space biology and its practical applications, including technical and logistical considerations, opportunities, and the unique advantages and limitations of conducting an experiment in space
U.S. NRC, DOE, national laboratories, professional organizations, and industry	Dosimetry
REAC/TS	Medical management of radiological/nuclear incidents; early evaluation and treatment of acute radiation syndrome; decontamination techniques
Radiation oncology departments	Fundamentals of radiation and radiation biology
MELODI (European Radiation Protection Week), EURADOS (winter school), and NEA/OECD (International Radiological Protection School)	Radiation biology, radiation measurements, radiation health effects, and radiation protection

NOTES: Descriptions of duration and periodicity are pre-pandemic. Adjustments to virtual learning during the pandemic are not reflected in this table. AFRRI = Armed Forces Radiobiology Research Institute; CDC = Centers for Disease Control and Prevention; DoD = Department of Defense; DOE = Department of Energy; EURADOS = European Radiation Dosimetry Group; MELODI = Multidisciplinary European Low-Dose Initiative; NASA = National Aeronautics and Space Administration; NCI = National Cancer Institute; NIAID = National Institute of Allergy and Infectious Diseases; NRC = U.S. Nuclear Regulatory Commission; NEA/OECD = Nuclear Energy Agency and Organisation for Economic Co-operation and Development; REAC/TS = Radiation Emergency Assistance Center/Training Site.

ESSENTIAL COMPONENTS OF THE LOW-DOSE RADIATION PROGRAM 203

Low-Dose Radiation Issues Coverage	Main Audience	Duration/Periodicity
Yes but not explicitly	Scientists, industry, medical practitioners, other	Week-long course provided once every 4 years at NCI's offices in Rockville, Maryland
Yes but not explicitly	Public health professionals	Annually at conferences and CDC campus in Atlanta, Georgia
No	DoD military and civilian personnel	3-day course provided annually at AFRRI's campus in Bethesda, Maryland
No	Radiation research community	Two to three times per year
No	Government partners only	Monthly
Yes but not explicitly	Principal investigators, senior research scientists, and postdoctoral scholars with interest in space radiation research	Virtual courses spread out over 6 months taking place annually
Yes but not explicitly	Federal, state, and local government officials	Varies
No	Health care professionals, emergency responders, and health physicists	2–3 days annually
Typically geared toward higher (therapeutic) radiation doses	Residents and graduate students	2–3 hours per semester
Yes	Radiation protection professionals and radiation researchers	3–5 days annually

targeted toward the radiation health research community. Although most of the international courses are available to interested participants and U.S. participants can benefit from them, especially via remote participation, there is an obvious need for easy access to in-person learning on low-dose radiation issues in the United States.

Training for individuals engaged in risk management and development of public policy related to low-dose and low-dose-rate radiation exposures will ensure that policies and guidelines are based on best available and current scientific information on the adverse effects of these exposures. Specific courses need to be developed that address scientific understanding and how this is incorporated in supporting analyses of risks and benefits associated with regulations and guidelines. Training in this area will be enhanced by funding mechanisms that support studies of radiation exposure in specific U.S. populations.

Improving communications about the adverse health effects of low-dose and low-dose-rate exposures is critical to building public trust. This requires establishing a community of experts trained to inform (a) the public in plain language about current knowledge about adverse health effects, knowledge gaps, ongoing research and public policy development through public meetings, traditional media and social media; (b) the scientific and medical communities about current knowledge, knowledge gaps, and ongoing research; (c) policy makers including Congress on current knowledge and processes for analyses of risks and benefits associated with regulations and guidelines that focus on specific impacted U.S. populations.

Trainers and curricula for these training activities will need to be developed and sustained. The low-dose radiation program needs to create a centralized database for cataloguing available training opportunities in radiation science with emphasis on low-dose radiation. These may include modules for research, communication, and policy making; formal training programs that emphasize and integrate all of these areas; and websites that curate information about low-dose and low-dose-rate radiation exposures, adverse health effects, and cost-benefit analyses that have been used during the development of public protection policies.

6.7 ENGAGEMENT AND COMMUNICATIONS WITH STAKEHOLDERS

The low-dose radiation program will interest diverse audiences and stakeholder groups including federal agencies with radiation protection or radiation research responsibilities and policy makers, the radiation research and other scientific communities both within the United States and internationally, members of impacted communities and advocacy groups, and members of the general public. The technical knowledge of low-dose and low-dose-rate radiation, the direct or indirect impacts of this research, and the acceptability of the findings will vary considerably across the different stakeholder groups. Therefore, the committee considers it important that the new low-dose radiation program dedicates resources to establish and maintain appropriate processes for stakeholder engagement and communication. Incorporating the concerns, views, and experiences of the diverse stakeholder communities while maintaining a high standard of scientific work will be essential to the program's success.

The committee held a 2-day meeting to receive information and perspectives from social scientists, government representatives, researchers, and members of the impacted communities and advocacy groups on how the low-dose radiation program can effectively engage and communicate with its stakeholders.

An invited speaker noted that low-dose radiation is not judged in the abstract but in the contexts where people encounter it. Each encounter shapes public beliefs and attitudes toward low-dose radiation research and the people and institutions responsible for it. The speaker noted that effective communication needs to be coordinated by creating a common picture, sharing knowledge and uncertainty accurately, being cogent by avoiding confusion and overload, and acting respectfully by accepting the right to know and to disagree. The speaker emphasized that the process for engaging stakeholders and the content—what stakeholders are told—reveals how well those responsible for communicating understand public concerns and are willing and able to address them.[19]

Those who attempt to communicate have limited knowledge about their diverse audiences and limited capacity for learning about their concerns; as a result, they often overestimate how well they understand others and are understood by them. Organizations without expertise in communication have difficulty either recognizing when they need help to convey their messages or finding help when they recognize the need. The speaker pointed to the work of the Institute of Medicine on risk communication (Fischhoff and Scheufele, 2013, 2014; NRC, 1989, 2009) and on community engagement in public health research for environmental justice issues (IOM, 1999). The 1999 report identified principles to guide the research (IOM, 1999). Relevant to this committee's task is the view that members of the impacted communities of concern need to participate in the design and execution of research.

The committee also heard presentations from the staff of federal (DOE, the U.S. Nuclear Regulatory Commission [U.S. NRC], EPA, and the Department of Homeland Security) and state agencies concerning their risk

---

[19] Baruch Fischhoff, Carnegie Mellon University, presentation to the committee on October 27, 2021.

communication and stakeholder interaction practices. The committee appreciated the general recognition of the ongoing challenges and the amount of effort that has been put into improving communications as well as the awareness of these staff members of the importance of working closely with stakeholders. But based on presentations from impacted communities and advocacy groups, the committee also saw that much effort is still needed to develop mutual trust and understanding. The committee also appreciates that a lack of public trust has been a longstanding challenge for DOE's radiation programs, originating from the Atomic Energy Commission's (AEC's) and later DOE's secrecy during the nuclear weapons program activities; such mistrust has persisted over multiple generations and hampers effective engagement (see Section 2.1.6).

Invited speakers from community and advocacy groups included leaders of the Navajo Nation, atomic veterans, nuclear workers, and those impacted by nuclear weapons testing and nuclear weapons production sites and nuclear waste cleanup. These speakers pointed the committee to several sources of information relevant to its task and also offered views on specific topics that need to be addressed by the low-dose radiation program. Many of these messages were also echoed in comments submitted to the committee by other members of the public in writing and are summarized in Box 6.1. The comments generally fell into one of the three categories: suggestions for research priorities, suggestions for program management, and suggestions for radiation protection policies. Although proposing changes or otherwise providing advice on radiation protection policies was outside the scope and expertise of this committee, these policy suggestions are also listed in Box 6.1.

Testimonies from community speakers included stories of personal and community member diseases considered attributable to radiation and expression of strong emotions—including frustration, feelings of betrayal, and distrust toward DOE—originating from DOE's and predecessor agencies' handling of releases from the nuclear weapons program. The committee heard repeatedly from the speakers about the conflict of interest that DOE has to both regulate radiation protection and lead research on radiation health effects. The history of conflicts is also documented in several reports (see, e.g., DOE-EHHS Openness, 1995; Geiger et al., 1992). The committee also received a strong message that impacted communities need to be meaningfully engaged in setting priorities for the low-dose radiation program because of the direct impact on their lives and that members of the impacted communities need to be invited to provide advice, and even oversight, to the research.[20]

---

[20] See Section 6.2 for the recommendation of the group of impacted community members and advocates about reinstitution of the MTA Fund or CIF to lead research that involves impacted communities.

> **BOX 6.1**
> **Summary of Comments Received from Members of Impacted Communities, Members of the Public, and Advocacy Groups**
>
> **Low-Dose and Low-Dose-Rate Radiation Research Priorities**
>
> - Health effects on women.
> - Prenatal and postnatal effects.
> - Transgenerational effects.
> - Precise quantification of risk per unit dose.
> - Associations of low-dose radiation exposures with non-cancer diseases including cardiovascular, neurological, kidney, immune system, and autoimmune diseases.
> - Effects of internal exposures (including from tritium[a]).
> - Biological factors that explain the effects of different types of radiation exposures.
> - Development of radiation biomarkers resulting from current and legacy exposures.
> - Role of social factors in low-dose radiation-induced disease.
> - Effects of low-dose radiation on populations in the United States that are disproportionally impacted, for example, Indigenous communities.
> - Accurate radiation dose reconstruction for exposed populations.
> - Establishment of a radioecology research line.
> - Establishment of a radiation risk communication research line.
>
> **Low-Dose Radiation Program Management**
>
> - The Department of Energy is not the appropriate agency to lead research on radiation health effects.
> - Impacted communities need to be meaningfully engaged in setting priorities for the low-dose radiation program because of the direct impact in their lives.
> - Low-dose radiation research needs to be driven and overseen by the community.
> - An external panel with independent experts and community member participation is needed to provide advice or oversight to low-dose radiation research.
>
> **Radiation Protection Policies and Other Considerations[b]**
>
> - Set standards based on the most vulnerable populations—for example, use the "land worker–mother" framework centered on Indigenous pregnant women as the standard for radiation protection.
> - Define standards for radiosensitive groups such as pregnant women, embryos, fetuses, infants, and children.
> - Develop "reference fetus," "reference child," "reference woman," "land worker–mother" radiation safety standards rather than continued dependence on use of "reference man."
> - Continue to use the linear no-threshold model in radiation protection.
> - Propose tightening of drinking water standards.
> - Address the people's right to a safe environment.
> - Devote resources to cleanup of nuclear legacy waste.
> - Compensate workers, downwinders, atomic veterans, uranium miners, and Native American communities for health effects from exposure to radiation.
>
> ---
>
> [a] Letter from Arjun Makhijani, Institute for Energy and Environmental Research, to the committee on January 7, 2022.
>
> [b] These issues were outside the scope of this committee's work, as specified in the Statement of Task (see Box S.1).

During the 2-day meeting and in subsequent meetings and public comments received in writing, the committee observed that—generally speaking—there was a noticeable difference between the perception of people with and without technical expertise about the certainty of adverse effects of low doses of radiation. Experts typically perceive low doses of radiation from nuclear power and nuclear waste as less risky than non-experts (Slovic, 2012).[21] However, experts may rate risks from medical X-rays and radon higher compared to non-experts (Slovic, 2012).

Experience over many years and in many fields, including the chemical and petrochemical industries, has shown that perceptions are not easily changed simply by presenting scientific facts and information. This understanding has led to a reformulation of the risk assessment/risk management paradigm to include stakeholder participation in every step of a six-step framework: problem formulation, risk assessment, options development, decisions, actions, and evaluation (Commission on Risk Assessment and Risk Management, 1997; NRC, 2009). The scientific uncertainties related to risks from low doses of radiation complicate non-experts' understanding of the risks, but existing research argues that these uncertainties need to be effectively communicated to allow informed decisions considering the risks and benefits of exposures to radiation (Allisy-Roberts and Day, 2008; Fischhoff and Davis, 2014; Osman et al., 2019).

The committee concluded that the success of the low-dose radiation program will depend not only on its scientific integrity but also on its ability to meaningfully engage and communicate with the stakeholders. The low-dose radiation program needs to do the following:

- Develop *transparent* processes for stakeholder identification, engagement, and communication.
- Identify stakeholders and solicit their perspectives and expectations related to the low-dose radiation program.
- Commit to engaging with all stakeholders, including those from the impacted communities, in meaningful ways.
- Include members of the impacted communities in the independent advisory committee (see Section 6.2) so that they may participate in various aspects of research planning and implementation.
- Set up additional advisory subcommittees with substantial stakeholder participation to advise on specific projects that involve human populations or populations exposed to low-dose radiation.

---

[21] One invited expert thought that the public attitude toward radiation from these sources is irrational fear and termed it radiophobia (Gerry Thomas, Imperial College London, presentation to the committee on October 27, 2021).

- Develop communication and engagement strategies for the diverse audiences and test them for their effectiveness. Specific activities may include but not be limited to maintaining a dedicated website with information on funded projects, links to scientific groups that carry out low-dose radiation research, links to scientific publications, and reports on research findings written in lay language. Communication and engagement strategies may also include collaborating with groups who have expertise in environmental risk communication even if they are not working on radiation issues and providing support for modest communication projects.
- Host public meetings, issue press releases, and take other opportunities for engagement to discuss aspects of the low-dose radiation program of interest to the stakeholders.
- Work with community educators such as school science teachers and local community-based organizations that are not usually involved in radiation-related activities.

Past experience indicates that studies that involve dose reconstruction and risk assessments of impacted communities are likely to be scrutinized (Hoffman et al., 2001; McEwan et al., 1997). The committee recognizes that even with the above-mentioned processes in place, acceptance of the program's credibility and trust toward its scientific findings will take substantial and sustained effort.

6.8 COORDINATION

Coordination is key to increasing innovative capacity, harnessing the expertise and competencies of specialized groups, avoiding unnecessary duplication of efforts, and ultimately meeting research goals faster while efficiently using available resources, including funds. In this section, the committee describes various mechanisms for coordination and a proposed model for leading the coordinated effort.

6.8.1 Mechanisms for Coordination

Coordination can occur in many ways—for example, by division of tasks, mutual awareness of activities to help exploit possible synergies, and sharing of resources such as facilities or data. For the low-dose radiation program to be successful and accomplish the scientific goals identified by this committee, it needs to establish mechanisms for coordination across federal agencies and other national and international organizations that carry out low-dose radiation research or have relevant expertise and entities that carry out relevant (non-radiation) research.

During the previous low-dose radiation program, there appeared to be little coordination between DOE and other federal organizations except the National Aeronautics and Space Administration. Most government representatives who briefed the committee, including those from NCI, NIAID, the Centers for Disease Control and Prevention, the National Institute for Occupational Safety and Health, and the Armed Forces Radiobiology Research Institute, described rather unplanned and spontaneous interactions with DOE staff, typically occurring during scientific conferences, as opposed to intentionally institutionalizing and scheduling coordinating efforts to look for opportunities for collaboration in radiation research. Similarly, little systematic coordination occurred with international organizations except when interested U.S. or foreign scientists happened to reach out for collaboration. Although these informal interactions are important, there is a need for more systematic efforts to institutionalize coordination.

During the committee's meetings, several representatives of federal agencies and other national and international organizations provided perspectives on opportunities for coordination with the new low-dose radiation program. These included the following:

- Hosting annual meetings or workshops with relevant agencies and national and international organizations, along with appropriate experts and funded researchers, to exchange views on research priorities; report progress; and identify areas of shared, overlapping, or closely related interests relevant to low-dose radiation research.
- Co-supporting technical sessions at scientific meetings organized by professional societies or other opportunities to increase awareness about the activities of common interest in low-dose radiation science.
- Making specific budget allocations to incentivize agencies and national and international organizations to work together on a variety of projects.
- Using MOUs and interagency agreements to divide tasks appropriately based on agency missions and expertise (see Section 4.1.3 for discussion of an MOU in support of radiation health research), and provide mechanisms for temporary assignment of personnel to learn new methodologies or use resources.
- Participating in national and international data sharing platforms to increase awareness about funded low-dose radiation research (see Section 4.5.4 for current NEA/OECD data sharing platform).
- Carrying out joint projects with international low-dose radiation programs and sharing costs.

- Providing access to study datasets to allow for meta-analysis and pooled analysis of archived data.
- Facilitating use of research infrastructure including facilities, computational capabilities, and dosimetry tools (see Section 5.4.4 for discussion of facilities).
- Leveraging expertise for input on requests for proposals, project review, service on advisory committees, and other activities.

The committee agrees that these opportunities for coordination will benefit the revitalized low-dose radiation program and there is a need to establish processes to allow for these coordinating mechanisms to succeed. Coordination can absorb substantial amounts of time and effort and requires sufficient resources. It can be instituted by Congress, interagency committees, task forces, or by the agencies and organizations themselves.

For example, the Consolidated Appropriations Act, 2021 specifically states, "The Secretary of Energy shall continue and strengthen collaboration with the Administrator of the National Aeronautics and Space Administration on basic research to understand the effects and risks of human exposure to ionizing radiation in low Earth orbit, and in the space environment." Also, the American Innovation and Competitiveness Act of 2017 tasked the National Science and Technology Council (NSTC) to coordinate government research within the U.S. government (NSTC, 2022). Finally, the Consolidated Appropriations Act, 2021 asks for coordination between the low-dose radiation program and the NSTC effort.

Today, there is no coordinating mechanism for low-dose radiation research in the United States. A historic model for radiation research and policy coordination, the Committee on Interagency Radiation Research and Policy Coordination (CIRRPC; see Section 4.1.6), which became a subcommittee of the Committee on Health, Safety and Food under NSTC (Young, 2020), was recently supported as a means to coordinate radiation biology research within the U.S. government (NSTC, 2022). CIRRPC was challenged by lack of consensus across federal agencies that constituted its membership and was terminated after 11 years of operation. NSTC in its recent report does not discuss to what extent a CIRRPC-type committee can engage with nongovernmental and international partners and meaningfully engage all stakeholders, including members of the impacted communities in its processes, and be seen as a trusted non-politicized scientific entity.

The U.S. Global Change Research Program (USGCRP) is an existing example of a large, complex, and multidisciplinary effort involving many agencies of the federal government that is coordinated through the NSTC. Established in 1989 by presidential initiative and mandated by Congress in the Global Change Research Act of 1990, USGCRP "assist[s] the Nation and the world to understand, assess, predict, and respond to human-induced and natural processes of global change."[22] USGCRP coordinates federal research and investments of 13 federal member agencies and has strong coordination with equivalent programs across the world. The National Academies provide advice and strategic direction to USGCRP by convening technical experts and decision-makers at semiannual meetings, and reviewing draft plans for the program (NASEM, 2021a).

There are several examples of successful multidisciplinary efforts coordinated at the agency level, albeit they involve a smaller number of participating agencies, with a few others peripherally engaged. Such was the Human Genome Project (Patrinos and Drell, 1997), involving NIH and DOE, with a well-defined objective, the delivery of the complete genetic sequence of the human genome. Given that DOE and NIH have traditionally supported most of the low-dose radiation research, this model for interagency coordination could be used as an alternative model to the NSTC-coordinated approach. For additional discussion, see Section 6.8.2.

6.8.2 Leadership

In addition to the agencies that have direct responsibility for radiation protection (e.g., EPA, the U.S. NRC, and DOE), other agencies within the U.S. government carry out or may carry out research in low-dose radiation, and there are other agencies whose work will benefit from a better understanding of adverse health effects from low levels of radiation exposure (see Figure 1.4 and Section 3.2). Therefore, the committee identified the need to establish leadership and scope of low-dose radiation research coordination.

The only entity at this point that Congress has tasked with a focused low-dose radiation program is DOE; therefore, the committee saw a role for DOE in coordinating low-dose radiation research within the United States. However, the committee also recognized the concerns raised by members of impacted communities about DOE's inherent conflicts with leading low-dose radiation research and by the research community on DOE's shortcomings related to management of the previous low-dose radiation program (see Section 6.9). In addition, the research agenda proposed by the committee extends beyond any single agency's capabilities, and a partnership with an agency whose mission is to enhance health would be warranted.

Among various federal agencies with missions to enhance or protect health, NIH is widely trusted by the scientific community and members of the public and does not have any regulatory responsibilities related to setting or implementing radiation protection standards; therefore, it has no perceived conflict of interest with leading low-dose radiation research

---

[22] See https://www.globalchange.gov/about/legal-mandate.

through a cross-institutional effort. In addition, it has well-established and transparent processes for soliciting, reviewing, and funding research. Within NIH, NIAID's Radiation and Nuclear Countermeasures Program (RNCP; see Section 4.1.3) could be suitable to support low-dose radiation research through a cross-institutional effort. Although RNCP currently supports research in moderate and high doses starting at about 1 gray and supports limited research on cancer (which is the primary focus of NCI), the committee was impressed with the program management's commitment and transparency as well as engagement with its stakeholder communities. NCI has processes similar to NIAID's and by virtue of its mission it focuses on cancer research. The Advanced Research Projects Agency for Health (ARPA-H), a proposed agency tasked with building high-risk, high-reward capabilities to drive biomedical breakthroughs, could also contribute to innovative low-dose radiation research.[23]

DOE and NIH have traditionally supported most of the low-dose radiation research in the United States, and there is a precedent for a successful coordination by the two agencies to complete the Human Genome Project (Patrinos and Drell, 1997). More recently, DOE and NCI launched the Joint Design of Advanced Computing Solutions for Cancer program to accelerate developments in precision oncology and advanced scientific computing.[24] The committee supports a similar approach to be used to lead the coordination of low-dose radiation research, with DOE leading a portion of the strategic research agenda (e.g., on genome biology, computational, and modeling research, and support for facilities for low-dose and low-dose-rate exposures), and NIH, through a cross-institutional effort that can involve NIAID and NCI, leading the epidemiological and biological research, but with mechanisms in place to allow for integration of the different research lines.

The committee recognizes the operational complexities of this arrangement and the interagency agreement between DOE and HHS, which was put in place in 1990 because of concerns regarding DOE's independence and objectivity in conducting research related to radiation health effects (see Section 4.1.4), provides some lessons learned. Factors that can help make interagency program management effective include (NRC, 2006b) (1) substantial support from the top, (2) effective communication and cooperation within each of the agencies and between the agencies at all levels, (3) a detailed agreement on what is to be accomplished and how, (4) continuous feedback mechanisms to ensure that priorities are agreed upon and funding

---

[23] See https://www.nih.gov/arpa-h. Currently, ARPA-H is included in the fiscal year 2022 budget as a component of the NIH.
[24] See https://datascience.cancer.gov/collaborations/nci-doe-capabilities.

is adequate, and (5) the ability of both agencies to take credit for the success of the program.

The committee also recognizes the organizational complexities of this arrangement. In Congress, DOE and NIH report to different authorization committees and appropriation subcommittees. In the executive branch, NIH's and DOE's research leadership report to different Cabinet secretaries. At the Office of Management and Budget, which is the White House lead on appropriation requests, NIH and DOE are overseen by different budget examiners. Given these complexities, adopting—and sustaining over decades—a workable DOE-NIH collaboration will require commitment from all entities involved in leading, providing oversight, and approving budgets for the two agencies.

6.9 DEPARTMENT OF ENERGY AND MANAGEMENT OF THE LOW-DOSE PROGRAM

Congress has assigned the management of the low-dose radiation program to DOE, but congressional staff told the committee that other government agencies could initiate their own low-dose radiation programs, carry out research that is dedicated to low-dose radiation, or have a low-dose radiation research component.[25] Following briefings by congressional staff,[26] DOE,[27] and members of the scientific[28] and impacted communities,[29] the committee observed that there are, in some cases, substantially different views and perspectives related to the suitability of DOE to manage the low-dose radiation program. These views and perspectives of the different

---

[25] Email communication from Alyse Huffman and Adam Rosenberg, Committee on Science, Space, and Technology, Energy Subcommittee, U.S. House of Representatives, to Ourania Kosti, National Academies, on January 24, 2022.

[26] Alyse Huffman and Adam Rosenberg, Committee on Science, Space, and Technology, Energy Subcommittee, U.S. House of Representatives, presentations to the committee on August 26, 2021.

[27] Todd Anderson, DOE, presentation to the committee on July 21, 2021.

[28] Panel discussion on August 26, 2021, with Edouard Azzam, Canadian Nuclear Laboratories; David Brenner, Columbia University; Albert Fornace, Jr., Georgetown University; Amy Kronenberg, Lawrence Berkeley National Laboratory; and Zhi-Min Yuan, Harvard T.H. Chan School of Public Health.

[29] Stakeholder engagement panel discussion on October 28, 2021, with President Jonathan Nez, Navajo Nation; Jill Jim, Navajo Nation Department of Health; Mary Dickson, representative of downwinders of U.S. nuclear tests; Keith Kiefer, National Commander of the National Association of Atomic Veterans; Benetick Maddison, Marshallese Educational Initiative (prerecorded presentation); Arjun Makhijani, Institute for Energy and Environmental Research; Trisha Pritikin, Hanford Downwinder, author of *The Hanford Plaintiffs: Voices from the Fight for Atomic Justice*; and Beata Tsosie-Peña, Environmental Health and Justice Program at Tewa Women United in New Mexico (prerecorded presentation).

ESSENTIAL COMPONENTS OF THE LOW-DOSE RADIATION PROGRAM   215

stakeholders as presented to the committee during the public meetings are summarized in the following sections.

6.9.1 Congress's Views

In the Consolidated Appropriations Act, 2021, Congress identifies DOE as the manager for the program primarily because of its history of managing the previous program and its overall responsibility on nuclear issues. However, DOE's Office of Science, where the previous program was housed, does not currently have in-house experts in radiation sciences who are experienced in the challenges of low-dose radiation health research or who interact with the radiation health research community on a regular basis. In addition, little infrastructure remains in the national laboratories from the previous low-dose program. Still, when asked, congressional staff members who briefed the committee reiterated the position that DOE needs to comply with the congressional directive and establish the new program. Congressional staff also noted that, although they would be interested in the committee's views on other government agencies that could be more suitable to manage the program, they would not support outsourcing management of the program to an independent nonprofit organization outside of the U.S. government,[30] such as the Health Effects Institute,[31] which is well recognized for its role in air pollution research.

6.9.2 DOE's Views

DOE's Office of Science briefed the committee twice during the study. At the first briefing, in July 2021, the DOE representative did not indicate an interest in or commitment to managing the new low-dose radiation program and noted that the program did not fit within the office's current research priorities and portfolio; moreover, the program's long-term sustainability was uncertain, and its adoption within the office would depend on leadership buy-in.[32] The representative also told the committee that the funds from the 2021 appropriation had been used to support a computational research program at national laboratories (see more information about the project in Section 4.1.1) but provided little detail about the project or its relevance to low-dose radiation research. At the second briefing, in January 2022,[33] the same DOE representative provided a stronger ra-

---

[30] Adam Rosenberg, Committee on Science, Space, and Technology, Energy Subcommittee, U.S. House of Representatives, presentation to the committee on August 26, 2021.
[31] See www.healtheffects.org.
[32] Todd Anderson, DOE, presentation to the committee on July 21, 2021.
[33] Todd Anderson, DOE, presentation to the committee on January 24, 2022.

tionale for supporting the computational and information science research capabilities at the national laboratories and argued that this research will contribute toward improved understanding of low-dose radiation health effects.

6.9.3 Views of Members of the Scientific Community

Members of the scientific community have expressed concerns about the unpredictable nature of DOE's management and funding of the previous low-dose radiation program.[34] In addition, some scientists involved in the program indicated a lack of cohesion in the portfolio of the funded work, and a lack of strategic direction and independent review by experts that could enhance the quality of the science selected for funding and the cohesiveness of the program. Frustration of the research community toward DOE has continued after termination of the previous low-dose program and following allocation of appropriated funds from the Energy Act of 2019 and Consolidated Appropriations Act, 2021 to support a single project carried out in three national laboratories for the exploration of the potential for artificial intelligence and machine learning (see Section 4.1.1).

6.9.4 Views of Members of the Impacted Communities

Members of the impacted communities and advocates have consistently criticized DOE for an inherent conflict of interest in conducting radiation health research and have repeatedly expressed their distrust toward DOE to manage the program because of its role as manager of radiation exposures in different settings. As noted in Section 2.1.6, much of this distrust that has persisted over multiple generations originates from the AEC's and DOE's secrecy during the nuclear weapons program activities and cleanup operations.

6.9.5 The Committee's Views

The committee was not tasked with assessing the suitability of DOE to manage the low-dose program or with recommending an alternative management structure. But congressional staff told the committee that it would be interested in its views and possible alternative options for the management of the low-dose program. The committee is concerned that DOE does not currently meet important criteria for an effective managing

---

[34] Observation of committee members who are also members of the radiation research community.

agency, namely commitment to the program and absence of perceived conflicts with the research it supports.

In Section 6.8, the committee described the merits of NIH as a trusted research institution. Congress's interest in transferring the responsibility for managing the program to NIH is currently unknown, and the committee is aware that enactment of relevant legislation could take years, potentially risking the loss of Congress's interest altogether to support the program. Given such uncertainty and risk, DOE is the most viable option for immediately reestablishing a low-dose radiation program. The committee has detailed a prioritized research agenda and organizational elements that, if adopted by DOE, would go a long way toward meeting the scientific goals as well as establishing trust. Also, as outlined in this report, DOE would need to coordinate with other agencies that are engaged in low-dose radiation research or have relevant capabilities; this would ensure that the capabilities at DOE on genome biology, computational, and modeling research are complemented by capabilities in other parts of the government.

The committee estimates that to initiate the new low-dose program, DOE could implement most of the essential elements identified in this chapter within about 2 years given adequate funding. However, it may take a longer time to convince the skeptics about DOE's long-term commitment to the program; therefore, DOE will need to take strong steps to mitigate the issues of distrust toward research that it manages.

DOE's progress with implementing the essential elements recommended by this committee needs to be formally and transparently assessed early in the process. For example, Congress may use the scheduled Government Accountability Office review of the low-dose program mandated in the Consolidated Appropriations Act, 2021, § 11001 (see Appendix A) to assess DOE's progress with implementing the recommended essential elements of the program. This review is scheduled to take place in 2023, 3 years after the enactment of the law. If Congress finds that DOE has failed to take steps to (1) initiate a low-dose radiation program of the scale and scope envisioned by Congress, (2) adopt the research agenda recommended by this committee, and (3) implement the essential elements recommended by this committee, it may consider alternatives for placement and management of the low-dose radiation program, for example within NIH, likely as a cross-institutional effort, for example, by NIAID and/or NCI and/or the newly conceptualized ARPA-H.

6.10 CHAPTER SUMMARY, FINDINGS, AND RECOMMENDATION

The committee identified eight essential elements of a robust, multidisciplinary low-dose radiation program: programmatic commitment, independent advice and evaluation, transparency, prioritized strategic research agenda, appropriate research-sponsorship mechanisms, training, engagement and communications with relevant stakeholder communities, and coordination. Recognizing that the research agenda proposed by the committee extends beyond the resources of a single federal agency and will require coordination across several agencies, these elements apply to any agency that is involved or will be involved in low-dose radiation research.

Long-term commitment to the low-dose radiation program is needed to address the research priorities discussed by the committee in this report and to take advantage of the continuing technological and biological advances. Congress has assigned the management of the low-dose radiation program to DOE, but congressional staff told the committee that other government agencies could initiate their own low-dose radiation programs, carry out research that is dedicated to low-dose radiation, or have a low-dose radiation research component. Because the only entity at this point that Congress has tasked with a focused low-dose radiation program is DOE, the committee saw a role for DOE in coordinating low-dose radiation research within the United States. However, the committee also recognized the concerns raised by members of impacted communities about DOE's inherent conflicts with leading low-dose radiation research and by the research community on DOE's shortcomings related to management of the previous low-dose radiation program. In addition, the research agenda proposed by the committee extends beyond any single agency's capabilities, and a partnership with an agency whose mission is to enhance health would be warranted.

Among various federal agencies with missions to enhance or protect health, NIH is widely trusted by the scientific community and members of the public and does not have any regulatory responsibilities related to setting or implementing radiation protection standards; therefore, it has no perceived conflict of interest with leading low-dose radiation research through a cross-institutional effort. In addition, it has well-established and transparent processes for soliciting, reviewing, and funding research. Within NIH, NIAID's RNCP could be suitable to support low-dose radiation research through a cross-institutional effort. Although RNCP currently supports research in moderate and high doses starting at about 1 gray and supports limited research on cancer (which is the primary focus of NCI), the committee was impressed with the program management's commitment and transparency as well as engagement with its stakeholder communities. NCI has processes similar to NIAID's and by virtue of its mission it focuses on cancer research. ARPA-H, a proposed agency tasked with building high-risk, high-reward capabilities to drive biomedical breakthroughs, could also contribute to innovative low-dose radiation research leadership.

DOE and NIH have traditionally supported most of the low-dose radiation research in the United States, and there is a precedent for a successful coordination by the two agencies to complete the Human Genome Project. The committee supports a similar approach to be used to lead the coordination of low-dose radiation research, with DOE leading a portion of the strategic research agenda (e.g., on genome biology, computational, and modeling research, and support for facilities for low-dose and low-dose-rate exposures), and NIH, through a cross-institutional effort, leading the epidemiological and biological research, but with mechanisms in place to allow for integration of the different research lines.

The committee was not tasked with assessing the suitability of DOE to manage the low-dose radiation program or with recommending an alternative management structure. But congressional staff was interested in views and possible alternative options for the management of the low-dose program.

DOE does not currently meet important criteria for an effective managing agency, namely commitment to the program and absence of perceived conflicts with the research it supports. Among various federal agencies with experience with research funding, NIH is an example of a federal organization that meets these criteria.

The committee estimates that to initiate the new low-dose program, DOE could implement most of the essential elements identified by the committee within about 2 years given adequate funding. DOE's progress with implementing the essential elements needs to be formally and transparently assessed. For example, Congress may use the scheduled Government Accountability Office review of the low-dose program mandated in the Consolidated Appropriations Act, 2021, § 11001. This review is scheduled to take place in 2023, 3 years after the enactment of the law. If Congress finds that DOE failed to adopt the research agenda and implement the essential elements recommended by this committee, it may consider alternatives for placement and management of the low-dose radiation program, for example within NIH, likely as a cross-institutional effort, for example, by NIAID and/or NCI and/or the newly conceptualized ARPA-H.

Finding 8: The Department of Energy's (DOE's) Office of Science has a long history leading and supporting radiation research at national laboratories and universities to advance knowledge of radiation health effects and mechanisms of these effects. However, since about 2016, the Office's focus has been directed away from radiation health effects research, resulting in a lack of leadership and scientific activity in this area. Separate offices within DOE and within other federal agencies and national and international organizations have relevant expertise and have supported and continue to support research in radiation health effects. Except for the National Aeronautics and Space Administration, radiation research carried out by these other entities has not been coordinated with that supported by DOE's Office of Science.

Finding 9: Impacted communities exposed to radiation as a result of activities carried out as part of the U.S. nuclear weapons program (1942–1991) have strongly objected to the Department of Energy's (DOE's) management of the low-dose radiation program. They assert that the agency's role in promoting nuclear technologies and its responsibility for management and cleanup of its nuclear sites conflict with its role as a manager of studies on low-dose and low-dose-rate radiation health effects that may serve as the basis for exposure management decisions. This conflict, and the legacy of DOE's history of problematic community interactions, is a source of distrust of the agency by these communities.

Recommendation B: Agencies responsible for the management of the multidisciplinary low-dose radiation program should incorporate the following elements:
1. Programmatic commitment to developing and maintaining a long-term multidisciplinary low-dose radiation research program that leverages the advances in U.S. research infrastructure and health effects research.
2. Independent scientific advice and program evaluation by a trusted entity.
3. Transparent management of the research process.
4. A prioritized strategic research agenda developed with input from all relevant scientific, regulatory, and impacted stakeholder communities nationally and internationally.
5. Research sponsorship mechanisms that support competitive research and infrastructure development projects and employ transparent peer review to select projects that are aligned with the program's strategic research agenda.
6. Training and research support for scientists of all career levels and relevant disciplines that promote equity, diversity, and inclusion.
7. Commitment to engagement and communication with all relevant stakeholder communities.
8. Coordination across federal agencies and other national and international organizations that carry out low-dose radiation research or have relevant expertise and entities that carry out relevant (non-radiation) research.

References

AAPM (American Association of Physicists in Medicine). (2021). AAPM/ACR/HPS Joint Statement on Proper Use of Radiation Dose Metric Tracking for Patients Undergoing Medical Imaging Exams. Policies and Procedures, PP 35-A. Alexandria, VA, American Association of Physicists in Medicine.

Aardema, M. J., and J. T. MacGregor. (2002). "Toxicology and genetic toxicology in the new era of "toxicogenomics": Impact of "-omics" technologies." Mutation Research 499(1): 13–25. doi: 10.1016/s0027-5107(01)00292-5.

Abalo, K. D., E. Rage, K. Leuraud, D. B. Richardson, H. D. Le Pointe, D. Laurier, and M. O. Bernier. (2021). "Early life ionizing radiation exposure and cancer risks: Systematic review and meta-analysis." Pediatric Radiology 51(1): 45–56. doi: 10.1007/s00247-020-04803-0. Erratum, Pediatric Radiology 51: 157–158 (2021).

Aceves, W. J. (2018). "Cost-benefit analysis and human rights." St. John's Law Review 92(3): 431–451. https://scholarship.law.stjohns.edu/cgi/viewcontent.cgi?article=7079&context=lawreview.

Acharya, M. M., J. E. Baulch, A. A. D. Baddour, L. A. Apodaca, L. Alikhani, C. Garcia, M. C. Angulo, R. S. Batra, C. L. Limoli, P. M. Klein, I. Soltesz, E. A. Kramar, C. E. L. Stark, M. A. Wood, C. M. Fallgren, T. B. Borak, and R. A. Britten. (2019). "New concerns for neurocognitive function during deep space exposures to chronic, low dose-rate, neutron radiation." eNeuro 6(5). doi: 10.1523/ENEURO.0094-19.2019.

ACS (American Cancer Society). (2020). Lifetime Risk of Developing or Dying from Cancer. Kennesaw, GA, American Cancer Society. https://www.cancer.org/cancer/cancer-basics/lifetime-probability-of-developing-or-dying-from-cancer.html.

Adhikari, S., E. C. Nice, E. W. Deutsch, L. Lane, G. S. Omenn, S. R. Pennington, Y. K. Paik, C. M. Overall, F. J. Corrales, I. M. Cristea, J. E. Van Eyk, M. Uhlén, C. Lindskog, D. W. Chan, A. Bairoch, J. C. Waddington, J. L. Justice, J. LaBaer, H. Rodriguez, F. He, M. Kostrzewa, P. Ping, R. L. Gundry, P. Stewart, S. Srivastava, S. Srivastava, F. C. S. Nogueira, G. B. Domont, Y. Vandenbrouck, M. P. Y. Lam, S. Wennersten, J. A. Vizcaino, M. Wilkins, J. M. Schwenk, E. Lundberg, N. Bandeira, G. Marko-Varga, S. T. Weintraub, C. Pineau, U. Kusebauch, R. L. Moritz, S. B. Ahn, M. Palmblad, M. P. Snyder, R. Aebersold, and M. S. Baker. (2020). "A high-stringency blueprint of the human proteome." Nature Communications 11(1): 5301. doi: 10.1038/s41467-020-19045-9.

AEC (Atomic Energy Commission). (1955). Atomic Test Effects in the Nevada Test Site Region. Washington, DC, U.S. Atomic Energy Commission.

Ahadi, S., W. Zhou, S. M. Schüssler-Fiorenza Rose, M. R. Sailani, K. Contrepois, M. Avina, M. Ashland, A. Brunet, and M. Snyder. (2020). "Personal aging markers and ageotypes revealed by deep longitudinal profiling." Nature Medicine 26(1): 83–90. doi: 10.1038/s41591-019-0719-5.

Ahn, Y.-S., R. M. Park, and D.-H. Koh. (2008). "Cancer admission and mortality in workers exposed to ionizing radiation in Korea." Journal of Occupational and Environmental Medicine 50(7): 791–803. doi: 10.1097/JOM.0b013e3181677551d.

Ainsbury, E. A., C. Dalke, N. Hamada, M. A. Benadjaoud, J. R. Jourdain, V. Chumak, M. Ginjaume, J. L. Kok, M. Mancuso, L. Sabatier, L. Struelens, and J. Thariat. (2021). "Radiation-induced lens opacities: Epidemiological, clinical and experimental evidence, methodological issues, research gaps and strategy." Environment International 146: 06213. doi: 10.1016/j.envint.2020.106213.

Ainsbury, E. A., C. Dalke, M. Mancuso, M. Kadhim, R. A. Quinlan, T. Azizova, L. T. Dauer, J. R. Dynlacht, R. Tanner, and N. Hamada. (2022). "Introduction to the special LD-LensRad focus issue. Radiation Research 197(1): 1–6. doi: 10.1667/RADE-21-00188.1.

AIP (American Institute of Physics). (2021). Academies Panel to Consider Future of Revived DOE Low-Dose Radiation Program. August 12. https://www.aip.org/fyi/2022/academies-panel-consider-future-revived-doe-low-dose-radiation-program.

Ajmal, S. (2021). "Contrast-enhanced ultrasonography: Review and applications." Cureus 13(9): e18243. doi: 10.7759/cureus.18243.

Akiba, S., and S. Mizuno. (2012). "The third analysis of cancer mortality among Japanese nuclear workers, 1991–2002: Estimation of excess relative risk per radiation dose." Journal of Radiological Protection 32(1): 73–83. doi: 10.1088/0952-4746/32/1/73.

Alexandrov, L. B., J. Kim, N. J. Haradhvala, M. N. Huang, A. W. Tian Ng, Y. Wu, A. Boot, K. R. Covington, D. A. Gordenin, E. N. Bergstrom, S. M. A. Islam, N. Lopez-Bigas, L. J. Klimczak, J. R. McPherson, S. Morganella, R. Sabarinathan, D. A. Wheeler, and V. Mustonen; PCAWG Mutational Signatures Working Group, G. Getz, S. G. Rozen, and M. R. Stratton; PCAWG Consortium. (2020). "The repertoire of mutational signatures in human cancer." Nature 578(7793): 94–101. doi: 10.1038/s41586-020-1943-3.

Ali, S. S. (2019). "Frantic parents fear for kids after radioactive contamination found at Ohio middle school." NBC News, May 15. https://www.nbcnews.com/news/us-news/frantic-parents-fear-kids-after-radioactive-contamination-found-ohio-middle-n1005771.

Allisy-Roberts, P., and P. Day. (2008). "Uncertainty evaluation and expression in dose and risk assessment." Journal of Radiological Protection 28(3): 265–269. doi: 10.1088/0952-4746/28/3/E02.

Almond, D., L. Edlund, and M. Palme. (2009). "Chernobyl's subclinical legacy: Prenatal exposure to radioactive fallout and school outcomes in Sweden." Quarterly Journal of Economics 124(4): 1729–1772. doi: 10.1162/qjec.2009.124.4.1729.

Amano, M. A., B. French, R. Sakata, M. Dekker, and A. V. Brenner. (2021). "Lifetime risk of suicide among survivors of the atomic bombings of Japan." Epidemiology and Psychiatric Sciences 30: e43. doi: 10.1017/S204579602100024X.

Amdur, R. J., and J. S. Bedford. (1994). "Dose-rate effects between 0.3 and 30 Gy/h in a normal and a malignant human cell line." International Journal of Radiation Oncology, Biology, Physics 30(1): 83–90. doi: 10.1016/0360-3016(94)90522-3.

Andersen, P. K., R. B. Geskus, T. de Witte, and H. Putter. (2012). "Competing risks in epidemiology: Possibilities and pitfalls." International Journal of Epidemiology 41(3): 861–870. doi: 10.1093/ije/dyr213.

Anderson, J. L., S. J. Bertke, J. Yiin, K. Kelly-Reif, and R. D. Daniels. (2021). "Ischaemic heart and cerebrovascular disease mortality in uranium enrichment workers." Occupational and Environmental Medicine 78(2): 105–111. doi: 10.1136/oemed-2020-106423.

Ando, K., Y. Muguruma, and T. Yahata. (2008). "Humanizing bone marrow in immune-deficient mice." Current Topics in Microbiology and Immunology 324: 77–86. doi: 10.1007/978-3-540-75647-7_4.

ANS (American Nuclear Society). (2017). ANS Nuclear Grand Challenges. http://cdn.ans.org/challenges/docs/nuclear_grand_challenges-report.pdf?_ga=2.171724192.1606616436.1643651604-1471315233.1613263563.

ANS. (2022). Risks of Exposure to Low-Level Ionizing Radiation. https://cdn.ans.org/policy/statements/docs/ps41-bi.pdf?_ga=2.185895085.564315287.1643141575-1468864878.1643141575.

Applegate, K. E., W. Rühm, A.Wojcik, M. Bourguignon, A. Brenner, K. Hamasaki, T. Imai, M. Imaizumi, T. Imaoka, S. Kakinuma, T. Kamada, N. Nishimura, N. Okonogi, K. Ozasa, C. E. Rübe, A. Sadakane, R. Sakata, Y. Shimada, K. Yoshida, and S. Bouffler. (2020). "Individual response of humans to ionising radiation: Governing factors and importance for radiological protection." Radiation and Environmental Biophysics 59: 185–209. doi: 10.1007/s00411-020-00837-y.

Applegate, K. E., Ú. Findlay, L. Fraser, Y. Kinsella, L. Ainsbury, and S. Bouffler. (2021). "Radiation exposures in pregnancy, health effects and risks to the embryo/foetus—information to inform the medical management of the pregnant patient." Journal of Radiological Protection 41(4). doi: 10.1088/1361-6498/ac1c95.

Armstrong, G. T., N. Jain, W. Liu, T. E. Merchant, M. Stovall, D. K. Srivastava, J. G. Gurney, R. J. Packer, L. L. Robison, and K. R. Krull. (2010). "Region-specific radiotherapy and neuropsychological outcomes in adult survivors of childhood CNS malignancies." Neuro-Oncology 12: 1173–1186. doi: 10.1093/neuonc/noq104.

Auxier, J. P., J. D. Auxier II, and H. L. Hall. (2017). "Review of current nuclear fallout codes." Journal of Environmental Radioactivity 171: 246–252. doi: 10.1016/j.jenvrad.2017.02.010.

Averbeck, D., S. Candéias, S. Chandna, N. Foray, A. A. Friedl, S. Haghdoost, P. A. Jeggo, K. Lumniczky, F. Paris, R. Quintens, and L. Sabatier. (2020). "Establishing mechanisms affecting the individual response to ionizing radiation." International Journal of Radiation Biology 96(3): 297–323. doi: 10.1080/09553002.2019.1704908.

Azizova, T. V., E. Batistatou, E. S. Grigorieva, R. McNamee, R. Wakeford, H. Liu, F. de Vocht, and R. M. Agius. (2018). "An assessment of radiation-associated risks of mortality from circulatory disease in the cohorts of Mayak and Sellafield nuclear workers." Radiation Research 189(4): 371–388. doi: 10.1667/RR14468.1.

Azizova, T. V., M. V. Bannikova, E. S. Grigoryeva, V. L. Rybkina, and N. Hamada. (2020). "Occupational exposure to chronic ionizing radiation increases risk of Parkinson's disease incidence in Russian Mayak workers." International Journal of Epidemiology 49(2): 435–447. https://doi.org/10.1093/ije/dyz230.

Batkins, S. (2016). "The costs and benefits of nuclear regulation." American Action Forum. September 8. https://www.americanactionforum.org/research/costs-benefits-nuclear-regulation.

Batkins, S., P. Rossetti, and P. Goldbeck. (2017). "Putting nuclear regulatory costs in context." American Action Forum. https://www.americanactionforum.org/research/putting-nuclear-regulatory-costs-context.

Bazyka, D., K. Loganovsky, I. Ilyenko, S. Chumak, and M. Bomko. (2015). "Gene expression, telomere and cognitive deficit analysis as a function of Chornobyl radiation dose and age: From in utero to adulthood." Problems of Radiation Medicine and Radiobiology 20: 283–310.

Bedford, J. S. (2001). "The radiobiology of low-dose-rate and fractionated irradiation." In Principles and Practice of Brachytherapy: Using Afterloading Systems (A. Flynn, E. J. Hall, and C. A. F. Joslin, eds.), pp. 161–179. New York, Arnold.

Bedford, J. S., and W. C. Dewey. (2002). "Historical and current highlights in radiation biology: Has anything important been learned by irradiating cells?" Radiation Research 158(3): 251–291. doi: 10.1667/0033-7587(2002)158[0251:hachir]2.0.co;2.

Behjati, S., G. Gundem, D. C. Wedge, N. D. Roberts, P. S. Tarpey, S. L. Cooke, P. Van Loo, L. B. Alexandrov, M. Ramakrishna, H. Davies, S. Nik-Zainal, C. Hardy, C. Latimer, K. M. Raine, L. Stebbings, A. Menzies, D. Jones, R. Shepherd, A. P. Butler, J. W. Teague, M. Jorgensen, B. Khatri, N. Pillay, A. Shlien, P. A. Futreal, C. Badie, U. McDermott, G. S. Bova, A. L. Richardson, A. M. Flanagan, M. R. Stratton, P. J. Campbell, and ICGC Prostate Group. (2016). "Mutational signatures of ionizing radiation in second malignancies." Nature Communications 7: 12605. doi: 10.1038/ncomms12605.

Bene, B. J., W. F. Blakely, D.M. Burmeister, L. Cary, S. J. Chhetri, C. M. Davis, S. P. Ghosh, G. P. Holmes-Hampton, S. Iordanskiy, J. F. Kalinich, J. G. Kiang, V. P. Kumar, R. J. Lowy, A. Miller, M. Naeem, D. A. Schauer, L. Senchak, V. K. Singh, A. J. Stewart, E. M. Velazquez, and M. Xiao. (2021). "Celebrating 60 years of accomplishments of the Armed Forces Radiobiology Research Institute." Radiation Research 196(2): 129–146. doi: 10.1667/21-00064.1.

Bennett, D. A., D. Landry, J. Little, and C. Minelli. (2017). "Systematic review of statistical approaches to quantify, or correct for, measurement error in a continuous exposure in nutritional epidemiology." BMC Medical Research Methodology 17(1): 146.

BERAC (Biological and Environmental Research Advisory Committee). (2016). Letter and Final Report. Low-Dose Radiation Expert Subcommittee, Biological and Environmental Research Advisory Committee, U.S. Department of Energy. https://science.osti.gov/-/media/ber/berac/pdf/charges/Low_Dose_letter_and_BERAC_report.pdf?la=en&hash=7BA54E931244BFA12829490B1636555D2C2FBD25.

Berlivet, J., D. Hémon, É. Cléro, G. Ielsch, D. Laurier, S. Guissou, B. Lacour, J. Clavel, and S. Goujon. (2020). "Ecological association between residential natural background radiation exposure and the incidence rate of childhood central nervous system tumors in France, 2000–2012." Journal of Environmental Radioactivity 211: 106071. doi: 10.1016/j.jenvrad.2019.106071.

Bernier, M. O., H. Baysson, M. S. Pearce, M. Moissonnier, E. Cardis, M. Hauptmann, L. Struelens, J. Dabin, C. Johansen, N. Journy, D. Laurier, M. Blettner, L. Le Cornet, R. Pokora, P. Gradowska, J. M. Meulepas, K. Kjaerheim, T. Istad, H. Olerud, A. Sovik, M. Bosch de Basea, I. Thierry-Chef, A. Kaijser, A. Nordenskjöld, A. Berrington de Gonzalez, R. W. Harbron, and A. Kesminiene. (2019). "Cohort Profile: The EPI-CT study: A European pooled epidemiological study to quantify the risk of radiation-induced cancer from paediatric CT." International Journal of Epidemiology 48(2): 379–381. doi: 10.1093/ije/dyy231.

Bernstein, B. E., J. A. Stamatoyannopoulos, J. F. Costello, B. Ren, A. Milosavljevic, A. Meissner, M. Kellis, M. A. Marra, A. L. Beaudet, J. R. Ecker, P. J. Farnham, M. Hirst, E. S. Lander, T. S. Mikkelsen, and J. A. Thomson. (2010). "The NIH Roadmap Epigenomics Mapping Consortium." Nature Biotechnology 28(10): 1045–1048. doi: 10.1038/nbt1010-1045.

Berrington de González, A., A. Bouville, P. Rajaraman, and M. Schubauer-Berigan. (2017). "Ionizing radiation." Chap. 13 in Cancer Epidemiology and Prevention (M. Thun, M. S. Linet, J. R. Cerhan, C. A. Haiman, and D. Schottenfeld, eds.). Oxford University Press.

REFERENCES

Berrington de González, A., R. D. Daniels, E. Cardis, H. M. Cullings, E. Gilbert, M. Hauptmann, G. Kendall, D. Laurier, M. S. Linet, M. P. Little, J. H. Lubin, D. L. Preston, D. B. Richardson, D. Stram, I. Thierry-Chef, and M. K. Schubauer-Berigan. (2020). "Epidemiological studies of low-dose ionizing radiation and cancer: Rationale and framework for the monograph and overview of eligible studies." Journal of the National Cancer Institute Monographs 56: 97–113. doi: 10.1093/jncimonographs/lgaa009.

Berrington de González, A., E. Pasqual, and L. Veiga. (2021). "Epidemiological studies of CT scans and cancer risk: The state of the science. British Journal of Radiology 94(1126): 20210471. doi: 10.1259/bjr.20210471.

Bhawal, R., A. L. Oberg, S. Zhang, and M. Kohli. (2020). "Challenges and opportunities in clinical applications of blood-based proteomics in cancer." Cancers (Basel) 12(9): 2428. doi: 10.3390/cancers12092428.

Bigbee, W. L., R. H. Jensen, T. Veidebaum, M. Tekkel, M. Rahu, A. Stengrevics, A. Auvinen, T. Hakulinen, K. Servomaa, T. Rytömaa, G. I. Obrams, and J. D. Boice, Jr. (1997). "Biodosimetry of Chernobyl cleanup workers from Estonia and Latvia using the glycophorin A in vivo somatic cell mutation assay." Radiation Research 147(2): 215–224.

Bissell, M. J., and W. C. Hines. (2011). "Why don't we get more cancer? A proposed role of the microenvironment in restraining cancer progression." Nature Medicine 17(3): 320–329. doi: 10.1038/nm.2328.

Bixler, N., and A. Nosek. (2021). MACCS Theory Manual. No. SAND2021-11535. Sandia National Laboratory, Albuquerque, NM.

Black, S. E., A. Butikofer, P. J. Devereux, and K. G. Salvanes. (2019). "This is only a test? Long-run and intergenerational impacts of prenatal exposure to radioactive fallout." Review of Economics and Statistics 101(3): 531–546.

Black, S., D. Phillips, J. W. Hickey, J. Kennedy-Darling, V. G. Venkataraaman, N. Samusik, Y. Goltsev, C. M. Schürch, and G. P. Nolan. (2021). "CODEX multiplexed tissue imaging with DNA-conjugated antibodies." Nature Protocols 16(8): 3802–3835. doi: 10.1038/s41596-021-00556-8.

Bleesing, J. J., M. R. Brown, C. Novicio, D. Guarraia, J. K. Dale, S. E. Straus, and T. A. Fleisher. (2002). "A composite picture of TcR α/β+ CD4-CD8- T Cells (α/β-DNTCs) in humans with autoimmune lymphoproliferative syndrome." Clinical Immunology 104(1): 21–30. doi: 10.1006/clim.2002.5225.

Blettner, M., H. Zeeb, A. Auvinen, T. J. Ballard, M. Caldora, H. Eliasch, M. Gundestrup, T. Haldorsen, N. Hammar, G. P. Hammer, D. Irvine, I. Langner, A. Paridou, E. Pukkala, V. Rafnsson, H. Storm, H. Tulinius, U. Tveten, and A. Tzonou. (2003). "Mortality from cancer and other causes among male airline cockpit crew in Europe." International Journal of Cancer 106(6): 946–952. doi: 10.1093/aje/kwg107.

Blomstrand, M., E. Holmberg, M. A. Aberg, M. Lundell, T. Björk-Eriksson, P. Karlsson, and K. Blomgren. (2014). "No clinically relevant effect on cognitive outcomes after low-dose radiation to the infant brain: A population-based cohort study in Sweden." Acta Oncologica 53(9): 1143–1150. doi: 10.3109/0284186X.2014.899434.

Blush, S. M., and T. H. Heitman. (1995). Train Wreck Along the River of Money: An Evaluation of the Hanford Cleanup, a Report for the U.S. Senate Committee on Energy and Natural Resources. Washington, DC, U.S. Government Printing Office.

Boerma, M., C. M. Davis, I. L. Jackson, D. Schaue, and J. P. Williams. (2022). "All for one, though not one for all: Team players in normal tissue radiobiology." International Journal of Radiation Biology 98(3): 346–366. doi: 10.1080/09553002.2021.1941383.

Boice, J. D., Jr., and R. W. Miller. (1999). "Childhood and adult cancer after intrauterine exposure to ionizing radiation." Teratology 59(4): 227–233. doi: 10.1002/(SICI)1096-9926(199904)59:4<227::AID-TERA7>3.0.CO;2-E.

Boice, J. D., Jr., S. S. Cohen, M. T. Mumma, E. D. Ellis, K. F. Eckerman, R. W. Leggett, B. B. Boecker, A. B. Brill, and B. E. Henderson. (2011). "Updated mortality analysis of radiation workers at Rocketdyne (Atomics International), 1948–2008." Radiation Research 176(2): 244–258. https://doi.org/10.1667/RR2487.1.

Boice, J. D., Jr., S. S. Cohen, M. T. Mumma, S. C. Howard, R. C. Yoder, and L. T. Dauer. (2021). "Mortality among medical radiation workers in the United States, 1965-2016." International Journal of Radiation Biology (Nov 3): 1–63. doi: 10.1080/09553002.2021.1967508.

Boice, J. D., Jr., A. Bouville, L. T. Dauer, A. P. Golden, and R. Wakeford. (2022a). "Introduction to the special issue on the US Million Person Study of health effects from low-level exposure to radiation." International Journal of Radiation Biology 98(4): 529–532. doi: 10.1080/09553002.2021.1989906.

Boice, J. D., Jr., S. S. Cohen, M. T. Mumma, and E. D. Ellis. (2022b). "The Million Person Study, whence it came and why." International Journal of Radiation Biology 98(4):537–550. doi: 10.1080/09553002.2019.1589015.

Boice, J. D., Jr., E. D. Ellis, A. P. Golden, L. B. Zablotska, M. T. Mumma, and S. S. Cohen. (2022c). "Sex-specific lung cancer risk among radiation workers in the Million Person Study and among TB fluoroscopy patients." International Journal of Radiation Biology 98(4): 769–780. doi: 10.1080/09553002.2018.1547441.

Borak, T. B., L. H. Heilbronn, N. Krumland, and M. M. Weil. (2021). "Design and dosimetry of a facility to study health effects following exposures to fission neutrons at low-dose rates for long durations." International Journal of Radiation Biology 97(8): 1063–1076. doi: 10.1080/09553002.2019.1688884.

Brackmann, L. K., A. Poplawski, C. L. Grandt, H. Schwarz, T. Hankeln, S. Rapp, S. Zahnreich, D. Galetzka, I. Schmitt, C. Grad, L. Eckhard, J. Mirsch, M. Blettner, P. Scholz-Kreisel, M. Hess, H. Binder, H. Schmidberger, and M. Marron. (2020). "Comparison of time and dose dependent gene expression and affected pathways in primary human fibroblasts after exposure to ionizing radiation. Molecular Medicine 26(1): 85. doi: 10.1186/s10020-020-00203-0.

Brambilla, M., J. Vassileva, A. Kuchcinska, and M. M. Rehani. (2020). "Multinational data on cumulative radiation exposure of patients from recurrent radiological procedures: Call for action." European Radiology 30(5): 2493–2501. doi: 10.1007/s00330-019-06528-7.

Brenner, A. V., D. L. Preston, R. Sakata, H. Sugiyama, A. Berrington de Gonzalez, B. French, M. Utada, E. K. Cahoon, A. Sadakane, K. Ozasa, E. J. Grant, and K. Mabuchi. (2018). "Incidence of breast cancer in the Life Span Study of Atomic Bomb Survivors: 1958–2009." Radiation Research 190(4): 433–444. doi: 10.1667/RR15015.1.

Brenner, A. V., H. Sugiyama, D. L. Preston, R. Sakata, B. French, A. Sadakane, E. K. Cahoon, M. Utada, K. Mabuchi, and K. Ozasa. (2020). "Radiation risk of central nervous system tumors in the Life Span Study of Atomic Bomb Survivors, 1958–2009." European Journal of Epidemiology 35(6): 591–600. doi: 10.1007/s10654-019-00599-y.

Brenner, A. V., D. L. Preston, R. Sakata, J. Cologne, H. Sugiyama, M. Utada, E. K. Cahoon, E. Grant, K. Mabuchi, and K. Ozasa. (2022). "Comparison of all solid cancer mortality and incidence dose-response in the Life Span Study of Atomic Bomb Survivors, 1958–2009." Radiation Research. doi: 10.1667/RADE-21-00059.1.

Brenner, D. J. (2014). "What we know and what we don't know about cancer risks associated with radiation doses from radiological imaging." British Journal of Radiology 87(1035): 20130629. doi: 10.1259/bjr.20130629.

Brenner, D. J., R. Doll, D. T. Goodhead, E. J. Hall, C. E. Land, J. B. Little, J. H. Lubin, D. L. Preston, R. J. Preston, J. S. Puskin, E. Ron, R. K. Sachs, J. M. Samet, R. B. Setlow, and M. Zaider. (2003). "Cancer risks attributable to low doses of ionizing radiation: Assessing what we really know." Proceedings of the National Academy of Sciences of the United States of America 100(24): 13761–13766. doi: 10.1073/pnas.2235592100.

Brodeur, G. M., K. E. Nichols, S. E. Plon, J. D. Schiffman, and D. Malkin. (2017). "Pediatric cancer predisposition and surveillance: An overview, and a tribute to Alfred G. Knudson Jr." Clinical Cancer Research 23(11): e1–e5. doi: 10.1158/1078-0432.CCR-17-0702.

Brooks, A. L. (2012). A History of the United States Department of Energy (DOE) Low-dose Radiation Research Program: 1998–2008. https://web.archive.org/web/20150906124027/http://lowdose.energy.gov/pdf/albRoughDraft/doeHistoryComplete09262012.pdf.

Bromet, E. J. (2011). "Lessons learned from radiation disasters." World Psychiatry 10: 83–84. doi: 10.1002/j.2051-5545.2011.tb00020.x.

Bromet, E. J. (2012). "Mental health consequences of the Chernobyl disaster." Journal of Radiological Protection 32: N71-5. doi: 10.1088/0952-4746/32/1/N71.

Bromet, E. J. (2014). "Emotional consequences of nuclear power plant disasters." Health Physics 106(2): 206–210. doi: 10.1097/HP.0000000000000012.

Bromet, E., and L. Litcher-Kelly. (2002). "Psychological response of mothers of young children to the Three Mile Island and Chernobyl nuclear plant accidents one decade later." In Toxic Turmoil (J. Havenaar, J. Cwikel, and E. Bromets, eds.), pp. 69–84. Springer.

Budgen, M. (2021). "Return to Fukushima, 10 years later," Lifegate, March 11. https://www.lifegate.com/fukushima-10-years.

Burger, J., M. Gochfeld, and K. Pletnikoff. (2009). "Collaboration versus communication: The Department of Energy's Amchitka Island and the Aleut Community." Environmental Research 109(4): 503–510. doi: 10.1016/j.envres.2009.01.002.

Bushnell, D. M. (2020). Space Tourism. NASA Technical Reports Server, National Aeronautics and Space Administration. https://ntrs.nasa.gov/citations/20205005651?utm_source=FBPAGE&utm_medium=NASA%20Scientific%20and%20Technical%20Information%20(STI)%20Program&utm_campaign=NASASocial&linkId=109243812.

Cahoon, E. K., D. L. Preston, D. A. Pierce, E. Grant, A. V. Brenner, K. Mabuchi, M. Utada, and K. Ozasa. (2017). "Lung, laryngeal and other respiratory cancer incidence among Japanese atomic bomb survivors: An updated analysis from 1958 through 2009." Radiation Research 187(5): 538–548. doi: 10.1667/RR14583.1.

Cahoon, E. K., R. Zhang, S. L. Simon, R. M. Pfeiffer, and A. Bouville. (2021). "Projected cancer risks to residents of New Mexico from exposure to trinity radioactive fallout: Erratum." Health Physics 120(1): 94–97. doi: 10.1097/01.HP.0000725236.16225.17.

Caldwell, G. G., D. B. Kelley, and C. W. Heath, Jr. (1980). "Leukemia among participants in military maneuvers at a nuclear bomb test. A preliminary report." Journal of the American Medical Association 244(14): 1575–1578. doi: 10.1001/jama.1980.03310140033025.

Campisi, J., J. K. Andersen, P. Kapahi, and S. Melov. (2011). "Cellular senescence: A link between cancer and age-related degenerative disease?" Seminars in Cancer Biology 21(6): 354–359. doi: 10.1016/j.semcancer.2011.09.001.

Cardarelli, J. J., II, and B. A. Ulsh. (2018). "It is time to move beyond the linear no-threshold theory for low-dose radiation protection." Dose-Response 16(3). doi: 10.1177/1559325818779651.

Carey, M. P. (2014). Cost-Benefit and Other Analysis Requirements in the Rulemaking Process. Washington, DC, Congressional Research Service.

Castillo, H., X. Li, and G. B. Smith. (2021). "*Deinococcus radiodurans* UWO298 dependence on background radiation for optimal growth." Frontiers in Genetics 12: 644292. doi: 10.3389/fgene.2021.644292.

CDC (Centers for Disease Control and Prevention) (2020). Radiation Response Briefing Manual: A Guide for Key Leaders and Public Health Decision Makers. Centers for Disease Control and Prevention.

Chakraborty, N., A. Gautam, G. P. Holmes-Hampton, V. P. Kumar, S. Biswas, R. Kumar, D. Hamad, G. Dimitrov, A. O. Olabisi, R. Hammamieh, and S. P. Ghosh. (2020). "microRNA and metabolite signatures linked to early consequences of lethal radiation." Scientific Reports 10(1): 5424. doi: 10.1038/s41598-020-62255-w.

Chaves, M., and H. de Jong. (2021). "Qualitative modeling, analysis and control of synthetic regulatory circuits." In Synthetic Gene Circuits, Vol. 2229: Methods in Molecular Biology (F. Menolascina, ed.), pp. 1–40. Humana, New York. doi: 10.1007/978-1-0716-1032-9_1.

Cheminfo Services Inc. (2012). Review of the Rare Earth Elements and Lithium Mining Sectors: Final Report, Cheminfo Services Inc.

Chen, J.-H., Y.-C. Yen, S.-H. Liu, F.-P. Lee, K.-C. Lin, M.-T. Lai, C.-C. Wu, T.-M. Chen, S.-P. Yuan, C.-L. Chang, and S.-Y. Wu. (2015). "Dementia risk in irradiated patients with head and neck cancer." Medicine (Baltimore) 94(45): e1983. doi: 10.1097/MD.0000000000001983.

Cheng, E. S., S. Egger, S. Hughes, M. Weber, J. Steinberg, B. Rahman, H. Worth, A. Ruano-Ravina, P. Rawstorne, and X. Q. Yu. (2021). "Systematic review and meta-analysis of residential radon and lung cancer in never-smokers." European Respiratory Review 30(159): 200230. doi: 10.1183/16000617.0230-2020.

Choudhury, P., and M. Gupta. (2017). "Personalized and precision medicine in cancer: A theranostic approach." Current Radiopharmaceuticals 10(3): 166–170. doi: 10.2174/1874471010666170728094008.

Chua, E. Y. D., J. H. Mendez, M. Rapp, S. L. Ilca, Y. Zi Tan, K. Maruthi, H. Kuang, C. M. Zimanyi, A. Cheng, E. T. Eng, A. J. Noble, C. S. Potter, and B. Carragher. (2022). "Better, faster, cheaper: Recent advances in cryo-electron microscopy." Annual Review of Biochemistry. doi: 10.1146/annurev-biochem-032620-110705.

Clement, C., W. Rühm, J. Harrison, K. Applegate, D. Cool, C. M. Larsson, C. Cousins, J. Lochard, S. Bouffler, K. Cho, M. Kai, D. Laurier, S. Liu, and S. Romanov. (2021). "Keeping the ICRP recommendations fit for purpose." Journal of Radiological Protection 41(4): 1390–1409. doi: 10.1088/1361-6498/ac1611.

Clewell, R. A., C. M. Thompson, and H. J. Clewell, III. (2019). "Dose-dependence of chemical carcinogenicity: Biological mechanisms for thresholds and implications for risk assessment." Chemico-Biological Interactions 301: 112–127. doi: 10.1016/j.cbi.2019.01.025.

Cochran, L. D., A. C. Eckert, B. Hunt, and T. Kraus. (2020). "Uncertainty analysis of consequence management data products." Health Physics 118(4): 382–395.

Cohen, B. (1987). Reducing the Hazards of Nuclear Power: Insanity in Action. Bethesda, MD, Atomic Industrial Forum, Public Affairs and Information Program.

Collaborative Cross Consortium. (2012). "The genome architecture of the Collaborative Cross mouse genetic reference population." Genetics 190(2): 389–401. doi: 10.1534/genetics.111.132639.

Collins, F. S., and A. D. Barker. (2007). "Mapping the cancer genome: Pinpointing the genes involved in cancer will help chart a new course across the complex landscape of human malignancies." Scientific American 296(3): 50–57.

COMARE (Committee on Medical Aspects of Radiation in the Environment). (2016). Seventeenth Report: Further Consideration of the Incidence of Cancers Around the Nuclear Installations at Sellafield and Dounreay. Wetherby, UK, COMARE. https://assets.publishing.service.gov.uk/government/uploads/system/uploads/attachment_data/file/554981/COMARE_17th_Report.pdf.

Commission on Risk Assessment and Risk Management. (1997). Symposium on a Public Health Approach to Environmental Health Risk Management, 8 August 1997, Washington, DC. https://cfpub.epa.gov/si/si_public_record_report.cfm?Lab=NCEA&count=10000&dirEntryId=55006&searchall=&showcriteria=2&simplesearch=0&timstype=.

Complex Trait Consortium. (2004). "The Collaborative Cross, a community resource for the genetic analysis of complex traits." Nature Genetics 36(11): 1133–1137. doi: 10.1038/ng1104-1133.

Cone, M. (1997). "Desert lands contaminated by toxic spills." Los Angeles Times. April 24. https://www.latimes.com/archives/la-xpm-1997-04-24-mn-51903-story.html.

Cook-Deegan, R. M. (1994). The Gene Wars: Science, Politics, and the Human Genome. New York, Norton.
Coskun, A. F., G. Han, S. Ganesh, S. Y. Chen, X. R. Clavé, S. Harmsen, S. Jiang, C. M. Schürch, Y. Bai, C. Hitzman, and G. P. Nolan. (2021). "Nanoscopic subcellular imaging enabled by ion beam tomography." Nature Communications 12(1): 789. doi: 10.1038/s41467-020-20753-5.
Court-Brown, W. M., and R. Doll. (1957). Leukaemia and Aplastic Anaemia in Patients Irradiated for Ankylosing Spondylitis, Vol. 295: Medical Research Council Special Report Series. London, Her Majesty's Stationery Office.
Cremer, P., R. Hachamovitch, and B. Tamarappoo. (2014). "Clinical decision making with myocardial perfusion imaging in patients with known or suspected coronary artery disease." Seminars in Nuclear Medicine 44(4): 320–329. doi: 10.1053/j.semnuclmed.2014.04.006.
Cullings, H. M., S. Fujita, S. Funamoto, E. J. Grant, G. D. Kerr, and D. L. Preston. (2006). "Dose estimation for atomic bomb survivor studies: Its evolution and present status." Radiation Research 166(1 Pt. 2): 219–254. doi: 10.1667/RR3546.1.
Cullings, H. M., E. J. Grant, S. D. Egbert, T. Watanabe, T. Oda, F. Nakamura, T. Yamashita, H. Fuchi, S. Funamoto, K. Marumo, R. Sakata, Y. Kodama, K. Ozasa, and K. Kodama. (2017). "DS02R1: Improvements to atomic bomb survivors' input data and implementation of Dosimetry System 2002 (DS02) and resulting changes in estimated doses." Health Physics 112(1): 56–97. doi: 10.1097/HP.0000000000000598.
Cuttler, J. M., and M. Pollycove. (2009). "Nuclear energy and health: And the benefits of low-dose radiation hormesis." Dose-Response 7(1): 52–89. doi: 10.2203/dose-response.08-024.Cuttler.
Daniels, R. D., G. M. Kendall, I. Thierry-Chef, M. S. Linet, and H. M. Cullings. (2020). "Strengths and weaknesses of dosimetry used in studies of low-dose radiation exposure and cancer." Journal of the National Cancer Institute 2020(56): 114–132. doi: 10.1093/jncimonographs/lgaa001.
Danzer, M., and N. Danzer. 2016. "The long-run consequences of Chernobyl: Evidence on subjective well-being, mental health, and welfare." Journal of Public Economics 135: 47–60. doi: 10.1016/j.jpubeco.2016.01.001.
Darby, S., D. Hill, A. Auvinen, J. M. Barros-Dios, H. Baysson, F. Bochicchio, H. Deo, R. Falk, F. Forastiere, M. Hakama, I. Heid, L. Kreienbrock, M. Kreuzer, F. Lagarde, I. Mäkeläinen, C. Muirhead, W. Oberaigner, G. Pershagen, A. Ruano-Ravina, E. Ruosteenoja, A. S. Rosario, M. Tirmarche, L. Tomášek, E. Whitley, H. E. Wichmann, and R. Doll. (2005). "Radon in homes and risk of lung cancer: Collaborative analysis of individual data from 13 European case-control studies." British Medical Journal 330(7485): 223–226. doi: 10.1136/bmj.38308.477650.63.
Datta, R., T. M. Heaster, J. T. Sharick, A. A. Gillette, and M. C. Skala. (2020). "Fluorescence lifetime imaging microscopy: Fundamentals and advances in instrumentation, analysis, and applications." Journal of Biomedical Optics 25(7): 1–43. doi: 10.1117/1.JBO.25.7.071203.
Dauer, L. T., N. Hamada, and E. A. Blakely. (2017). "National Council on Radiation Protection and Measurements Commentary Number 26: Impact of revised guidance on radiation protection for the lens of the eye." Journal of the American College of Radiology 14(7): 980–982. doi: 10.1016/j.jacr.2017.05.003.
Davis, S., K. J. Kopecky, and T. Hamilton. (2002). Hanford Thyroid Disease Study: Final report. Seattle, Fred Hutchinson Cancer Research Center.
Dawson, S. E. (1992). "Navajo uranium workers and the effects of occupational illnesses: A case study." Human Organization 51(4): 389–397. doi: 10.17730/humo.51.4.e02484g513501t35.

Dawson, T. M., T. E. Golde, and C. Lagier-Tourenne. (2018). "Animal models of neurodegenerative diseases." Nature Neuroscience 21: 1370–1379. doi: 10.1038/s41593-018-0236-8.

Denkinger, M. D., H. Leins, R. Schirmbeck, M. C. Florian, and H. Geiger. (2015). "HSC aging and senescent immune remodeling." Trends in Immunology 36(12): 815–824. doi: 10.1016/j.it.2015.10.008.

Dhingra, R., and R. S. Vasan. (2017). "Biomarkers in cardiovascular disease: Statistical assessment and section on key novel heart failure biomarkers." Trends in Cardiovascular Medicine 27(2): 123–133. doi: 10.1016/j.tcm.2016.07.005.

DHS (Department of Homeland Security). (2016). Nuclear/Radiological Incident Annex to the Response and Recovery Federal Interagency Operational Plans. Washington, DC, Department of Homeland Security. https://www.fema.gov/sites/default/files/2020-07/fema_incident-annex_nuclear-radiological.pdf.

DiCarlo, A. L., A. C. Bandremer, B. A. Hollingsworth, S. Kasim, A. Laniyonu, N. F. Todd, S.-J. Wang, E. R. Wertheimer, and C. I. Rios. (2020). "Cutaneous radiation injuries: Models, assessment and treatments." Radiation Research 194(3): 315–344. doi: 10.1667/RADE-20-00120.1.

Dindaoğlu, T. (2014). "The use of the GIS Kriging technique to determine the spatial changes of natural radionuclide concentrations in soil and forest cover." Journal of Environmental Health Science and Engineering 12(1): 130. doi: 10.1186/s40201-014-0130-6.

Dobrzyński, L., K. W. Fornalski, and L. E. Feinendegen. (2015). "Cancer mortality among people living in areas with various levels of natural background radiation." Dose-Response 13(3): 1–10. doi: 10.1177/1559325815592391.

DOE (Department of Energy). (2020a). Report on the Status of the Runit Dome in the Marshall Islands: Report to Congress. https://www.energy.gov/sites/prod/files/2020/06/f76/DOE-Runit-Dome-Report-to-Congress.pdf.

DOE. (2020b). U.S. Department of Energy Announces $160 Million in First Awards Under Advanced Reactor Demonstration Program. https://www.energy.gov/ne/articles/us-department-energy-announces-160-million-first-awards-under-advanced-reactor.

DOE. (2021a). Biological Systems Science Division Strategic Plan. Washington, DC, DOE/SC-0205. U.S. Department of Energy Office of Science. https://science.osti.gov/-/media/ber/pdf/bssd/BSSD_Strategic_Plan_2021_HR.pdf.

DOE. (2021b). Science/Biological and Environmental Research FY 2022 Congressional Budget Request: Science. Washington, DC, Department of Energy. https://www.energy.gov/sites/default/files/2021-06/03%20BER%20Program%20Narrative%206_16_21.pdf.

DOE and EPA (Environmental Protection Agency). (1995). Policy on Decommissioning Department of Energy Facilities Under CERCLA. https://www.etec.energy.gov/Library/Main/1995DOE-EPAD&DMemo.pdf.

DOE EHHS Openness. (1995). Human Radiation Experiments: Oral Histories. https://ehss.energy.gov/ohre/roadmap/histories/0457/0457toc.html.

Doll, R., and R. Wakeford. (1997). "Risk of childhood cancer from fetal irradiation." British Journal of Radiology 70(830): 130–139. doi: 10.1259/bjr.70.830.9135438.

Donaubauer, A. J., I. Becker, T. Weissmann, B. M. Fröhlich, L. E. Muñoz, T. Gryc, M. Denzler, O. J. Ott, R. Fietkau, U. S. Gaipl, and B. Frey. (2021). "Low dose radiation therapy induces long-lasting reduction of pain and immune modulations in the peripheral blood—Interim analysis of the IMMO-LDRT01 Trial." Frontiers in Immunology 12: 740742. doi: 10.3389/fimmu.2021.740742. Erratum, Frontiers in Immunology 13: 859489 (2022). doi: 10.3389/fimmu.2022.859489.

DOT (Department of Transportation). (2021). Departmental Guidance on Valuation of a Statistical Life in Economic Analysis. Transportation Policy. https://www.transportation.gov/office-policy/transportation-policy/revised-departmental-guidance-on-valuation-of-a-statistical-life-in-economic-analysis.

Doudna, J. A. (2020). "The promise and challenge of therapeutic genome editing." Nature 578: 229–236. doi: 10.1038/s41586-020-1978-5.

Dron, L., A. Dillman, M. J. Zoratti, J. Haggstrom, E. J. Mills, and J. J. H. Park. (2021). "Clinical trial data sharing for COVID-19-related research." Journal of Medical Internet Research 23(3): e26718. doi: 10.2196/26718.

Duyx, B., M. J. E. Urlings, G. H. M. Swaen, L. M. Bouter, and M. P. Zeegers. (2017). "Scientific citations favor positive results: A systematic review and meta-analysis." Journal of Clinical Epidemiology 88: 92–101. doi: 10.1016/j.jclinepi.2017.06.002.

Dwivedi, R., D. Mehrotra, and S. Chandra. (2022). "Potential of Internet of Medical Things (IoMT) applications in building a smart healthcare system: A systematic review." Journal of Oral Biology and Craniofacial Research 12(2): 302–318. doi: 10.1016/j.jobcr.2021.11.010.

Ellis, M. J., and C. M. Perou. (2013). "The genomic landscape of breast cancer as a therapeutic roadmap." Cancer Discovery 3(1): 27–34. doi: 10.1158/2159-8290.CD-12-0462.

Ellis, M. J., M. Gillette, S. A. Carr, A. G. Paulovich, R. D. Smith, K. K. Rodland, R. R. Townsend, C. Kinsinger, M. Mesri, H. Rodriguez, D. C. Liebler, and Clinical Proteomic Tumor Analysis Consortium. (2013). "Connecting genomic alterations to cancer biology with proteomics: The NCI Clinical Proteomic Tumor Analysis Consortium." Cancer Discovery 3(10): 1108–1112. doi: 10.1158/2159-8290.CD-13-0219.

Elmaraezy, A., M. Ebraheem Morra, A. Tarek Mohammed, A. Al-Habaa, A. Elgebaly, A. Abdelmotaleb Ghazy, A. M. Khalil, N. Tien Huy, and K. Hirayama. (2017). "Risk of cataract among interventional cardiologists and catheterization lab staff: A systematic review and meta-analysis." Catheterization and Cardiovascular Interventions 90(1): 1–9. doi: 10.1002/ccd.27114.

EPA (Environmental Protection Agency). (1999). "Radon in drinking water health risk reduction and cost analysis." Federal Register 64: 9560–9599. https://www.govinfo.gov/content/pkg/FR-1999-02-26/pdf/99-4416.pdf.

EPA. (2003). EPA Assessment of Risks from Radon in Homes. Washington, DC, Office of Air and Radiation, Environmental Protection Agency. https://www.epa.gov/sites/default/files/2015-05/documents/402-r-03-003.pdf.

EPA. (2008). Technical Report on Technologically Enhanced Naturally Occurring Radioactive Materials from Uranium Mining, Vol. 1: Mining and Reclamation Background, and Vol. 2, Investigation of Potential Health, Geographic, and Environmental Issues of Abandoned Uranium Mines. https://nepis.epa.gov/Exe/ZyPDF.cgi/9100I3Y4.PDF?Dockey=9100I3Y4.PDF.

EPA. (2010). Guidelines for Preparing Economic Analyses. Washington, DC, Environmental Protection Agency. https://www.epa.gov/environmental-economics/guidelines-preparing-economic-analyses.

EPA. (2014). Distribution of the "Radiation Risk Assessment at CERCLA Sites: Q&A." https://nepis.epa.gov/Exe/ZyPDF.cgi/P100K3TC.PDF?Dockey=P100K3TC.PDF.

EPA. (2017). PAG Manual: Protective Action Guides and Planning Guidance for Radiological Incidents. Washington, DC, Office of Radiation and Indoor Air, Radiation Protection Division, Environmental Protection Agency. https://www.epa.gov/sites/default/files/2017-01/documents/epa_pag_manual_final_revisions_01-11-2017_cover_disclaimer_8.pdf.

EPA. (2018a). Home Buyer's and Seller's Guide to Radon. https://www.epa.gov/sites/default/files/2015-05/documents/hmbuygud.pdf.

EPA. (2018b). Working Together: FY 2018–2022 U.S. EPA Strategic Plan. Washington, DC, Office of Planning, Analysis, and Accountability, Office of the Chief Financial Officer, Environmental Protection Agency. https://www.epa.gov/sites/default/files/2018-02/documents/fy-2018-2022-epa-strategic-plan.pdf.

EPA. (2021). Notification of Evaluation: Process for Updating Federal Radiation Policies and Guidance Project No. OSRE-FY21-0208. https://www.epa.gov/system/files/documents/2021-07/_epaoig_notificationmemo_7-8-21_radiation.pdf.

EPA. (2022). Hotline: EPA Is Taking Steps to Update Its Federal Radiation Guidance Report No. 22-E-0016. https://www.epa.gov/system/files/documents/2022-01/_epaoig_20220106-22-e-0016.pdf.

EPRI (Electric Power Research Institute). (2011). Technical Considerations for NRC/National Academy Proposed Study of Cancer Risks in Populations Living Near Nuclear Facilities. Palo Alto, CA, Electric Power Research Institute.

EPRI. (2014). Epidemiology and Mechanistic Effects of Radiation on the Lens of the Eye: Review and Scientific Appraisal of the Literature. Palo Alto, CA, Electric Power Research Institute.

EPRI. (2020). Cardiovascular Risks from Low-Dose Radiation Exposure: Review and Scientific Appraisal of the Literature. Palo Alto, CA, Electric Power Research Institute.

FAA (Federal Aviation Administration). 2003. What Aircrews Should Know About Their Occupational Exposure to Ionizing Radiation. https://www.faa.gov/data_research/research/med_humanfacs/oamtechreports/2000s/media/0316.pdf.

Fantuzzi, E., M.-A. Chevallier, R. Cruz-Suarez, M. Luszik-Bhadra, S. Mayer, D. J. Thomas, R. Tanner, and F. Vanhavere. (2014). "EURADOS Intercomparison 2012 for Neutron Dosemeters." EURADOS Report 2014-02. Braunschweig, Germany, European Radiation Dosimetry Group. doi: 10.12768/kfkq-g944.

FDA (Food and Drug Administration). (1977). Chemical Compounds in Food Producing Animals: Criteria and Procedures for Evaluating Assays for Carcinogenic Residues in Edible Products of Animals. Federal Register 42: 10,412.

FDA. (1998). Mammography Quality Standards Act (MQSA) (As Amended by MQSRA of 1998 and 2004), Title 42—The Public Health and Welfare, Chapter 6A—Public Health Service, Subchapter II—General Powers and Duties, Part F—Licensing of Biological Products and Clinical, Laboratories, Subpart 3—Mammography Facilities. https://www.fda.gov/media/74251/download.

Feinberg, A. P., M. A. Koldobskiy, and A. Göndör. (2016). "Epigenetic modulators, modifiers and mediators in cancer aetiology and progression." Nature Reviews Genetics 17(5): 284–299. doi: 10.1038/nrg.2016.13.

Fernandez-Antoran, D., G. Piedrafita, K. Murai, S. H. Ong, A. Herms, C. Frezza, and P. H. Jones. (2019). "Outcompeting p53-mutant cells in the normal esophagus by redox manipulation." Cell Stem Cell 25(3): 329–341. doi: 10.1016/j.stem.2019.06.011.

Field, R. W., D. J. Steck, B. J. Smith, C. P. Brus, E. L. Fisher, J. S. Neuberger, C. E. Platz, R. A. Robinson, R. F. Woolson, and C. F. Lynch. (2000). "Residential radon gas exposure and lung cancer: The Iowa Radon Lung Cancer Study." American Journal of Epidemiology 151(11): 1091–1102. doi: 10.1093/oxfordjournals.aje.a010153.

Fischhoff, B., and A. L. Davis. (2014). "Communicating scientific uncertainty." Proceedings of the National Academy of Sciences of the United States of America 111: 13664–13671. doi: 10.1073/pnas.1317504111.

Fischhoff, B., and D. A. Scheufele. (2013). "The science of science communication: Introduction." Proceedings of the National Academy of Sciences of the United States of America 110(Suppl. 3): 14031–14032. doi: 10.1073/pnas.1312080110.

Fischhoff, B., and D. A. Scheufele. (2014). "The science of science communication II." Proceedings of the National Academy of Sciences of the United States of America 111(Suppl. 4): 13583–13584. doi: 10.1073/pnas.1414635111.

Fisher, D. R. (2021). "Perspectives on internal dosimetry for optimized radionuclide therapy." Cancer Biotherapy and Radiopharmaceuticals 37(3). doi: 10.1089/cbr.2021.0318.

Foox, J., J. Nordlund, C. Lalancette, T. Gong, M. Lacey, S. Lent, B. W. Langhorst, V. K. C. Ponnaluri, L. Williams, K. R. Padmanabhan, R. Cavalcante, A. Lundmark, D. Butler, C. Mozsary, J. Gurvitch, J. M. Greally, M. Suzuki, M. Menor, M. Nasu, A. Alonso, C. Sheridan, A. Scherer, S. Bruinsma, G. Golda, A. Muszynska, P. P. Łabaj, M. A. Campbell, F. Wos, A. Raine, U. Liljedahl, T. Axelsson, C. Wang, Z. Chen, Z. Yang, J. Li, X. Yang, H. Wang, A. Melnick, S. Guo, A. Blume, V. Franke, I. Ibanez de Caceres, C. Rodriguez-Antolin, R. Rosas, J. W. Davis, J. Ishii, D. B. Megherbi, W. Xiao, W. Liao, J. Xu, H. Hong, B. Ning, W. Tong, A. Akalin, Y. Wang, Y. Deng, and C. E. Mason. (2021). "The SEQC2 epigenomics quality control (EpiQC) study. Genome Biology 22(1): 332. doi: 10.1186/s13059-021-02529-2. Erratum, Genome Biology 22(1): 3502021 (2021). doi: 10.1186/s13059-021-02573-y.

Fournier, L., O. Laurent, E. Samson, S. Caër-Lorho, P. Laroche, B. Le Guen, D. Laurier, and K. Leuraud. (2016). "External radiation dose and cancer mortality among French nuclear workers: Considering potential confounding by internal radiation exposure." International Archives of Occupational and Environmental Health 89(8): 1183–1191. doi: 10.1007/s00420-016-1152-4.

FPG (Fukushima Prefectural Government). 2021. Fukushima Today: Steps for Reconstruction and Revitalization in Fukushima Prefecture. http://www.pref.fukushima.lg.jp/site/portal-english/ayumi-en-15.html.

Franceschi, C., R. Ostan, S. Mariotti, D. Monti, and G. Vitale. (2019). "The aging thyroid: A reappraisal within the geroscience integrated perspective." Endocrine Reviews 40(5): 1250–1270. doi: 10.1210/er.2018-00170.

Fulop, T., J. M. Witkowski, F. Olivieri, and A. Larbi (2018). "The integration of inflammaging in age-related diseases." Seminars in Immunology 40: 17–35. doi: 10.1016/j.smim.2018.09.003.

Fulwyler, M. J. (1965). "Electronic separation of biological cells by volume." Science 150(3698): 910–911. doi: 10.1126/science.150.3698.910.

Fulwyler, M. J. (1980). "Flow cytometry and cell sorting." Blood Cells 6(2): 173–184. PMID: 6155162.

GAO (Government Accountability Office). (1994). Report to the Chairman, Committee on Governmental Affairs, U.S. Senate—Nuclear Health and Safety: Consensus on Acceptable Radiation Risk to the Public Is Lacking. Washington, DC, General Accounting Office. https://www.gao.gov/assets/rced-94-190.pdf.

GAO. (2000). Radiation Standards: Scientific Basis Inconclusive, and EPA and NRC Disagreement Continues. https://www.gao.gov/products/rced-00-152.

GAO. (2017). Low-Dose Radiation: Interagency Collaboration on Planning Research Could Improve Information on Health Effects. https://www.gao.gov/assets/gao-17-546.pdf.

GAO. (2019). Department of Energy: Program-wide Strategy and Better Reporting Needed to Address Growing Environmental Cleanup Liability. Washington, DC, U.S. Government Publishing Office. https://www.gao.gov/assets/gao-19-28.pdf.

GAO. (2021). Department of Energy: Environmental Liability Continues to Grow, But Opportunities May Exist to Reduce Costs and Risks. https://www.gao.gov/assets/gao-21-585r.pdf.

Garnett, R. (2020). "A comprehensive review of dual-energy and multi-spectral computed tomography." Clinical Imaging 67: 160–169. doi: 10.1016/j.clinimag.2020.07.030.

Garty, G., Y. Xu, G. W. Johnson, L. B. Smilenov, S. K. Joseph, M. Pujol-Canadell, H. C. Turner, S. A. Ghandhi, Q. Wang, R. Shih, R. C. Morton, D. E. Cuniberti, S. R. Morton, C. Bueno-Beti, T. L. Morgan, P. F. Caracappa, E. C. Laiakis, A. J. Fornace, Jr., S. A. Amundson, and D. J. Brenner. (2020). "VADER: A variable dose-rate external 137Cs irradiator for internal emitter and low dose rate studies." Scientific Reports 10(1): 19899. doi: 10.1038/s41598-020-76941-2.

Garty, G., R. Obaid, N. Deoli, E. Royba, A. D. Harken, and D. J. Brenner. (2022). "FLASH irradiator at the Radiological Research Accelerator Facility." Scientific Reports. Available at https://www.researchsquare.com/article/rs-1281287/v1.

Geiger H. J. (1992). Dead Reckoning: A Critical Review of the Department of Energy's Epidemiologic Research. Washington, DC, Physicians for Social Responsibility.

Gessel, M. M., J. L. Norris, and R. M. Caprioli. (2014). "MALDI imaging mass spectrometry: Spatial molecular analysis to enable a new age of discovery." Journal of Proteomics 107: 71–82. doi: 10.1016/j.jprot.2014.03.021.

Gibbs, R. A. (2020). "The Human Genome Project changed everything." Nature Reviews Genetics 21: 575–576. doi: 10.1038/s41576-020-0275-3.

Gilbert, E. S., M. P. Little, D. L. Preston, and D. O. Stram. (2020). "Issues in interpreting epidemiologic studies of populations exposed to low-dose, high-energy photon radiation." JNCI Monographs 2020(56): 176–187. doi: 10.1093/jncimonographs/lgaa004.

Gillies, M., D. B. Richardson, E. Cardis, R. D. Daniels, J. A. O'Hagan, R. Haylock, D. Laurier, K. Leuraud, M. Moissonnier, M. K. Schubauer-Berigan, I. Thierry-Chef, and A. Kesminiene. (2017). "Mortality from circulatory diseases and other non-cancer outcomes among nuclear workers in France, the United Kingdom and the United States (INWORKS)." Radiation Research 188(3): 276–290. doi: 10.1667/RR14608.1.

Glionna, J. M. (2012). "A year after tsunami, a cloud of distrust hangs over Japan." Los Angeles Times, March 11.

Goecks, J., V. Jalili, L. M. Heiser, and J. W. Gray. (2020). "How machine learning will transform biomedicine." Cell 181(1): 92–101. doi: 10.1016/j.cell.2020.03.022.

Goldstein, B. D., M. Demak, M. Northridge, and D. Wartenberg. (1992). "Risk to groundlings of death due to airplane accidents: A risk communication tool." Risk Analysis 12(3): 339–341. doi: 10.1111/j.1539-6924.1992.tb00685.x.

Goldstein, B. D., C. Powers, J. Moore, and E. Faustman. (1999). "CRESP: A new approach to stakeholder-responsive, cost-effective research." European Journal of Oncology 4(5): 537–541.

Gomolka, M., B. Blyth, M. Bourguignon, C. Badie, A. Schmitz, C. Talbot, C. Hoeschen, and S. Salomaa. (2020). "Potential screening assays for individual radiation sensitivity and susceptibility and their current validation state." International Journal of Radiation Biology 96(3): 280–296. doi: 10.1080/09553002.2019.1642544.

Graham, J. D. (2021). The Global Rise of the Modern Plug-in Electric Vehicle: Public Policy, Innovation and Strategy. Northampton, MA, Edward Elgar.

Graham, J. D., L. Green, and M. J. Roberts. (1988). In Search of Safety: Chemicals and Cancer Risk. Cambridge, MA, Harvard University Press.

Graham, J. D. E., J. B. E. Wiener, E. Hatziandreu, C. Williams, M. E. Adams, H. Chang, H. S. Frazier, P. D. Anderson, S. W. Putnam, K. Walker, and G. M. Gray. (1995). Risk vs. Risk: Tradeoffs in Protecting Health and the Environment. Cambridge, MA, Harvard University Press.

Grajewski, B., E. A. Whelan, C. C. Lawson, M. J. Hein, M. A. Waters, J. L. Anderson, L. A. MacDonald, C. J. Mertens, C. Y. Tseng, R. T. Cassinelli II, and L. Luo. (2015). "Miscarriage among flight attendants." Epidemiology 26(2): 192–203. doi: 10.1097/EDE.0000000000000225.

Grajewski, B., L. C. Yong, S. J. Bertke, P. Bhatti, M. P. Little, M. J. Ramsey, J. D. Tucker, E. M. Ward, E. A. Whelan, A. J. Sigurdson, and M. A. Waters. (2018). "Chromosome translocations and cosmic radiation dose in male U.S. commercial airline pilots." Aerospace Medicine and Human Performance 89(7): 616–625. doi: 10.3357/AMHP.4502.2018.

Grant, E. J., K. Furukawa, R. Sakata, H. Sugiyama, A. Sadakane, I. Takahashi, M. Utada, Y. Shimizu, and K. Ozasa. (2015). "Risk of death among children of atomic bomb survivors after 62 years of follow-up: A cohort study." The Lancet: Oncology 16(13): 1316–1323. doi: 10.1016/S1470-2045(15)00209-0.

Grant, E. J., A. Brenner, H. Sugiyama, R. Sakata, A. Sadakane, M. Utada, E. K. Cahoon, C. M. Milder, M. Soda, H. M. Cullings, D. L. Preston, K. Mabuchi, and K. Ozasa. (2017). "Solid cancer incidence among the Life Span Study of atomic bomb survivors: 1958–2009." Radiation Research 187(5): 513–537. doi: 10.1667/RR14492.1.

Grant, E. J., M. Yamamura, A. V. Brenner, D. L. Preston, M. Utada, H. Sugiyama, R. Sakata, K. Mabuchi, and K. Ozasa. (2020). "Radiation risks for the incidence of kidney, bladder and other urinary tract cancers: 1958–2009." Radiation Research 195(2): 140–148. doi: 10.1667/RADE-20-00158.1.

Gray, J. W., P. N. Dean, J. C. Fuscoe, D. C. Peters, B. J. Trask, G. J. van den Engh, and M. A. Van Dilla. (1987). "High-speed chromosome sorting." Science 238(4825): 323–329. doi: 10.1126/science.2443974. PMID: 2443974.

Gray, J. W., J. N. Lucas, D. Pinkel, and A. Awa. (1992). "Structural chromosome analysis by whole chromosome painting for assessment of radiation-induced genetic damage." Journal of Radiation Research 33(Suppl.): 80–86. doi: 10.1269/jrr.33.supplement_80.

Greco, L., G. Percannella, P. Ritrovato, F. Tortorella, and M. Vento. (2020). "Trends in IoT based solutions for health care: Moving AI to the edge." Pattern Recognition Letters 135: 346–353. doi: 10.1016/j.patrec.2020.05.016.

Grilj, V., M. Buonanno, D. Welch, and D. J. Brenner. (2020). "Proton irradiation platforms for preclinical studies of high-dose-rate (FLASH) effects at RARAF." Radiation Research 194(6): 646–655.

Grosche, B., M. Kreuzer, M. Kreisheimer, M. Schnelzer, and A. Tschense. (2006). "Lung cancer risk among German male uranium miners: A cohort study, 1946–1998." British Journal of Cancer 95(9): 1280–1277. https://doi.org/10.1038/sj.bjc.6603403.

Gross, C. (2021). Estimate of EEOICPA Liabilities. https://www.dol.gov/sites/dolgov/files/owcp/energy/regs/compliance/public_reading_room/actuarial_report_fy21.pdf.Gross Consulting.

Gudzenko, N., K. Mabuchi, A. V. Brenner, M. P. Little, M. Hatch, V. Drozdovitch, V. Vij, V. Chumak, E. Bakhanova, N. Trotsyuk, V. Kryuchkov, I. Golovanov, D. Bazyka, and E. K. Cahoon. (2022). "Risk of thyroid cancer in Ukrainian cleanup workers following the Chornobyl accident." European Journal of Epidemiology 37(1): 67–77. doi: 10.1007/s10654-021-00822-9.

Gupta, K., M. C. Nowlin, J. T. Ripberger, H. C. Jenkins-Smith, and C. L. Silva. (2019). "Tracking the nuclear "mood" in the United States: Introducing a long term measure of public opinion about nuclear energy using aggregate survey data." Energy Policy 133: 110888. doi: 10.1016/j.enpol.2019.110888.

Haerer, H. A., M. D. Freshley, R. O. Gilbert, L. G. Morgan, B. A. Napier, R. E. Rhoads, and R. K. Woodruff. (1989). The Hanford Environmental Dose Reconstruction Project: Overview. https://www.osti.gov/servlets/purl/5478757.

Hamada, N., M. Maeda, K. Otsuka, and M. Tomita. (2011). "Signaling pathways underpinning the manifestations of ionizing radiation-induced bystander effects." Current Molecular Pharmacology 4: 79–95. doi: 10.2174/1874467211104020079.

Hamada, N., T. V. Azizova, and M. P. Little. (2020). "An update on effects of ionizing radiation exposure on the eye." British Journal of Radiology 93(1115): 20190829. doi: 10.1259/bjr.20190829.

Hammer, G. P., M. Blettner, and H. Zeeb. (2009). "Epidemiological studies of cancer in aircrew." Radiation Protection Dosimetry 136(4): 232–239. doi: 10.1093/rpd/ncp125.

Hampel, H., A. Vergallo, F. Caraci, A. C. Cuello, P. Lemercier, B. Vellas, K. V. Giudici, F. Baldacci, B. Hänisch, M. Haberkamp, K. Broich, R. Nisticò, E. Emanuele, F. Llavero, J. L. Zugaza, A. Lucía, E. Giacobini, and S. Lista; Alzheimer Precision Medicine Initiative. (2021). "Future avenues for Alzheimer's disease detection and therapy: Liquid biopsy, intracellular signaling modulation, systems pharmacology drug discovery." Neuropharmacology 185: 108081. doi: 10.1016/j.neuropharm.2020.108081.

Hanahan, D. (2022). "Hallmarks of cancer: New dimensions." Cancer Discovery 12(1): 31–46. doi: 10.1158/2159-8290.CD-21-1059.

Hanahan, D., and R. A. Weinberg. (2011). "Hallmarks of cancer: The next generation." Cell 144(5): 646–674. doi: 10.1016/j.cell.2011.02.013.

Hansson, O. (2021). "Biomarkers for neurodegenerative diseases." Nature Medicine 27(6): 954–963. doi: 10.1038/s41591-021-01382-x.

Harding, S. M., J. L. Benci, J. Irianto, D. E. Discher, A. J. Minn, and R. A. Greenberg. (2017). "Mitotic progression following DNA damage enables pattern recognition within micronuclei." Nature 548(7668): 466–470. doi: 10.1038/nature23470.

Härtlova, A., S. F. Erttmann, F. A. Raffi, A. M. Schmalz, U. Resch, S. Anugula, S. Lienenklaus, L. M. Nilsson, A. Kröger, J. A. Nilsson, T. Ek, S. Weiss, and N. O. Gekara. (2015). "DNA damage primes the type I interferon system via the cytosolic DNA sensor STING to promote anti-microbial innate immunity." Immunity 42(2): 332–343. doi: 10.1016/j.immuni.2015.01.012. PMID: 25692705.

Hauptmann, M., R. D. Daniels, E. Cardis, H. M. Cullings, G. M. Kendall, D. Laurier, M. S. Linet, M. P. Little, J. H. Lubin, D. L. Preston, D. B. Richardson, D. O. Stram, I. Thierry-Chef, M. K. Schubauer-Berigan, E. S. Gilbert, and A. Berrington de Gonzalez. (2020). "Epidemiological studies of low-dose ionizing radiation and cancer: Summary bias assessment and meta-analysis." Journal of the National Cancer Institute Monographs 2020(56): 188–200. doi: 10.1093/jncimonographs/lgaa010.

Hayashi, T., H. E. Lynch, S. Geyer, K. Yoshida, K. Furudoi, K. Sasaki, Y. Morishita, H. Nagamura, M. Maki, Y. Hu, I. Hayashi, S. Kyoizumi, Y. Kusunoki, W. Ohishi, S. Fujiwara, M. Misumi, I. Shterev, J. Nikolich-Žugich, D. Murasko, L. P. Hale, G. D. Sempowski, and K. Nakachi. (2018). "Impact of early life exposure to ionizing radiation on influenza vaccine response in an elderly Japanese cohort." Vaccine 36(45): 6650–6659. doi: 10.1016/j.vaccine.2018.09.054.

Hayata, I., C. Wang, W. Zhang, D. Chen, M. Minamihisamatsu, H. Morishima, L. Wei, and T. Sugahara. (2004). "Effect of high-level natural radiation on chromosomes of residents in southern China." Cytogenetic and Genome Research 104(1–4): 237–239. doi: 10.1159/000077496.

Haylock, R. G. E., M. Gillies, N. Hunter, W. Zhang, and M. Phillipson. (2018). "Cancer mortality and incidence following external occupational radiation exposure: An update of the 3rd analysis of the UK national registry for radiation workers." British Journal of Cancer 119: 631–637. doi: 10.1038/s41416-018-0184-9.

Heeb, C. M., S. P. Gydesen, J. C. Simpson, and D. J. Bates. (1996). "Reconstruction of radionuclide releases from the Hanford Site, 1944–1972." Health Physics 71(4): 545–555. doi: 10.1097/00004032-199610000-00012.

Heinävaara, S., S. Toikkanen, K. Pasanen, P. K. Verkasalo, P. Kurttio, and A. Auvinen (2010). "Cancer incidence in the vicinity of Finnish nuclear power plants: An emphasis on childhood leukemia." Cancer Causes and Control 21(4): 587–595. doi: 10.1007/s10552-009-9488-7.

Hendry, J. H., M. Sohrabi, W. Burkart, S. L. Simon, A. Wojcik, E. Cardis, D. Laurier, M. Tirmarche, and I. Hayata. (2009). "Human exposure to high natural background radiation: What can it teach us about radiation risks?" Journal of Radiological Protection 29(2): A29–A42. doi: 10.1088/0952-4746/29/2A/S03.

Herzenberg, L. A., R. G. Sweet, and L. A. Herzenberg. (1976). "Fluorescence-activated cell sorting." Scientific American 234(3): 108–117. doi: 10.1038/scientificamerican0376-108.

HHS (Department of Health and Human Services). (2016). Guidelines for Regulatory Impact Analysis. Washington, DC, Department of Health and Human Services.

Hladik, D., and S. Tapio. (2016). "Effects of ionizing radiation on the mammalian brain." Mutation Research: Reviews in Mutation Research 770(Pt. B): 219–230. doi: 10.1016/j.mrrev.2016.08.003.

Hoadley, K. A., C. Yau, T. Hinoue, D. M. Wolf, A. J. Lazar, E. Drill, R. Shen, A. M. Taylor, A. D. Cherniack, V. Thorsson, R. Akbani, R. Bowlby, C. K. Wong, M. Wiznerowicz, F. Sanchez-Vega, A. G. Robertson, B. G. Schneider, M. S. Lawrence, H. Noushmehr, and T. M. Malta, Cancer Genome Atlas Network; J. M. Stuart, C. C. Benz, and P. W. Laird. (2018). "Cell-of-origin patterns dominate the molecular classification of 10,000 tumors from 33 types of cancer." Cell 173(2): 291–304. doi: 10.1016/j.cell.2018.03.022.

Hoffman, F. O., A. I. Apostoae, and B. A. Thomas. (2001). "A perspective on public concerns about exposure to fallout from the production and testing of nuclear weapons." Presented at 2001 Annual Meeting of the National Council on Radiation Protection and Measurements. https://www3.nd.edu/~kshrader/interest/NCRP.pdf.

Holaday, D. A., and H. N. Doyle. (1964). "Environmental studies in the uranium mines." Radiological Health and Safety in Mining and Milling of Nuclear Materials (Vienna, 26–31 Aug. 1963), Proceeding Series—International Atomic Energy Agency, pp. 9–20. Vienna, Austria, International Atomic Energy Agency.

Hornhardt, S., M. Gomolka, L. Walsh, and T. Jung. (2006). "Comparative investigations of sodium arsenite, arsenic trioxide and cadmium sulphate in combination with gamma-radiation on apoptosis, micronuclei induction and DNA damage in a human lymphoblastoid cell line." Mutation Research: Fundamental and Molecular Mechanisms of Mutagenesis 600(1): 165–176. doi: 10.1016/j.mrfmmm.2006.04.002.

Howell, E. (2021). "Space tourism took a giant leap in 2021: Here's 10 milestones from the year." https://www.space.com/space-tourism-giant-leap-2021-milestones.

HPA (Health Protection Agency). (2010). Circulatory Disease Risk Report of the Independent Advisory Group on Ionising Radiation. https://eprints.whiterose.ac.uk/86824/1/RCE-16_for_web.pdf.

HPS (Health Physics Society). (2021). Report of the Health Physics Society Research Needs Task Force. Herndon, VA, Health Physics Society.

Hu, A. E., B. French, R. Sakata, P. Bhatti, B. Bockwoldt, E. J. Grant, and A. I. Phipps. (2021). "The possible impact of passive smoke exposure on radiation-related risk estimates for lung cancer among women: The Life Span Study of Atomic Bomb Survivors." International Journal of Radiatiation Biology 97(11): 1548–1554. doi: 10.1080/09553002.2021.1976863.

Huang, C., Y. R. Neupane, X. C. Lim, R. Shekhani, B. Czarny, M. G. Wacker, G. Pastorin, and J. W. Wang. (2021). "Extracellular vesicles in cardiovascular disease." Advances in Clinical Chemistry 103: 47–95. doi: 10.1016/bs.acc.2020.08.006.

Huang, Q., F. Li, X. Liu, W. Li, W. Shi, F. F. Liu, B. O'Sullivan, Z. He, Y. Peng, A. C. Tan, L. Zhou, J. Shen, G. Han, X. J. Wang, J. Thorburn, A. Thorburn, A. Jimeno, D. Raben, J. S. Bedford, and C. Y. Li. (2011). "Caspase 3-mediated stimulation of tumor cell repopulation during cancer radiotherapy." Nature Medicine 17(7): 860–866. doi: 10.1038/nm.2385.

Huang, Y. F., K. Aoki, S. Akase, M. Ishihara, Y. S. Liu, G. Yang, Y. Kizuka, S. Mizumoto, M. Tiemeyer, X. D. Gao, K. F. Aoki-Kinoshita, and M. Fujita. (2021). "Global mapping of glycosylation pathways in human-derived cells." Developmental Cell 56(8): 1195–1209. doi: 10.1016/j.devcel.2021.02.023.

HuBMAP Consortium. (2019). "The human body at cellular resolution: The NIH Human Biomolecular Atlas Program." Nature 574(7777): 187–192. doi: 10.1038/s41586-019-1629-x.

Hussmann, J. A., J. Ling, P. Ravisankar, J. Yan, A. Cirincione, A. Xu, D. Simpson, D. Yang, A. Bothmer, C. Cotta-Ramusino, J. S. Weissman, and B. Adamson. (2021). "Mapping the genetic landscape of DNA double-strand break repair. Cell 184(22): 5653–5669. doi: 10.1016/j.cell.2021.10.002.

IAEA (International Atomic Energy Agency). (2018). Radiation Protection and Safety in Medical Uses of Ionizing Radiation. https://www-pub.iaea.org/MTCD/Publications/PDF/PUB1775_web.pdf.

IAEA. (2021). Patient Radiation Exposure Monitoring in Medical Imaging. Safety Report Series. Vienna, Austria, International Atomic Energy Agency.

IARC (International Agency for Research on Cancer). (2018). Thyroid Health Monitoring After Nuclear Accidents. IARC Technical Publication No. 46. http://publications.iarc.fr/Book-And-Report-Series/Iarc-Technical-Publications/Thyroid-Health-Monitoring-AfterNuclear-Accidents-2018.

ICGC (International Cancer Genome Consortium). (2010). "International network of cancer genome projects." Nature 464(7291): 993–998. doi: 10.1038/nature08987. Erratum, Nature 465(7300): 966 (2010).

ICRP (International Commission on Radiological Protection). (1975). Report of the Task Group on Reference Man. ICRP Publication 23. Oxford, UK, Pergamon Press.

ICRP. (1977). "Recommendations of the International Commission on Radiological Protection (ICRP Publication 26)." Annals of the ICRP 1(3).

ICRP. (1979). "Limits for intakes of radionuclides by workers (ICRP Publication 30, Part 1, including addendum)." Annals of the ICRP 2(3–4).

ICRP. (1991). "1990 Recommendations of the International Commission on Radiological Protection (ICRP Publication 60)." Annals of the ICRP 21(1–3).

ICRP. (1994). "Human respiratory tract model for radiological protection: A report of a task group of the International Commission on Radiological Protection (ICRP Publication 66)." Annals of the ICRP 24(1–3).

ICRP. (1995). "Age-dependent doses to members of the public from intake of radionuclides—Part 3, ingestion dose coefficients (ICRP Publication 69)." Annals of the ICRP 25(1).

ICRP. (1996). "Radiological protection and safety in medicine (ICRP Publication 73)." Annals of the ICRP 26(2).

ICRP. (2007). "The 2007 recommendations of the International Commission on Radiological Protection (ICRP Publication 103)." Annals of the ICRP 37(2–4). https://journals.sagepub.com/doi/pdf/10.1177/ANIB_37_2-4.

ICRP. (2009). "Adult reference computational phantoms (ICRP Publication 110)." Annals of the ICRP 39(2).

ICRP. (2012). "ICRP statement on tissue reactions/early and late effects of radiation in normal tissues and organs: Threshold doses for tissue reactions in a radiation protection context (ICRP Publication 118)." Annals of the ICRP 41(1–2). http://journals.sagepub.com/doi/pdf/10.1177/ANIB_41_1–2.

ICRP. (2015). "Occupational intakes of radionuclides: Part 1 (ICRP Publication 130)." Annals of the ICRP 44(2).

ICRP. (2016a). "Occupational intakes of radionuclides: Part 2 (ICRP Publication 134)." Annals of the ICRP 45(3/4): 1–352.

ICRP. (2016b). "The ICRP computational framework for internal dose assessment for reference adults: Specific absorbed fractions (ICRP Publication 133)." Annals of the ICRP 45(2): 1–74.

ICRP. (2020). "Adult mesh-type reference computational phantoms (ICRP Publication 145)." Annals of the ICRP 49(3).

Ilienko, I. M., N. A. Golyarnik, O. V. Lyaskivska, O. A. Belayev, and D. A. Bazyka. (2018). "Expression of biological markers induced by ionizing radiation at the late period after exposure in a wide range of doses." Problems of Radiation Medicine and Radiobiology 23: 331–350. doi: 10.33145/2304-8336-2018-23-331-350.

Ingólfsson, H. I., C. Neale, T. S. Carpenter, R. Shrestha, C. A. López, T. H. Tran, T. Oppelstrup, H. Bhatia, L. G. Stanton, X. Zhang, S. Sundram, F. Di Natale, A. Agarwal, G. Dharuman, S. I. L. Kokkila Schumacher, T. Turbyville, G. Gulten, Q. N. Van, D. Goswami, F. Jean-Francois, C. Agamasu, D. Chen, J. J. Hettige, T. Travers, S. Sarkar, M. P. Surh, Y. Yang, A. Moody, S. Liu, B. C. Van Essen, A. F. Voter, A. Ramanathan, N. W. Hengartner, D. K. Simanshu, A. G. Stephen, P. T. Bremer, S. Gnanakaran, J. N. Glosli, F. C. Lightstone, F. McCormick, D. V. Nissley, and F. H. Streitz. (2022). "Machine learning-driven multiscale modeling reveals lipid-dependent dynamics of RAS signaling proteins." Proceedings of the National Academy of Sciences of the United States of America 119(1): e2113297119. doi: 10.1073/pnas.2113297119.

IOM (Institute of Medicine). (1999). Toward Environmental Justice: Research, Education, and Health Policy Needs. Washington, DC, National Academy Press. doi: 10.17226/6034.

IOM. (2006). Valuing Health for Regulatory Cost-Effectiveness Analysis. Washington, DC, The National Academies Press.

IOM and NRC (National Research Council). (2014). Research on Health Effects of Low-Level Ionizing Radiation Exposure: Opportunities for the Armed Forces Radiobiology Research Institute. Washington, DC, The National Academies Press.

Ishida, Y., T. Takabatake, S. Kakinuma, K. Doi, K. Yamauchi, M. Kaminishi, S. Kito, Y. Ohta, Y. Amasaki, H. Moritake, T. Kokubo, M. Nishimura, T. Nishikawa, O. Hino, and Y. Shimada. (2010). "Genomic and gene expression signatures of radiation in medulloblastomas after low-dose irradiation in Ptch1 heterozygous mice." Carcinogenesis 31(9): 1694–1701. doi: 10.1093/carcin/bgq145.

Jablon, S., Z. Hrubec, and J. D. Boice, Jr. (1991). "Cancer in populations living near nuclear facilities: A survey of mortality nationwide and incidence in two states." Journal of the American Medical Association 265(11): 1403–1408. doi: 10.1001/jama.1991.03460110069026.

JCER (Japan Center for Economic Research). (2019). Follow Up Report of Public Financial Burden of the Fukushima Nuclear Accident. Tokyo, Japan Center for Economic Research. https://www.jcer.or.jp/english/accident-cleanup-costsrising-to-35-80-trillion-yen-in-40-years.

Jenkins-Smith, H. C., C. L. Silva, K. Gupta, and R. P. Rechard. (2017). Public Preferences Related to Radioactive Waste Management in the United States: Methodology and Response Reference Report for the 2016 Energy and Environment Survey, Sandia National Laboratories.

Jenuwein, T., and C. D. Allis. (2001). "Translating the histone code." Science 293(5532): 1074–1080. doi: 10.1126/science.1063127.

Jeong, M., Y.-W. Jin, K.H. Yang, Y.-O. Ahn, and C.-Y. Cha. (2010). "Radiation exposure and cancer incidence in a cohort of nuclear power industry workers in the Republic of Korea, 1992–2005." Radiation and Environmental Biophysics 49(1): 47–55. doi: 10.1007/s00411-009-0247-7.

Jeukens, C. R. L. P. N., H. Boere, B. A. J. M. Wagemans, P. J. Nelemans, E. C. Nijssen, R. Smith-Bindman, J. E. Wildberger, and A. M. Sailer (2021). "Probability of receiving a high cumulative radiation dose and primary clinical indication of CT examinations: A 5-year observational cohort study." BMJ Open 11(1): e041883. doi: 10.1136/bmjopen-2020-041883.

Jia, T., C. Wang, Z. Han, X. Wang, M. Ding, and Q. Wang. (2020). "Experimental rodent models of cardiovascular diseases." Frontiers in Cardiovascular Medicine 7: 588075. doi: 10.3389/fcvm.2020.588075.

Jiang, J. X., M. A. Makary, and G. Bai. (2022). "Commercial negotiated prices for CMS-specified shoppable radiology services in U.S. hospitals." Radiology 302(3): 622–624. doi: 10.1148/radiol.2021211948.

Johnson, B. E., A. L. Creason, J. M. Stommel, J. M. Keck, S. Parmar, C. B. Betts, A. Blucher, C. Boniface, E. Bucher, E. Burlingame, T. Camp, K. Chin, J. Eng, J. Estabrook, H. S. Feiler, M. B. Heskett, Z. Hu, A. Kolodzie, B. L. Kong, M. Labrie, J. Lee, P. Leyshock, S. Mitri, J. Patterson, J. L. Riesterer, S. Sivagnanam, J. Somers, D. Sudar, G. Thibault, B. R. Weeder, C. Zheng, X. Nan, R. F. Thompson, L. M. Heiser, P. T. Spellman, G. Thomas, E. Demir, Y. H. Chang, L. M. Coussens, A. R. Guimaraes, C. Corless, J. Goecks, R. Bergan, Z. Mitri, G. B. Mills, and J. W. Gray. (2022). "An omic and multidimensional spatial atlas from serial biopsies of an evolving metastatic breast cancer." Cell Reports Medicine 3(2): 100525. doi: 10.1016/j.xcrm.2022.100525.

Johnson, J. (2019). "Can nuclear power help save us from climate change?" Chemical and Engineering News 97(37): 18–19. https://pubs.acs.org/doi/10.1021/cen-09737-feature2.

Jones, C. B., C. M. Davis, and K. S. Sfanos. (2020). "The potential effects of radiation on the gut-brain axis." Radiation Research 193(3): 209–222. doi: 10.1667/RR15493.1.

Jumper, J., R. Evans, A. Pritzel, T. Green, M. Figurnov, O. Ronneberger, K. Tunyasuvunakool, R. Bates, A. Žídek, A. Potapenko, A. Bridgland, C. Meyer, S. A. A. Kohl, A. J. Ballard, A. Cowie, B. Romera-Paredes, S. Nikolov, R. Jain, J. Adler, T. Back, S. Petersen, D. Reiman, E. Clancy, M. Zielinski, M. Steinegger, M. Pacholska, T. Berghammer, S. Bodenstein, D. Silver, O. Vinyals, A. W. Senior, K. Kavukcuoglu, P. Kohli, and D. Hassabis. (2021). "Highly accurate protein structure prediction with AlphaFold." Nature 596(7873): 583–589. doi: 10.1038/s41586-021-03819-2.

Kaatsch, P., C. Spix, R. Schulze-Rath, S. Schmiedel, and M. Blettner. (2008). "Leukaemia in young children living in the vicinity of German nuclear power plants." International Journal of Cancer 122(4): 721–726. doi: 10.1002/ijc.23330.

Kaiser, J. C., R. Meckbach, and P. Jacob. (2014). "Genomic instability and radiation risk in molecular pathways to colon cancer." PLoS ONE 9(10): e111024. doi: 10.1371/journal.pone.0111024.

Kataoka, M., M. Honda, A. Ohashi, K. Yamaguchi, N. Mori, M. Goto, T. Fujioka, M. Mori, Y. Kato, H. Satake, M. Iima, and K. Kubota. (2022). "Ultrafast dynamic contrast-enhanced MRI of the breast: How is it used?" Magnetic Resonance in Medical Sciences 21(1): 83–94. doi: 10.2463/mrms.rev.2021-0157.

Kato, T. A., H. Nagasawa, M. M. Weil, J. B. Little, and J. S. Bedford. (2006). "Levels of γ-H2AX foci after low-dose-rate irradiation reveal a DNA DSB rejoining defect in cells from human ATM heterozygotes in two AT families and in another apparently normal individual." Radiation Research 166(3): 443–453. doi: 10.1667/RR3604.1.

Kato, T. A., P. F. Wilson, H. Nagasawa, M. M. Fitzek, M. M. Weil, J. B. Little, and J. S. Bedford. (2007). "A defect in DNA double strand break processing in cells from unaffected parents of retinoblastoma patients and other apparently normal humans." DNA Repair 6: 818–829. doi: 10.1016/j.dnarep.2007.01.008.

Keenan, A. B., S. L. Jenkins, K. M. Jagodnik, S. Koplev, E. He, D. Torre, Z. Wang, A. B. Dohlman, M. C. Silverstein, A. Lachmann, M. V. Kuleshov, A. Ma'ayan, V. Stathias, R. Terryn, D. Cooper, M. Forlin, A. Koleti, D. Vidovic, C. Chung, S. C. Schürer, J. Vasiliauskas, M. Pilarczyk, B. Shamsaei, M. Fazel, Y. Ren, W. Niu, N. A. Clark, S. White, N. Mahi, L. Zhang, M. Kouril, J. F. Reichard, S. Sivaganesan, M. Medvedovic, J. Meller, R. J. Koch, M. R. Birtwistle, R. Iyengar, E. A. Sobie, E. U. Azeloglu, J. Kaye, J. Osterloh, K. Haston, J. Kalra, S. Finkbiener, J. Li, P. Milani, M. Adam, R. Escalante-Chong, K. Sachs, A. Lenail, D. Ramamoorthy, E. Fraenkel, G. Daigle, U. Hussain, A. Coye, J. Rothstein, D. Sareen, L. Ornelas, M. Banuelos, B. Mandefro, R. Ho, C. N. Svendsen, R. G. Lim, J. Stocksdale, M. S. Casale, T. G. Thompson, J. Wu, L. M. Thompson, V. Dardov, V. Venkatraman, A. Matlock, J. E. Van Eyk, J. D. Jaffe, Malvina Papanastasiou, A. Subramanian,

T. R. Golub, S. D. Erickson, M. Fallahi-Sichani, M. Hafner, N. S. Gray, J.-R. Lin, C. E. Mills, J. L. Muhlich, M. Niepel, C. E. Shamu, E. H Williams, D. Wrobel, P. K. Sorger, L. M. Heiser, J. W. Gray, J. E. Korkola, G. B. Mills, M. LaBarge, H. S. Feiler, M. A. Dane, E. Bucher, M. Nederlof, D. Sudar, S. Gross, D. F. Kilburn, R. Smith, K. Devlin, R. Margolis, L. Derr, A. Lee, and A. Pillai. (2018). "The Library of Integrated Network-Based Cellular Signatures NIH Program: System-Level Cataloging of Human Cells Response to Perturbations." Cell Systems 6(1): 13–24. doi: 10.1016/j.cels.2017.11.001.

Kendall, G. M., M. P. Little, R. Wakeford, K. J. Bunch, J. C. Miles, T. J. Vincent, J. R. Meara, and M. F. Murphy (2013). "A record-based case-control study of natural background radiation and the incidence of childhood leukaemia and other cancers in Great Britain during 1980–2006." Leukemia 27(1): 3–9. doi: 10.1038/leu.2012.151.

Keogh, R. H., P. A. Shaw, P. Gustafson, R. J. Carroll, V. Deffner, K. W. Dodd, H. Küchenhoff, J. A. Tooze, M. P. Wallace, V. Kipnis, and L. S. Freedman. (2020). "STRATOS guidance document on measurement error and misclassification of variables in observational epidemiology: Part 1—Basic theory and simple methods of adjustment." Statistics in Medicine 39(16): 2197–2231. doi: 10.1002/sim.8532.

Kim, R. S. (2015). "A new comparison of nested case-control and case-cohort designs and methods." European Journal of Epidemiology 30(3): 197–207. doi: 10.1007/s10654-014-9974-4.

Kim, S. H., J. M. Park, and H. Kim. (2020). "The prevalence of stroke according to indoor radon concentration in South Koreans: Nationwide cross section study." Medicine (Baltimore) 99(4): e18859. doi: 10.1097/MD.0000000000018859.

Kitahara, C. M., M. S. Linet, P. Rajaraman, E. Ntowe, and A. Berrington de González. (2015). "A new era of low-dose radiation epidemiology." Current Environmental Health Reports 2(3): 236–249. doi: 10.1007/s40572-015-0055-y.

Kitahara, C. M., D. L. Preston, G. Neta, M. P. Little, M. M. Doody, S. L. Simon, A. J. Sigurdson, B. H. Alexander, and M. S. Linet. (2018). "Occupational radiation exposure and thyroid cancer incidence in a cohort of U.S. radiologic technologists, 1983–2013." International Journal of Cancer 143(9): 2145–2149. doi: 10.1002/ijc.31270.

Kitamura, H., T. Okubo, K. Kodama, and the Nuclear Emergency Workers Study Group. (2018). "Epidemiological study of health effects in Fukushima nuclear emergency workers—Study design and progress report." Radiation Protection Dosimetry 182(1): 40–48. doi: 10.1093/rpd/ncy136.

Kocakavuk, E., K. J. Anderson, F. S. Varn, K. C. Johnson, S. B. Amin, E. P. Sulman, M. P. Lolkema, F. P. Barthel, and R. G. W. Verhaak. (2021). "Radiotherapy is associated with a deletion signature that contributes to poor outcomes in patients with cancer." Nature Genetics 53(7): 1088–1096. doi: 10.1038/s41588-021-00874-3.

Kodaira, M., H. Ryo, N. Kamada, N. Takahashi, H. Nakajima, T. Nomura, and N. Nakamura. (2010). "No evidence of increased mutation rates at microsatellite loci in offspring of A-bomb survivors." Radiation Research 173: 205–213. doi: 10.1667/RR1991.1.

Kreuzer, M., and S. Bouffler. (2021). "Guest editorial: Non-cancer effects of ionizing radiation—Clinical implications, epidemiological and mechanistic evidence and research gaps." Environment International 149: 106286. doi: 10.1016/j.envint.2020.106286.

Kreuzer, M., C. Sobotzki, M. Schnelzer, and N. Fenske. (2018). "Factors modifying the radon-related lung cancer risk at low exposures and exposure rates among German uranium miners. Radiation Research 189(2): 165–176. doi: 10.1667/RR14889.1.

Krewski, D., J. H. Lubin, J. M. Zielinski, M. Alavanja, V. S. Catalan, R. W. Field, J. B. Klotz, E. G. Létourneau, C. F. Lynch, J. L. Lyon, D. P. Sandler, J. B. Schoenberg, D. J. Steck, J. A. Stolwijk, C. Weinberg, and H. B. Wilcox. (2006). "A combined analysis of North American case-control studies of residential radon and lung cancer." Journal of Toxicology and Environmental Health Part A: Current Issues 69(7): 533–597. doi: 10.1080/15287390500260945.

Kungulovski, G., and A. Jeltsch. (2016). "Epigenome editing: State of the art, concepts, and perspectives." Trends in Genetics 32(2): 101–113. doi: 10.1016/j.tig.2015.12.001.

Kuntz, R. E., E. M. Antman, R. M. Califf, J. R. Ingelfinger, H. M. Krumholz, A. Ommaya, E. D. Peterson, J. S. Ross, J. Waldstreicher, S. V. Wang, D. A. Zarin, D. M. Whicher, S. M. Siddiqi, and M. Hamilton Lopez. (2019). "Individual patient-level data sharing for continuous learning: A strategy for trial data sharing." NAM Perspectives. Discussion Paper, Washington, DC, National Academy of Medicine, doi: 10.31478/201906b.

Kusunoki, Y., and T. Hayashi. (2008). "Long-lasting alterations of the immune system by ionizing radiation exposure: Implications for disease development among atomic bomb survivors." International Journal of Radiation Biology 84(1): 1–14. doi: 10.1080/09553000701616106.

Kusunoki, Y., M. Yamaoka, F. Kasagi, T. Hayashi, D. G. MacPhee, and S. Kyoizumi. (2003). "Long-lasting changes in the T-cell receptor V beta repertoires of CD4 memory T-cell populations in the peripheral blood of radiation-exposed people." British Journal of Haematology 122(6): 975–984. doi: 10.1046/j.1365-2141.2003.04520.x.

Kwan, M. L., D. L. Miglioretti, E. C. Marlow, E. J. Aiello Bowles, S. Weinmann, S. Y. Cheng, K. A. Deosaransingh, P. Chavan, L. M. Moy, W. E. Bolch, J. R. Duncan, R. T. Greenlee, L. H. Kushi, J. D. Pole, A. K. Rahm, N. K. Stout, and R. Smith-Bindman; Radiation-Induced Cancers Study Team. (2019). "Trends in medical imaging during pregnancy in the United States and Ontario, Canada, 1996 to 2016." JAMA Network Open 2(7): e197249. doi: 10.1001/jamanetworkopen.2019.7249.

Kwon, D., F. O. Hoffman, B. E. Moroz, and S. L. Simon. (2016). "Bayesian dose-response analysis for epidemiological studies with complex uncertainty in dose estimation." Statistics in Medicine 35(3): 399–423. doi: 10.1002/sim.6635.

Kyoizumi, S., M. Yamaoka, Y. Kubo, K. Hamasaki, T. Hayashi, K. Nakachi, F. Kasagi, and Y. Kusunoki. (2010). "Memory CD4 T-cell subsets discriminated by CD43 expression level in A-bomb survivors." International Journal of Radiation Biology 86(1): 56–62. doi: 10.3109/09553000903272641.

La Tessa, C., M. Sivertz, I. H. Chiang, D. Lowenstein, and A. Rusek. (2016). "Overview of the NASA space radiation laboratory." Life Sciences in Space Research 11: 18–23. doi: 10.1016/j.lssr.2016.10.002.

Lanekoff, I., V. V. Sharma, and C. Marques. (2022). "Single-cell metabolomics: Where are we and where are we going?" Current Opinion in Biotechnology 75: 102693. doi: 10.1016/j.copbio.2022.102693.

Langholz, B., and D. C. Thomas. (1990). "Nested case-control and case-cohort methods of sampling from a cohort: A critical comparison. American Journal of Epidemiology 131(1): 169–176. doi: 10.1093/oxfordjournals.aje.a115471.

Larsen, S. B., C. J. Cowley, S. M. Sajjath, D. Barrows, Y. Yang, T. S. Carroll, and E. Fuchs. (2021). "Establishment, maintenance, and recall of inflammatory memory." Cell Stem Cell 28(10): 1758–1774. doi: 10.1016/j.stem.2021.07.001.

Laurier, D., W. Rühm, F. Paquet, K. Applegate, D. Cool, C. Clement, and International Commission on Radiological Protection. (2021). "Areas of research to support the system of radiological protection." Radiation and Environmental Biophysics 60(4): 519–530. doi: 10.1007/s00411-021-00947-1.

Lave, L. B. (1981). The Strategy of Social Regulation. Washington, DC, Brookings Institution.

Lee, B., J. Sung, M. Yoon, and S. Lee. (2014). "Radiotherapy-induced secondary cancer risk for breast cancer: 3D conformal therapy versus IMRT versus VMAT." Journal of Radiological Protection 34(2): 325–331. doi: 10.1088/0952-4746/34/2/325.

Lei, X., Y. Cao, B. Ma, Y. Zhang, L. Ning, J. Qian, L. Zhang, Y. Qu, T. Zhang, D. Li, Q. Chen, J. Shi, X. Zhang, C. Ma, Y. Zhang, and E. Duan. (2020). "Development of mouse preimplantation embryos in space." National Science Review 7(9): 1437–1446. doi: 10.1093/nsr/nwaa062.

Leung, C. T., Y. Yang, K. N. Yu, N. Tam, T. F. Chan, X. Lin, R. Y. C. Kong, J. M. Y. Chiu, A. S. T. Wong, W. Y. Lui, K. W. Y. Yuen, K. P. Lai, and R. S. S. Wu. (2021). "Low-dose radiation can cause epigenetic alterations associated with impairments in both male and female reproductive cells." Frontiers in Genetics 12: 710143. doi: 10.3389/fgene.2021.710143.

Leuraud, K., D. B. Richardson, E. Cardis, R. D. Daniels, M. Gillies, R. Haylock, M. Moissonnier, M. K. Schubauer-Berigan, I. Thierry-Chef, A. Kesminiene, and D. Laurier. (2021). "Risk of cancer associated with low-dose radiation exposure: Comparison of results between the INWORKS nuclear workers study and the A-bomb survivors study. Radiation and Environmental Biophysics 60(1): 23–39. doi: 10.1007/s00411-020-00890-7.

Lewis, J., J. Hoover, and D. MacKenzie. (2017). "Mining and environmental health disparities in Native American communities." Current Environmental Health Reports 4(2): 130–141. doi: 10.1007/s40572-017-0140-5.

Li, L., A. J. Blomberg, J. D. Spengler, B. A. Coull, J. D. Schwartz, and P. Koutrakis. (2020). "Unconventional oil and gas development and ambient particle radioactivity." Nature Communications 11: 1–8. doi: 10.1038/s41467-020-18226-w.

Li, R., L. Di, J. Li, W. Fan, Y. Liu, W. Guo, W. Liu, L. Liu, Q. Li, L. Chen, Y. Chen, C. Miao, H. Liu, Y. Wang, Y. Ma, D. Xu, D. Lin, Y. Huang, J. Wang, F. Bai, and C. Wu. (2021). "A body map of somatic mutagenesis in morphologically normal human tissues." Nature 597(7876): 398–403. doi: 10.1038/s41586-021-03836-1.

Liao, J., W. Huang, and G. Liu. (2015). "Animal models of coronary heart disease. Journal of Biomedical Research 30(1): 3–10. doi: 10.7555/JBR.30.20150051.

Lim, H., A. J. Agopian, L. W. Whitehead, C. W. Beasley, P. H. Langlois, R. J. Emery, and D. K. Waller. (2015). "Maternal occupational exposure to ionizing radiation and major structural birth defects." Birth Defects Research Part A: Clinical and Molecular Teratology 103(4): 243–254. doi: 10.1002/bdra.23340.

Lin, J. R., M. Fallahi-Sichani, and P. K. Sorger. (2015). "Highly multiplexed imaging of single cells using a high-throughput cyclic immunofluorescence method." Nature Communications 6: 8390. doi: 10.1038/ncomms9390.

Linet, M. S., C. M. Kitahara, E. Ntowe, R. A. Kleinerman, E. S. Gilbert, N. Naito, R. S. Lipner, D. L. Miller, A. Berrington de Gonzalez, and Multi-Specialty Occupational Health Group. (2017). "Mortality in U.S. physicians likely to perform fluoroscopy-guided interventional procedures compared with psychiatrists, 1979 to 2008." Radiology 284(2): 482–494. doi: 10.1148/radiol.2017161306.

Litkowski, P. E., G. W. Smetana, M. L. Zeidel, and M. S. Blanchard. (2016). "Curbing the urge to image." American Journal of Medicine 129(10): 1131–1135. doi: 10.1016/j.amjmed.2016.06.020.

Little, M. P., T. V. Azizova, D. Bazyka, S. D. Bouffler, E. Cardis, S. Chekin, V. V. Chumak, F. A. Cucinotta, F. de Vathaire, P. Hall, J. D. Harrison, G. Hildebrandt, V. Ivanov, V. V. Kashcheev, S. V. Klymenko, M. Kreuzer, O. Laurent, K. Ozasa, T. Schneider, S. Tapio, A. M. Taylor, I. Tzoulaki, S. Bouffler, W. L. Vandoolaeghe, R. Wakeford, L. B. Zablotska, W. Zhang, and S. E. Lipshultz. (2012). "Systematic review and meta-analysis of circulatory disease from exposure to low-level ionizing radiation and estimates of potential population mortality risks." Environmental Health Perspectives 120(11): 1503–1511. doi: 10.1289/ehp.1204982.

Little, M. P., R. Wakeford, D. Borrego, B. French, L. B. Zablotska, M. J. Adams, R. Allodji, F. de Vathaire, C. Lee, A. V. Brenner, J. S. Miller, D. Campbell, M. S. Pearce, M. M. Doody, E. Holmberg, M. Lundell, S. Sadetzki, M. S. Linet, and A. Berrington de González. (2018). "Leukaemia and myeloid malignancy among people exposed to low doses (<100 mSv) of ionising radiation during childhood: A pooled analysis of nine historical cohort studies. The Lancet: Haematology 5(8): e346–e358. doi: 10.1016/S2352-3026(18)30092-9.

Little, M. P., E. K. Cahoon, C. M. Kitahara, S. L. Simon, N. Hamada, and M. S. Linet. (2020a). "Occupational radiation exposure and excess additive risk of cataract incidence in a cohort of US radiologic technologists." Occupational and Environmental Medicine 77(1): 1–8. doi: 10.1136/oemed-2019-105902.

Little, M. P., A. Patel, N. Hamada, and P. Albert. (2020b). "Analysis of cataract in relationship to occupational radiation dose accounting for dosimetric uncertainties in a cohort of U.S. radiologic technologists." Radiation Research 194(2): 153–161. doi: 10.1667/RR15529.1.

Little, M. P., T. V. Azizova, and N. Hamada. (2021a). "Low- and moderate-dose non-cancer effects of ionizing radiation in directly exposed individuals, especially circulatory and ocular diseases: A review of the epidemiology." International Journal of Radiation Biology 97(6): 782–803. doi: 10.1080/09553002.2021.1876955.

Little, M. P., T. Lee, M. G. Kimlin, C. M. Kitahara, R. Zhang, B. H. Alexander, M. S. Linet, and E. K. Cahoon. (2021b). "Lifetime ambient UV radiation exposure and risk of basal cell carcinoma by anatomic site in a nationwide U.S. cohort, 1983–2005." Cancer Epidemiology, Biomarkers and Prevention 30(10): 1932–1946. doi: 10.1158/1055-9965.EPI-20-1815.

Little, M. P., A. Patel, C. Lee, M. Hauptmann, A. Berrington de Gonzalez, and P. Albert. (2022a). "Impact of reverse causation on estimates of cancer risk associated with radiation exposure from computerized tomography: A simulation study modeled on brain cancer." American Journal of Epidemiology 191(1): 173–181. doi: 10.1093/aje/kwab247.

Little, M. P., R. Wakeford, S. D. Bouffler, K. Abalo, M. Hauptmann, N. Hamada, and G. M. Kendall. (2022b). "Review of the risk of cancer following low and moderate doses of sparsely ionising radiation received in early life in groups with individually estimated doses." Environment International 159: 106983. doi: 10.1016/j.envint.2021.106983.

Liu, Z., L. D. Lavis, and E. Betzig. (2015). "Imaging live-cell dynamics and structure at the single-molecule level." Molecular Cell 58(4): 644–659. doi: 10.1016/j.molcel.2015.02.033.

López, C. S., C. Bouchet-Marquis, C. P. Arthur, J. L. Riesterer, G. Heiss, G. Thibault, L. Pullan, S. Kwon, and J. W. Gray. (2017). "A fully integrated, three-dimensional fluorescence to electron microscopy correlative workflow." Methods in Cell Biology 140: 149–164. doi: 10.1016/bs.mcb.2017.03.008.

Lorenzo-Gonzalez, M., A. Ruano-Ravina, M. Torres-Duran, K. T. Kelsey, M. Provencio, I. Parente-Lamelas, V. Leiro-Fernández, I. Vidal-García, O. Castro-Añón, C. Martínez, A. Golpe-Gómez, M. Zapata-Cachafeiro, M. Piñeiro-Lamas, M. Pérez-Ríos, J. Abal-Arca, C. Montero-Martínez, A. Fernández-Villar, and J. M. Barros-Dios. (2019). "Lung cancer and residential radon in never-smokers: A pooling study in the northwest of Spain." Environmental Research 172: 713–718. doi: 10.1016/j.envres.2019.03.011.

Low, L. A., and M. A. Giulianotti. (2019). "Tissue chips in space: Modeling human diseases in microgravity." Pharmaceutical Research 37(1): 8. doi: 10.1007/s11095-019-2742-0.

Low, L. A., and D. A. Tagle. (2017). "Tissue chips—Innovative tools for drug development and disease modeling." Lab on a Chip 17(18): 3026–3036. doi: 10.1039/c7lc00462a.

Lumniczky, K., N. Impens, G. Armengol, S. Candéias, A. G. Georgakilas, S. Hornhardt, O. A. Martin, F. Rödel, and D. Schaue. (2021). "Low-dose ionizing radiation effects on the immune system." Environment International 149: 106212. doi: 10.1016/j.envint.2020.106212.

Lun, X. K., and B. Bodenmiller. (2020). "Profiling cell signaling networks at single-cell resolution." Molecular and Cellular Proteomics 19(5): 744–756. doi: 10.1074/mcp.R119.001790.

Lundgren, B., and H. O. Stefánsson. (2020). "Against the de minimis principle." Risk Analysis 40(5): 908–914. doi: 10.1111/risa.13445.

Lynge, E. (1996). "Risk of breast cancer is also increased among Danish female airline cabin attendants." British Medical Journal 312(7025): 253. doi: 10.1136/bmj.312.7025.253.

Lyon, J. L., S. C. Alder, M. B. Stone, A. Scholl, J. C. Reading, R. Holubkov, X. Sheng, G. L. White, Jr., K. T. Hegmann, L. Anspaugh, F. O. Hoffman, S. L. Simon, B. Thomas, R. Carroll, and A. W. Meikle. (2006). "Thyroid disease associated with exposure to the Nevada nuclear weapons test site radiation: A reevaluation based on corrected dosimetry and examination data." Epidemiology 17(6): 604–614. doi: 10.1097/01.ede.0000240540.79983.7f.

Mabuchi, K., D. L. Preston, A. V. Brenner, H. Sugiyama, M. Utada, R. Sakata, A. Sadakane, E. J. Grant, B. French, E. K. Cahoon, and K. Ozasa. (2020). "Risk of prostate cancer incidence among atomic bomb survivors: 1958–2009." Radiation Research 195(1): 66–76. doi: 10.1667/RR15481.1.

Machado, S. G., C. E. Land, and F. W. McKay. (1987). "Cancer mortality and radioactive fallout in southwestern Utah." American Journal of Epidemiology 125(1): 44–61. doi: 10.1093/oxfordjournals.aje.a114511.

Mackenzie, K. J., P. Carroll, L. Lettice, Ž. Tarnauskaitė, K. Reddy, F. Dix, A. Revuelta, E. Abbondati, R. E. Rigby, B. Rabe, F. Kilanowski, G. Grimes, A. Fluteau, P. S. Devenney, R. E. Hill, M. A. Reijns, and A. P. Jackson. (2016). "Ribonuclease H2 mutations induce a cGAS/STING-dependent innate immune response." EMBO Journal 35(8): 831–844. doi: 10.15252/embj.201593339.

Makkia, R., K. Nelson, H. Zaidi, and M. Dingfelder. (2019). Construction of realistic hybrid computational fetal phantoms from radiological images in three gestational ages for radiation dosimetry applications." Physics in Medicine and Biology 64(20): 205003. doi: 10.1088/1361-6560/ab44f8.

Marino, S. A. (2017). "50 years of the Radiological Research Accelerator Facility (RARAF)." Radiation Research 187(4): 413–423. doi: 10.1667/RR002CC.1.

Marshall, B. D. L., and S. Galea. (2015). "Formalizing the role of agent-based modeling in causal inference and epidemiology." American Journal of Epidemiology 181(2): 92–99. doi: 10.1093/aje/kwu274.

Martinez, N. E., D. W. Jokisch, L. T. Dauer, K. F. Eckerman, R. E. Goans, J. D. Brockman, S. Y. Tolmachev, M. Avtandilashvili, M. T. Mumma, J. D. Boice, Jr., and R. W. Leggett. (2022). "Radium dial workers: Back to the future." International Journal of Radiation Biology 98(4): 750–768. doi: 10.1080/09553002.2021.1917785.

Marx, V. (2021). "Method of the Year: Spatially resolved transcriptomics." Nature Methods (1): 9–14. doi: 10.1038/s41592-020-01033-y. Erratum, Nature Methods 18(2): 219 (2021).

Masur, J. S., and E. A. Posner. (2018). "Cost-benefit analysis and the judicial role." University of Chicago Law Review 85(4): 935–986.

Matzinger, P. (1994). "Tolerance, danger, and the extended family." Annual Review of Immunology 12(1): 991–1045. doi: 10.1146/annurev.iy.12.040194.005015.

Mayer, S., M.-A. Chevallier, E. Fantuzzi, M. Hajek, M. Luszik-Bhadra, R. Tanner, D. J. Thomas, and F. Vanhavere. (2021). EURADOS Intercomparison IC2017n for Neutron Dosemeters. Neuherberg, European Radiation Dosimetry Group. doi: 10.12768/wxyx-yz95.

Maynard, L. H., O. Humbert, C. W. Peterson, and H. P. Kiem. (2021). "Genome editing in large animal models." Molecular Therapy 29(11): 3140–3152. doi: 10.1016/j.ymthe.2021.09.026.

Maynard, M. R., J. W. Geyer, J. P. Aris, R. Y. Shifrin, and W. Bolch. (2011). "The UF family of hybrid phantoms of the developing human fetus for computational radiation dosimetry." Physics in Medicine and Biology 56(15): 4839–4379. doi: 10.1088/0031-9155/56/15/014.

Maynard, M. R., N. S. Long, N. S. Moawad, R. Y. Shifrin, A. M. Geyer, G. Fong, and W. E. Bolch. (2014). "The UF family of hybrid phantoms of the pregnant female for computational radiation dosimetry." Physics in Medicine and Biology 59(15): 4325–4343. doi: 10.1088/0031-9155/59/15/4325.

Maynard, M. R., N. B. Shagina, E. I. Tolstykh, M. O. Degteva, T. P. Fell, and W. E. Bolch. (2015a). "Fetal organ dosimetry for the Techa River and Ozyorsk offspring cohorts, part 1: A Urals-based series of fetal computational phantoms." Radiation and Environmental Biophysics 54(1): 37–46. doi: 10.1007/s00411-014-0571-4.

Maynard, M. R., N. B. Shagina, E. I. Tolstykh, M. O. Degteva, T. P. Fell, and W. E. Bolch. (2015b). "Fetal organ dosimetry for the Techa River and Ozyorsk Offspring Cohorts, part 2: Radionuclide S values for fetal self-dose and maternal cross-dose." Radiation and Environmental Biophysics 54(1): 47–59. doi: 10.1007/s00411-014-0570-5.

Mazzei-Abba, A., C. L. Folly, A. Coste, R. Wakeford, M. P. Little, O. Raaschou-Nielsen, G. Kendall, D. Hémon, A. Nikkilä, C. Spix, A. Auvinen, and B. D. Spycher. (2020). "Epidemiological studies of natural sources of radiation and childhood cancer: Current challenges and future perspectives." Journal of Radiological Protection 40(1): R1–R23. doi: 10.1088/1361-6498/ab5a38.

Mazzei-Abba, A., C. L. Folly, C. Kreis, R. A. Ammann, C. Adam, E. Brack, M. Egger, C. E. Kuehni, and B. D. Spycher. (2021). "External background ionizing radiation and childhood cancer: Update of a nationwide cohort analysis." Journal of Environmental Radioactivity 238–239: 106734. doi: 10.1016/j.jenvrad.2021.106734.

McBride, W. H., H. Ji-Hong, C.-S. Chiang, J. L. Olson, C.-C. Wang, F. Pajonk, G. J. Dougherty, K. S. Iwamoto, M. Pervan, and Y.-P. Liao. (2004). "A sense of danger from radiation." Radiation Research 162(1): 1–19. doi: 10.1667/rr3196.

McEwan, A. C., S. L. Simon, K. F. Baverstock, K. R. Trott, K. Sankaranarayanan, and H. G. Paretzke. (1997). "Some reflections on the role of the Scientific Advisory Panel to the Marshall Islands nationwide radiological study." Health Physics 73(1): 265–269. doi: 10.1097/00004032-199707000-00023.

McKenna, M. J., E. Robinson, L. Taylor, C. Tompkins, M. N. Cornforth, S. L. Simon, and S. M. Bailey. (2019). "Chromosome translocations, inversions and telomere length for retrospective biodosimetry on exposed U.S. atomic veterans." Radiation Research 191(4): 311–322. doi: 10.1667/RR15240.1.

MELODI (Multidisciplinary European Low Dose Initiative). (2021). Strategic Research Agenda of the Multidisciplinary European Low Dose Initiative (MELODI)—2021. https://melodi-online.eu/wp-content/uploads/2021/10/MELODI-SRA-2021-FINAL-post-consultation.pdf.

Menzel, P. T. (2021). "How should willingness-to-pay values of quality-adjusted life years be updated and according to whom?" AMA Journal of Ethics 23(8): E601–E606. doi: 10.1001/amajethics.2021.601.

Merzenich, H., G. P. Hammer, K. Tröltzsch, K. Ruecker, J. Buncke, F. Fehringer, and M. Blettner. (2014). "Mortality risk in a historical cohort of nuclear power plant workers in Germany: Results from a second follow-up." Radiation and Environmental Biophysics 53(2): 405–416. doi: 10.1007/s00411-014-0523-z.

Mettler, F. A., Jr., M. Mahesh, M. Bhargavan-Chatfield, C. E. Chambers, J. G. Elee, D. P. Frush, D. L. Miller, H. D. Royal, M. T. Milano, D. C. Spelic, A. J. Ansari, W. E. Bolch, G. M. Guebert, R. H. Sherrier, J. M. Smith, and R. J. Vetter. (2020). "Patient exposure from radiologic and nuclear medicine procedures in the United States: Procedure volume and effective dose for the period 2006-2016." Radiology 295(2): 418–427. doi: 10.1148/radiol.2020192256.

Metzcar, J., Y. Wang, R. Heiland, and P. Macklin. (2019). "A review of cell-based computational modeling in cancer biology." JCO Clinical Cancer Informatics 3: 1–13. doi: 10.1200/CCI.18.00069.

Micke, O., M. H. Seegenschmiedt, I. A. Adamietz, G. Kundt, K. Fakhrian, U. Schaefer, and R. Muecke; German Cooperative Group on Radiotherapy for Nonmalignant Diseases. (2017). "Low-dose radiation therapy for benign painful skeletal disorders: The typical treatment for the elderly patient? International Journal of Radiation Oncology, Biology, Physics 98(4): 958–963. doi: 10.1016/j.ijrobp.2016.12.012.

Miller, R. C., G. Randers-Pehrson, C. R. Geard, E. J. Hall, and D. J. Brenner. (1999). "The oncogenic transforming potential of the passage of single alpha particles through mammalian cell nuclei." Proceedings of the National Academy of Sciences of the United States of America 96(1): 19–22. doi: 10.1073/pnas.96.1.19.

Mintz, B., and K. Illmensee. (1975). "Normal genetically mosaic mice produced from malignant teratocarcinoma cells." Proceedings of the National Academy of Sciences of the United States of America 72(9): 3585–3589. doi: 10.1073/pnas.72.9.3585.

Miousse, I. R., C. M. Skinner, V. Sridharan, J. W. Seawright, P. Singh, R. D. Landes, A. K. Cheema, M. Hauer-Jensen, M. Boerma, and I. Koturbash. (2019). "Changes in one-carbon metabolism and DNA methylation in the hearts of mice exposed to space environment-relevant doses of oxygen ions (^{16}O)." Life Sciences in Space Research 22: 8–15. doi: 10.1016/j.lssr.2019.05.003.

Moore, L., D. Leongamornlert, T. H. H. Coorens, M. A. Sanders, P. Ellis, S. C. Dentro, K. J. Dawson, T. Butler, R. Rahbari, T. J. Mitchell, F. Maura, J. Nangalia, P. S. Tarpey, S. F. Brunner, H. Lee-Six, Y. Hooks, S. Moody, K. T. Mahbubani, M. Jimenez-Linan, J. J. Brosens, C. A. Iacobuzio-Donahue, I. Martincorena, K. Saeb-Parsy, P. J. Campbell, and M. R. Stratton. (2020). "The mutational landscape of normal human endometrial epithelium." Nature 580(7805): 640–646. doi: 10.1038/s41586-020-2214-z.

Morgan, W. F. (2003a). "Non-targeted and delayed effects of exposure to ionizing radiation. I. Radiation-induced genomic instability and bystander effects in vitro." Radiation Research 159: 567–580. doi: 10.1667/0033-7587(2003)159[0567:nadeoe]2.0.co;2.

Morgan, W. F. (2003b). "Non-targeted and delayed effects of exposure to ionizing radiation. II. Radiation-induced genomic instability and bystander effects in vivo, clastogenic factors and transgenerational effects. Radiation Research 159: 581–596. doi: 10.1667/0033-7587(2003)159[0581:nadeoe]2.0.co;2.

Morton, L. M., D. M. Karyadi, C. Stewart, T. I. Bogdanova, E. T. Dawson, M. K. Steinberg, J. Dai, S. W. Hartley, S. J. Schonfeld, J. N. Sampson, Y. E. Maruvka, V. Kapoor, D. A. Ramsden, J. Carvajal-Garcia, C. M. Perou, J. S. Parker, M. Krznaric, M. Yeager, J. F. Boland, A. Hutchinson, B. D. Hicks, C. L. Dagnall, J. M. Gastier-Foster, J. Bowen, O. Lee, M. J. Machiela, E. K. Cahoon, A. V. Brenner, K. Mabuchi, V. Drozdovitch, S. Masiuk, M. Chepurny, L. Y. Zurnadzhy, M. Hatch, A. Berrington de Gonzalez, G. A. Thomas, M. D. Tronko, G. Getz, and S. J. Chanock. (2021). "Radiation-related genomic profile of papillary thyroid carcinoma after the Chernobyl accident." Science 372(6543): eabg2538. doi: 10.1126/science.abg2538.

Moses, L., and L. Pachter. (2022). "Museum of spatial transcriptomics." Nature Methods 19: 534–546. doi: 10.1038/s41592-022-01409-2.

Mukherjee, P., M. Zhou, E. Lee, A. Schicht, Y. Balagurunathan, S. Napel, R. Gillies, S. Wong, A. Thieme, A. Leung, and O. Gevaert. (2020). "A shallow convolutional neural network predicts prognosis of lung cancer patients in multi-institutional CT-image data. Nature Machine Intelligence 2(5): 274–282. doi: 10.1038/s42256-020-0173-6.

Mukherjee, S., E. C. Laiakis, A. J. Fornace, Jr., and S. A. Amundson. (2019). "Impact of inflammatory signaling on radiation biodosimetry: Mouse model of inflammatory bowel disease." BMC Genomics 20(1): 329. doi: 10.1186/s12864-019-5689-y.

Muller, H. J. (1927). Artificial transmutation of the gene. Science 6(1699): 84–87. doi: 10.1126/science.66.1699.84.

Murakami, M., K. Ono, M. Tsubokura, S. Nomura, T. Oikawa, T. Oka, M. Kami, and T. Oki. (2015). "Was the risk from nursing-home evacuation after the Fukushima accident higher than the radiation risk?" PLoS ONE 10(9): e0137906. doi: 10.1371/journal.pone.0137906.

Nagle, P. W., and R. P. Coppes. (2020). "Current and future perspectives of the use of organoids in radiobiology." Cells 9(12): 2649. doi: 10.3390/cells9122649.

Nair, R. R., B. Rajan, S. Akiba, P. Jayalekshmi, M. K. Nair, P. Gangadharan, T. Koga, H. Morishima, S. Nakamura, and T. Sugahara. (2009). "Background radiation and cancer incidence in Kerala, India-Karanagappally cohort study." Health Physics 96(1): 55–66. doi: 10.1097/01.HP.0000327646.54923.11.

Napier, B. A. (2002). "A re-evaluation of the ^{131}I atmospheric releases from the Hanford site." Health Physics 83(2): 204–226. doi: 10.1097/00004032-200208000-00006.

NASA (National Aeronautics and Space Administration). (2021). Human Research Program Integrated Research Plan. https://humanresearchroadmap.nasa.gov/Documents/IRP_Rev-Current.pdf.

NASA. (2022). NASA Space Flight Human-System Standard: Volume 1: Crew Health. https://standards.nasa.gov/sites/default/files/standards/NASA/B/2022-01-05-NASA-STD-3001-Vol1-Rev-B-Final-Draft-Signature-010522.pdf.

NASEM (National Academies of Sciences, Engineering, and Medicine). (2019a). Independent Assessment of Science and Technology for the Department of Energy's Defense Environmental Cleanup Program. Washington, DC, The National Academies Press.

NASEM. (2019b). Long-Term Health Monitoring of Populations Following a Nuclear or Radiological Incident in the United States: Proceedings of a Workshop. Washington, DC, The National Academies Press.

NASEM. (2019c). The Future of Low-Dose Radiation Research in the United States: Proceedings of a Symposium. Washington, DC, The National Academies Press.

NASEM. (2021a). 2021 Global Change Research Needs and Opportunities for 2022–2031. Washington, DC, The National Academies Press.

NASEM. (2021b). Radioactive Sources: Applications and Alternative Technologies. Washington, DC, The National Academies Press.

NASEM. (2021c). Space Radiation and Astronaut Health: Managing and Communicating Cancer Risks. Washington, DC, The National Academies Press.

Natesan, V., and S. J. Kim. (2021). "Lipid metabolism, disorders and therapeutic drugs—Review. Biomolecular Therapy (Seoul) 29(6): 596–604. doi: 10.4062/biomolther.2021.122.

Navaranjan, G., C. Berriault, M. Do, P. J. Villeneuve, and P. A. Demers. (2016). Cancer incidence and mortality from exposure to radon progeny among Ontario uranium miners. Occupational and Environmental Medicine 73(12): 838–845. doi: 10.1136/oemed-2016-103836.

NCI (National Cancer Institute). (1997). Estimated Exposures and Thyroid Doses Received by the American People from Iodine-131 in Fallout Following Nevada Atmospheric Nuclear Bomb Tests: Appendices to the Report. Bethesda, MD, National Cancer Institute.

NCRP (National Council on Radiation Protection and Measurements). (2009a). Ionizing Radiation Exposure of the Population of the United States. Bethesda, MD, National Council on Radiation Protection and Measurements.

NCRP. (2009b). Report 164: Uncertainties in Internal Radiation Dose Assessment. Bethesda, MD, National Council on Radiation Protection and Measurements.

NCRP. (2013). Report No. 174: Preconception and Prenatal Radiation Exposure: Health Effects and Protective Guidance. Bethesda, MD, National Council on Radiation Protection and Measurements.

NCRP. (2015a). Health Effects of Low Doses of Radiation: Perspectives on Integrating Radiation Biology and Epidemiology (NCRP Commentary No. 24). Bethesda, MD, National Council on Radiation Protection and Measurements.

NCRP. (2015b). Where Are the Radiation Professionals? (WARP). Bethesda, MD, National Council on Radiation Protection and Measurements.

NCRP. (2016). Guidance on Radiation Dose Limits for the Lens of the Eye. Bethesda, MD, National Council on Radiation Protection and Measurements.

NCRP. (2018a). Implications of Recent Epidemiologic Studies for the Linear-Nonthreshold Model and Radiation Protection (NCRP Commentary No. 27). Bethesda, MD, National Council on Radiation Protection and Measurements.

NCRP. (2018b). Report 178: Deriving Organ Doses and Their Uncertainty for Epidemiologic Studies (with a Focus on the One Million U.S. Workers and Veterans Study of Low-Dose Radiation Health Effects). Bethesda, MD, National Council on Radiation Protection and Measurements.

NCRP. (2019). Medical Radiation Exposure of Patients in the United States: Recommendations of the National Council on Radiation Protection and Measurements. Bethesda, MD, National Council on Radiation Protection and Measurements.

NCRP. (2020a). Report No. 186: Approaches for Integrating Information from Radiation Biology and Epidemiology to Enhance Low-Dose Health Risk Assessment: Recommendations of the National Council on Radiation Protection and Measurements. Bethesda, MD, National Council on Radiation Protection and Measurements.

NCRP. (2020b). Overview of Naturally Occurring Radioactive Material/Technologically Enhanced Naturally Occurring Radioactive Material from the Contemporary Oil and Gas Industry (NCRP Commentary No. 29). Bethesda, MD, National Council on Radiation Protection and Measurements.

Neel, J. V. (1998). "Genetic studies at the Atomic Bomb Casualty Commission–Radiation Effects Research Foundation: 1946–1997." Proceedings of the National Academy of Sciences of the United States of America 95: 5432–5436. doi: 10.1073/pnas.95.10.5432.

Neel, J. V., and W. J. Schull. (1956). "Studies on the potential genetic effects of the atomic bombs." Acta Genetica et Statistica Medica 6(2): 183–196. doi: 10.1159/000150821.

Neill, R. H., L. Chaturvedi, W. W.-L. Lee, T. M. Clemo, M. K. Silva, J. W. Kenney, W. T. Bartlett, and B. A. Walker. (1996). Review of the WIPP Draft Application to Show Compliance with EPA Transuranic Waste Disosal Standards. Albuquerque, NM, Environmental Evaluation Group. https://inis.iaea.org/collection/NCLCollectionStore/_Public/27/057/27057244.pdf.

Nelson, C. M., and M. J. Bissell. (2006). "Of extracellular matrix, scaffolds, and signaling: Tissue architecture regulates development, homeostasis, and cancer." Annual Review of Cell and Development Biology 22: 287–309. doi: 10.1146/annurev.cellbio.22.010305.104315.

Neriishi, K., E. Nakashima, A. Minamoto, S. Fujiwara, M. Akahoshi, H. K. Mishima, T. Kitaoka, and R. E. Shore. (2007). "Postoperative cataract cases among atomic bomb survivors: Radiation dose response and threshold." Radiation Research 168(4): 404–408. doi: 10.1667/RR0928.1.

Nickerson, A., T. Huang, L. J. Lin, and X. Nan. (2014). "Photoactivated localization microscopy with bimolecular fluorescence complementation (BiFC-PALM) for nanoscale imaging of protein-protein interactions in cells." PLoS ONE 9(6): e100589. doi: 10.1371/journal.pone.0100589.

Nikolova, M. P., and M. S. Chavali. (2019). "Recent advances in biomaterials for 3D scaffolds: A review." Bioactive Materials 4: 271–292. doi: 10.1016/j.bioactmat.2019.10.005.

Noda, A., K. Kato, C. Tamura, L. G. Biesecker, M. Imaizumi, Y. Inoue, G. E. Henderson, B. Wilfond, K. Muto, M. Naito, and J. Kayukawa. (2021). "Ethical, legal and social implications of human genome studies in radiation research: A workshop report for studies on atomic bomb survivors at the Radiation Effects Research Foundation." Journal of Radiation Research 62(4): 656–661. doi: 10.1093/jrr/rrab043.

Noe, P. R., and J. D. Graham. (2020). "The ascendancy of the cost-benefit state?" Administrative Law Review Accord 5(3): 85–152.

Nomura, S., S. Gilmour, M. Tsubokura, D. Yoneoka, A. Sugimoto, T. Oikawa, M. Kami, and K. Shibuya. (2013). "Mortality risk amongst nursing home residents evacuated after the Fukushima nuclear accident: A retrospective cohort study." PLoS ONE 8: e60192 doi: 10.1371/journal.pone.0060192.

Normile, D. (2021). "Japan plans to release Fukushima's wastewater into the ocean: Government says treatment and dilution will minimize risk to marine life and the environment." ScienceInsider, April 13. doi: 10.1126/science.abi9880.

NRC (National Research Council). (1989). Improving Risk Communication. Washington, DC, National Academy Press.

NRC. (1994). Science and Judgment in Risk Assessment. Washington, DC, National Academy Press.

NRC. (1998a). Research Priorities for Airborne Particulate Matter: I. Immediate Priorities and a Long-Range Research Portfolio. Washington, DC, National Academy Press.

NRC. (1998b). Serving Science and Society in the New Millennium: DOE's Biological and Environmental Research Program. Washington, DC, National Academy Press.

NRC. (1999a). Health Effects of Exposure to Radon: BEIR VI. Washington, DC, National Academy Press.

NRC. (1999b). Research Priorities for Airborne Particulate Matter: II. Evaluating Research Progress and Updating the Portfolio. Washington, DC, National Academy Press.

NRC. (2000). Review of the Hanford Thyroid Disease Study Draft Final Report. Washington, DC, National Academy Press. https://doi.org/10.17226/9738.

NRC. (2001). Research Priorities for Airborne Particulate Matter: III. Early Research Progress. Washington, DC, National Academy Press.

NRC. (2004). Research Priorities for Airborne Particulate Matter: IV. Continuing Research Progress. Washington, DC, The National Academies Press.

NRC. (2005). Assessment of the Scientific Information for the Radiation Exposure Screening and Education Program. Washington, DC, The National Academies Press.

NRC. (2006a). Health Risks from Exposure to Low Levels of Ionizing Radiation: BEIR VII Phase 2. Washington, DC, The National Academies Press.

NRC. (2006b). Review of the Worker and Public Health Activities Program Administered by the Department of Energy and the Department of Health and Human Services. Washington, DC, The National Academies Press.

NRC. (2009). Science and Decisions: Advancing Risk Assessment. Washington, DC, The National Academies Press.

NRC. (2012). Analysis of Cancer Risks in Populations Near Nuclear Facilities: Phase 1. Washington, DC, The National Academies Press.

NRC. (2014). Analysis of Cancer Risks in Populations Near Nuclear Facilities: Phase 2: Pilot Planning. Washington, DC, The National Academies Press.

NSTC (National Science and Technology Council). (2022). Radiation Biology: A Response to the American Innovation and Competitiveness Act. A Report by the Subcommittee on Physical Sciences Committee on Science of the National Science and Technology Council. https://www.whitehouse.gov/wp-content/uploads/2022/01/LDR-Report-2022.pdf.

Nuclear Safety Council and Carlos III Institute of Health. (2009). Epidemiological Study of the Possible Effect of Ionising Radiations Deriving from the Operation of Spanish Nuclear Fuel Cycle Facilities on the Health of the Population Living in Their Vicinity. Environmental and Cancer Epidemiology Unit, National Centre for Epidemiology, Nuclear Safety Council.

Nurk, S., S. Koren, A. Rhie, M. Rautiainen, A. V. Bzikadze, A. Mikheenko, M. R. Vollger, N. Altemose, L. Uralsky, A. Gershman, S. Aganezov, S. J. Hoyt, M. Diekhans, G. A. Logsdon, M. Alonge, S. E. Antonarakis, M. Borchers, G. G. Bouffard, S. Y. Brooks, G. V. Caldas, N. C. Chen, H. Cheng, C. S. Chin, W. Chow, L. G. de Lima, P. C. Dishuck, R. Durbin, T. Dvorkina, I. T. Fiddes, G. Formenti, R. S. Fulton, A. Fungtammasan, E. Garrison, P. G. S. Grady, T. A. Graves-Lindsay, I. M. Hall, N. F. Hansen, G. A. Hartley, M. Haukness, K. Howe, M. W. Hunkapiller, C. Jain, M. Jain, E. D. Jarvis, P. Kerpedjiev, M. Kirsche, M. Kolmogorov, J. Korlach, M. Kremitzki, H. Li, V. V. Maduro, T. Marschall, A. M. McCartney, J. McDaniel, D. E. Miller, J. C. Mullikin, E. W. Myers, N. D. Olson, B. Paten, P. Peluso, P. A. Pevzner, D. Porubsky, T. Potapova, E. I. Rogaev, J. A. Rosenfeld, S. L. Salzberg, V. A. Schneider, F. J. Sedlazeck, K. Shafin, C. J. Shew, A. Shumate, Y. Sims, A. F. A. Smit, D. C. Soto, I. Sović, J. M. Storer, A. Streets, B. A. Sullivan, F. Thibaud-Nissen, J. Torrance, J. Wagner, B. P. Walenz, A. Wenger, J. M. D. Wood, C. Xiao, S. M. Yan, A. C. Young, S. Zarate, U. Surti, R. C. McCoy, M. Y. Dennis, I. A. Alexandrov, J. L. Gerton, R. J. O'Neill, W. Timp, J. M. Zook, M. C. Schatz, E. E. Eichler, K. H. Miga, and A. M. Phillippy. (2022). "The complete sequence of a human genome." Science 376(6588): 44–53. doi: 10.1126/science.abj6987.

Nussbaum, R., P. Hoover, C. Grossman, and F. Nussbaum. (2004). "Community-based participatory health survey of Hanford, WA, downwinders: A model for citizen empowerment." Society and Natural Resources 17(6): 547–559. doi: 10.1080/08941920490452526.

Nuta, O., J. Moquet, S. Bouffler, D. Lloyd, O. Sepai, and K. Rothkamm. (2014). "Impact of long-term exposure to sodium arsenite on cytogenetic radiation damage." Mutagenesis 29(2): 123–129. doi: 10.1093/mutage/get070.

Ochola, D. O., R. Sharif, J. S. Bedford, T. J. Keefe, T. A. Kato, C. M. Fallgren, P. Demant, S. V. Costes, and M. M. Weila. (2019). "Persistence of gamma-H2AX foci in bronchial cells correlates with susceptibility to radiation associated lung cancer in mice." Radiation Research 191(1): 67–75. doi: 10.1667/RR14979.1.

Olney, R. (2021). "The geospatial economy: A flood of geospatial data is here to lift all boats." Forbes, September 1. https://www.forbes.com/sites/forbestechcouncil/2021/09/01/the-geospatial-economy-a-flood-of-geospatial-data-is-here-to-lift-all-boats/?sh=3d413b474982.

Oradovskaia, I. V., I. G. Pashchenkova, V. V. Feoktistov, M. F. Nikonova, G. K. Vikulov, N. V. Bozheskaia, and N. N. Smirnova. (2011). "The epidemiological analysis of monitoring of the immune status in liquidators of consequences of the Chernobyl accident for early identification of risk groups and diagnostics of oncological diseases. Report 2. Dependence of frequency and changes in the immune status on risk factors of radiation accident." Radiatsionnaia Biologiia, Radioecologiia 51(1): 117–133.

OSHA (Occupational Safety and Health Administration). (1977). "Occupational exposure to benzene: Emergency temporary standards." Federal Register 42: 22516–22529. Washington, DC, Occupational Safety and Health Administration, Department of Labor.

Osman, M., P. Ayton, F. Bouder, N. Pidgeon, and R. Lofstedt. (2019). "Evidence based uncertainty: What is needed now?" Journal of Risk Research 24(5): 1–7. doi: 10.1080/13669877.2019.1646316.

Otake, M., and W. J. Schull. (1998). "Radiation-related brain damage and growth retardation among the prenatally exposed atomic bomb survivors." International Journal of Radiation Biology 74(2): 159–171. doi: 10.1080/095530098141555.

Otake, M., W. J. Schull, and J. V. Neel. (1990). "Congenital malformations, stillbirths, and early mortality among the children of atomic bomb survivors: A reanalysis." Radiation Research 122(1): 1–11. doi: 10.2307/3577576.

Ozasa, K., Y. Shimizu, A. Suyama, F. Kasagi, M. Soda, E. J. Grant, R. Sakata, H. Sugiyama, and K. Kodama. (2012). "Studies of the mortality of atomic bomb survivors, Report 14, 1950-2003: An overview of cancer and noncancer diseases." Radiation Research 177(3): 229–243. doi: 10.1667/rr2629.1.

Ozasa, K., E. J. Grant, and K. Kodama. (2018). "Japanese legacy cohorts: The Life Span Study of Atomic Bomb Survivor cohort and survivors' offspring." Journal of Epidemiology 28: 162–169. doi: 10.2188/jea.JE20170321.

Ozasa, K., H. M., Cullings, W. Ohishi, A. Hida, and E. J. Grant. (2019). "Epidemiological studies of atomic bomb radiation at the Radiation Effects Research Foundation." International Journal of Radiation Biology 95(7): 879–891. doi: 10.1080/09553002.2019.1569778.

Park, J. J. H., R. Mogg, G. E. Smith, E. Nakimuli-Mpungu, F. Jehan, C. R. Rayner, J. Condo, E. H. Decloedt, J. B. Nachega, G. Reis, and E. J. Mills. (2021). "How COVID-19 has fundamentally changed clinical research in global health." The Lancet: Global Health 9(5): e711–e720. doi: 10.1016/S2214-109X(20)30542-8.

Pasqual, E., F. Boussin, D. Bazyka, A. Nordenskjold, M. Yamada, K. Ozasa, S. Pazzaglia, L. Roy, I. Thierry-Chef, F. de Vathaire, M. Abderrafi, and E. C. Benotmane. (2021). "Cognitive effects of low dose of ionizing radiation—Lessons learned and research gaps from epidemiological and biological studies." Environment International 147: 106295. doi: 10.1016/j.envint.2020.106295.

Patrinos, A., and D. W. Drell. (1997). "The Human Genome Project: View from the Department of Energy." Journal of the American Medical Women's Association 52(1): 8–10.

Paul, S., N. J. Kleiman, and S. A. Amundson. (2019). "Transcriptomic responses in mouse blood during the first week after in vivo gamma irradiation." Scientific Reports 9(1): 18364. doi: 10.1038/s41598-019-54780-0.

Paunesku, T., and G. Woloschak. (2018). "Reflections on basic science studies involving low doses of ionizing radiation. Health Physics 115(5): 623–627. doi: 10.1097/HP.0000000000000937.

Paunesku, T., A. Stevanović, J. Popović, and G. E. Woloschak. (2021). "Effects of low dose and low dose rate low linear energy transfer radiation on animals—Review of recent studies relevant for carcinogenesis." International Journal of Radiation Biology 97(6): 1–22. doi: 10.1080/09553002.2020.1859155.

Pearce, M. S., J. A. Salotti, M. P. Little, K. McHugh, C. Lee, K. P. Kim, N. L. Howe, C. M. Ronckers, P. Rajaraman, A. W. Sir Craft, L. Parker, and A. Berrington de González. (2012). "Radiation exposure from CT scans in childhood and subsequent risk of leukaemia and brain tumours: A retrospective cohort study." The Lancet 380(9840): 499–505. doi: 10.1016/S0140-6736(12)60815-0.

Peng, Y., H. Nagasawa, C. Warner, and J. S. Bedford. (2012). "Genetic susceptibility: Radiation effects relevant to space travel." Health Physics 103(5): 607–620. doi: 10.1097/HP.0b013e31826945b9.

Penn, I., and E. Lipton. (2021). "The lithium gold rush: Inside the rush to power electric vehicles." The New York Times, May 6. https://www.nytimes.com/2021/05/06/business/lithium-mining-race.html.

Perez, R. E., S. Younger, E. Bertheau, C. M. Fallgren, M. M. Weil, and J. Raber. (2020). "Effects of chronic exposure to a mixed field of neutrons and photons on behavioral and cognitive performance in mice." Behavioural Brain Research 379: 112377. doi: 10.1016/j.bbr.2019.112377.

Perez Horta, Z. P., C. M. Case, Jr., and A. L. DiCarlo. (2019). "Use of growth factors and cytokines to treat injuries resulting from a radiation public health emergency." Radiation Research 192(1): 92–97. doi: 10.1667/RR15383.1.

Pernot, E., J. Hall, S. Baatout, M.A. Benotmane, E. Blanchardon, S. Bouffler, H. El Saghire, M. Gomolka, A. Guertler, M. Harms-Ringdahl, P. Jeggo, M. Kreuzer, D. Laurier, C. Lindholm, R. Mkacher, R. Quintens, K. Rothkamm, L. Sabatier, S. Tapio, F. de Vathaire, and E. Cardis. (2012). "Ionizing radiation biomarkers for potential use in epidemiological studies." Mutation Research 751(2): 258–286. doi: 10.1016/j.mrrev.2012.05.003.

Peterson, A., and M. Cooke. (2019). "CANDLE illuminates new pathways in fight against cancer." energy.gov, August 14. https://www.energy.gov/articles/candle-illuminates-new-pathways-fight-against-cancer.

Petoussi-Henss, N., D. Satoh, H. Schlattl, M. Zankl, and V. Spielmann. (2021). "Organ doses of the fetus from external environmental exposures." Radiation and Environmental Biophysics 60(1): 93–113. doi: 10.1007/s00411-020-00891-6.

Pinkerton, L. E., M. J. Hein, J. L. Anderson, A. Christianson, M. P. Little, A. J. Sigurdson, and M. K. Schubauer-Berigan. (2018). "Melanoma, thyroid cancer, and gynecologic cancers in a cohort of female flight attendants." American Journal of Industrial Medicine 61(7): 572–581. doi: 10.1002/ajim.22854.

Pollard, J. M., and R. A. Gatti. (2009). "Clinical radiation sensitivity with DNA repair disorders: An overview." International Journal of Radiation Oncology, Biology, Physics 74(5): 1323–1331. doi: 10.1016/j.ijrobp.2009.02.057.

Popov, V. V., E. V. Kudryavtseva, N. Kumar Katiyar, A. Shishkin, S. I. Stepanov, and S. Goel. (2022). "Industry 4.0 and digitalisation in healthcare." Materials (Basel) 15(6): 2140. doi: 10.3390/ma15062140.

Preston, D. L., H. Cullings, A. Suyama, S. Funamoto, N. Nishi, M. Soda, K. Mabuchi, K. Kodama, F. Kasagi, and R. E. Shore. (2008). "Solid cancer incidence in atomic bomb survivors exposed in utero or as young children." Journal of the National Cancer Institute 100(6): 428–436. doi: 10.1093/jnci/djn045.

Preston, D. L., C. M. Kitahara, D. M. Freedman, A. J. Sigurdson, S. L. Simon, M. P. Little, E. K. Cahoon, P. Rajaraman, J. S. Miller, B. H. Alexander, M. M. Doody, and M. S. Linet. (2016). "Breast cancer risk and protracted low-to-moderate dose occupational radiation exposure in the US Radiologic Technologists Cohort, 1983–2008. British Journal of Cancer 115:1105. https://doi.org/10.1038/bjc.2016.292.

Pukkala, E., A. Auvinen, and G. Wahlberg. (1995). "Incidence of cancer among Finnish airline cabin attendants, 1967–92." British Medical Journal 311(7006): 649–652. doi: 10.1136/bmj.311.7006.649.

Puskin, J. S. (2009). "Perspective on the use of LNT for radiation protection and risk assessment by the U.S. Environmental Protection Agency." Dose-Response 7(4): 284–291. doi: 10.2203/dose-response.09-005.Puskin.

Putnam, F. W. (1998). "The Atomic Bomb Casualty Commission in retrospect." Proceedings of the National Academy of Sciences of the United States of America 95(10):5426–5431. doi: 10.1073/pnas.95.10.5426.

Quake, S. R. (2022). "A decade of molecular cell atlases." Trends in Genetics 29:S0168-9525(22)00004-X. doi: 10.1016/j.tig.2022.01.004.

Quigley, D., J. J. Alumkal, A. W. Wyatt, V. Kothari, A. Foye, P. Lloyd, R. Aggarwal, W. Kim, E. Lu, J. Schwartzman, K. Beja, M. Annala, R. Das, M. Diolaiti, C. Pritchard, G. Thomas, S. Tomlins, K. Knudsen, C. J. Lord, C. Ryan, J. Youngren, T. M. Beer, A. Ashworth, E. J. Small, and F. Y. Feng. (2017). "Analysis of circulating cell-free DNA identifies multiclonal heterogeneity of *BRCA2* reversion mutations associated with resistance to PARP Inhibitors." Cancer Discovery 7(9): 999–1005. doi: 10.1158/2159-8290.CD-17-0146.

Radisky, D. C., and M. J. Bissell. (2004). "Cancer. Respect thy neighbor!" Science 303(5659): 775–777. doi: 10.1126/science.1094412.

Rage, E., S. Caër-Lorho, D. Drubay, S. Ancelet, P. Laroche, and D. Laurier. (2015). "Mortality analyses in the updated French cohort of uranium miners (1946–2007)." International Archives of Occupational and Environmental Health 88(6): 717–730. doi: 10.1007/s00420-014-0998-6.

Rage, E., D. B. Richardson, P. A. Demers, M. Do, N. Fenske, M. Kreuzer, J. Samet, C. Wiggins, M. K. Schubauer-Berigan, K. Kelly-Reif, L. Tomasek, L. B. Zablotska, and D. Laurier. (2020). "PUMA—Pooled Uranium Miners Analysis: Cohort profile." Occupational and Environmental Medicine 77(3): 194–200. doi: 10.1136/oemed-2019-105981.

Rajaraman, P., M. M. Doody, C. L. Yu, D. L. Preston, J. S. Miller, A. J. Sigurdson, D. M. Freedman, B. H. Alexander, M. P. Little, D. L. Miller, and M. S. Linet. (2016). "Incidence and mortality risks for circulatory diseases in US radiologic technologists who worked with fluoroscopically guided interventional procedures, 1994–2008." Occupational and Environmental Medicine 73(1): 21–27. doi: 10.1136/oemed-2015-102888.

Rajaraman, P., M. Hauptmann, S. Bouffler, and A. Wojcik. (2018). "Human individual radiation sensitivity and prospects for prediction." Annals of the ICRP 47(3–4): 126–141. doi: 10.1177/0146645318764091.

Randers-Pehrson, G., G. W. Johnson, S. A. Marino, Y. Xu, A. D. Dymnikov, and D. J. Brenner. (2009). "The Columbia University sub-micron charged particle beam." Nuclear Instruments and Methods in Physics Research: Section A, Accelerators, Spectrometers, Detectors and Associated Equipment 609(2): 294–299. doi: 10.1016/j.nima.2009.08.041.

Rehani, M. M., K. Yang, E. R. Melick, J. Heil, D. Šalát, W. F. Sensakovic, and B. Liu. (2020). "Patients undergoing recurrent CT scans: Assessing the magnitude." European Radiology 30(4): 1828–1836. doi: 10.1007/s00330-019-06523-y.

Reid, J. R., and L. J. States. (2018). "Ionizing radiation use and cancer predisposition syndromes in children." Journal of the American College of Radiologists 15(9): 1238–1239. doi: 10.1016/j.jacr.2018.04.011.

Richardson, D. B., E. Cardis, R. D. Daniels, M. Gillies, J. A. O'Hagan, G. B. Hamra, R. Haylock, D. Laurier, K. Leuraud, K. Moissonnier, M. K. Schubauer-Berigan, I. Thierry-Chef, and A. Kesminiene. (2015). "Risk of cancer from occupational exposure to ionising radiation: Retrospective cohort study of workers in France, the United Kingdom, and the United States (INWORKS)." BMJ (Clinical Research ed.) 351: h5359. doi: 10.1136/bmj.h5359. Erratum, BMJ (Clinical Research ed.) 351: h6634.

Richardson, D. B., E. Rage, P. A. Demers, M. T. Do, N. DeBono, N. Fenske, V. Deffner, M. Kreuzer, J. Samet, C. Wiggins, M. K. Schubauer-Berigan, K. Kelly-Reif, L. Tomasek, L. B. Zablotska, and D. Laurier. (2021). "Mortality among uranium miners in North America and Europe: The Pooled Uranium Miners Analysis (PUMA)." International Journal of Epidemiology 50(2): 633–643. https://doi.org/10.1093/ije/dyaa195.

Riesterer, J. L., C. S. López, E. S. Stempinski, M. Williams, K. Loftis, K. Stoltz, G. Thibault, C. Lanicault, T. Williams, and J. W. Gray. (2020). "A workflow for visualizing human cancer biopsies using large-format electron microscopy." Methods in Cell Biology 158: 163–181. doi: 10.1016/bs.mcb.2020.01.005.

Rizki, A., and M. J. Bissell. (2004). "Homeostasis in the breast: It takes a village." Cancer Cell 6(1): 1–2. doi: 10.1016/j.ccr.2004.06.019.

Rodier, F., J. P. Coppe, C. K. Patil, W. A. Hoeijmakers, D. P. Munoz, S. R. Raza, A. Freund, E. Campeau, A. R. Davalos, and J. Campisi. (2009). "Persistent DNA damage signalling triggers senescence-associated inflammatory cytokine secretion." Nature Cell Biology 11(8): 973–979. doi: 10.1038/ncb1909.

Rodrigues-Moreira, S., S. G. Moreno, G. L. Ghinatti, D. Lewandowski, F. Hoffschir, F. Ferri, A.-S. Gallouet, D. Gay, H. Motohashi, M. Yamamoto, M. C. Joiner, N. Gault, and P.-H. Romeo. (2017). "Low-dose irradiation promotes persistent oxidative stress and decreases self-renewal in hematopoietic stem cells." Cell Reports 20: 3199–3211. doi: 10.1016/j.celrep.2017.09.013.

Rola, R., V. Sarkissian, A. Obenaus, G. A. Nelson, S. Otsuka, C. L. Limoli, and J. R. Fike. (2005). "High-LET radiation induces inflammation and persistent changes in markers of hippocampal neurogenesis." Radiation Research 164(4 Pt. 2): 556–560. doi: 10.1667/rr3412.1.

Rothkamm, K., and M. Löbrich. (2003). "Evidence for a lack of DNA double-strand break repair in human cells exposed to very low x-ray doses." Proceedings of the National Academy of Sciences of the United States of America 100(9): 5057–5062. doi: 10.1073/pnas.0830918100.

Rozenblatt-Rosen, O., A. Regev, P. Oberdoerffer, T. Nawy, A. Hupalowska, J. E. Rood, O. Ashenberg, E. Cerami, R. J. Coffey, E. Demir, L. Ding, E. D. Esplin, J. M. Ford, J. Goecks, S. Ghosh, J. W. Gray, J. Guinney, S. E. Hanlon, S. K. Hughes, E. S. Hwang, C. A. Iacobuzio-Donahue, J. Jané-Valbuena, B. E. Johnson, K. S. Lau, T. Lively, S. A. Mazzilli, D. Pe'er, S. Santagata, A. K. Shalek, D. Schapiro, M. P. Snyder, P. K. Sorger, A. E. Spira, S. Srivastava, K. Tan, R. B. West, and E. H. Williams; Human Tumor Atlas Network. (2020). "The Human Tumor Atlas Network: Charting tumor transitions across space and time at single-cell resolution." Cell 181(2): 236–249. doi: 10.1016/j.cell.2020.03.053.

Rubin, G. D. (2014). "Computed tomography: Revolutionizing the practice of medicine for 40 years." Radiology 273(2 Suppl.): S45–S74. doi: 10.1148/radiol.14141356.

Rühm, W., M. Eidemüller, and J. C. Kaiser. (2017). "Biologically-based mechanistic models of radiation-related carcinogenesis applied to epidemiological data." International Journal of Radiation Biology 93(10): 1093–1117. doi: 10.1080/09553002.2017.1310405.

Rühm, W., D. Laurier, and R. Wakeford. (2022). "Cancer risk following low doses of ionising radiation—Current epidemiological evidence and implications for radiological protection." Mutation Research: Genetic Toxicology and Environmental Mutagenesis 873: 503436. doi: 10.1016/j.mrgentox.2021.503436.

Russell, W. L. (1951). "X-ray-induced mutations in mice." Cold Spring Harbor Symposia on Quantitative Biology 16: 327–336. doi: 10.1101/sqb.1951.016.01.024.

Sadakane, A., B. French, A. V. Brenner, D. L. Preston, H. Sugiyama, E. J. Grant, R. Sakata, M. Utada, E. K. Cahoon, K. Mabuchi, and K. Ozasa. (2019). "Radiation and risk of liver, biliary tract, and pancreatic cancers among atomic bomb survivors in Hiroshima and Nagasaki: 1958–2009." Radiation Research 192(3): 299–310. doi: 10.1667/RR15341.1.

Sadowitz, M., and J. D. Graham. (1995). "A survey of residual cancer risks permitted by health, safety and environmental policy." Risk: Health, Safety and Environment 6(1): 17–35.

Saenko, V., V. Ivanov, A. Tsyb, T. Bogdanova, M. Tronko, Y. Demidchik, and S. Yamashita. (2011). "The Chernobyl accident and its consequences." Clinical Oncology 23(4): 234–243. doi: 10.1016/j.clon.2011.01.502.

Sakata, R., D. L. Preston, A. V. Brenner, H. Sugiyama, E. J. Grant, P. Rajaraman, A. Sadakane, M. Utada, B. French, E. K. Cahoon, K. Mabuchi, and K. Ozasa. (2019). "Radiation-related risk of cancers of the upper digestive tract among Japanese atomic bomb survivors." Radiation Research 192(3): 331–344. doi: 10.1667/RR15386.1.

Samet, J. M., D. R. Pathak, M. V. Morgan, C. R. Key, A. A. Valdivia, and J. H. Lubin. (1991). "Lung cancer mortality and exposure to radon progeny in a cohort of New Mexico underground uranium miners." Health Physics 61: 745–752. doi: 10.1097/00004032-199112000-00005.

Sato, T., S. Funamoto, C. Paulbeck, K. Griffin, C. Lee, H. Cullings, S. D. Egbert, A. Endo, N. Hertel, and W. E. Bolch. (2020). "Dosimetric impact of a new computational voxel phantom series for the Japanese atomic bomb survivors: Methodological improvements and organ dose response functions." Radiation Research 194(4): 390–402. doi: 10.1667/RR15546.1.

Save the Children. (2012). Fukushima Families: Children and Families Affected by Fukushima's Nuclear Crisis Share Their Concerns One Year on. http://www.savethechildren.org/atf/cf/%7B9def2ebe-10ae432c-9bd0-df91d2eba74a%7D/JAPAN_FUKUSHIMA_FAMILIES_REPORT.PDF.

Sawano, T., Y. Nishikawa, A. Ozaki, C. Leppold, and M. Tsubokura. (2018). "The Fukushima Daiichi Nuclear Power Plant accident and school bullying of affected children and adolescents: The need for continuous radiation education." Journal of Radiation Research 59(3): 381–384. doi: 10.1093/jrr/rry025.

Schapiro, D., C. Yapp, A. Sokolov, S. M. Reynolds, Y. A. Chen, D. Sudar, Y. Xie, J. Muhlich, R. Arias-Camison, S. Arena, A. J. Taylor, M. Nikolov, M. Tyler, J. R. Lin, E. A. Burlingame, Human Tumor Atlas Network; Y. H. Chang, S. L. Farhi, V. Thorsson, N. Venkatamohan, J. L. Drewes, D. Pe'er, D. A. Gutman, M. D. Herrmann, N. Gehlenborg, P. Bankhead, J. T. Roland, J. M. Herndon, M. P. Snyder, M. Angelo, G. Nolan, J. R. Swedlow, N. Schultz, D. T. Merrick, S. A. Mazzili, E. Cerami, S. J. Rodig, S. Santagata, and P. K. Sorger. (2022). "MITI minimum information guidelines for highly multiplexed tissue images." Nature Methods 19(3): 262–267. doi: 10.1038/s41592-022-01415-4.

Schimmerling, W. (2011). NASA Space Radiation Program Interagency Collaboration. https://three.jsc.nasa.gov/articles/InteragencyCollaboration030211.pdf.

Schonfeld, S. J., L. Y. Krestinina, S. Epifanova, M. O. Degteva, A. V. Akleyev, and D. L. Preston. (2013). Solid cancer mortality in the Techa River cohort (1950–2007). Radiation Research 179(2): 183–189. doi: 10.1667/RR2932.1.

Schubauer-Berigan, M. K., R. D. Daniels, and L. E. Pinkerton. (2009). "Radon exposure and mortality among White and American Indian uranium miners: An update of the Colorado Plateau cohort." American Journal of Epidemiology 169(6): 718–730. doi: 10.1093/aje/kwn406.

Schubauer-Berigan, M. K., R. D. Daniels, S. J. Bertke, C.-Y. Tseng, and D. B. Richardson. (2015). "Cancer mortality through 2005 among a pooled cohort of U.S. nuclear workers exposed to external ionizing radiation." Radiation Research 183(6): 620–631. doi: 10.1667/RR13988.1.

Schubauer-Berigan, M. K., A. Berrington de Gonzalez, E. Cardis, D. Laurier, J. H. Lubin, M. Hauptmann, and D. B. Richardson. (2020). "Evaluation of confounding and selection bias in epidemiological studies of populations exposed to low-dose, high-energy photon radiation." Journal of the National Cancer Institute Monographs 2020(56): 133–153. doi: 10.1093/jncimonographs/lgaa008.

Schull, W. J., M. Otake, and J. V. Neel. (1981). "Genetic effects of the atomic bombs: A reappraisal." Science 213(4513): 1220–1227.

Seibold, P., A. Auvinen, D. Averbeck, M. Bourguignon, J. M. Hartikainen, C. Hoeschen, O. Laurent, G. Noël, L. Sabatier, S. Salomaa, and M. Blettner. (2020). "Clinical and epidemiological observations on individual radiation sensitivity and susceptibility." International Journal of Radiation Biology 96(3): 324–339. doi: 10.1080/09553002.2019.1665209.

Seltser, R., and P. E. Sartwell. (1965). "The influence of occupational exposure to radiation on the mortality of American radiologists and other medical specialists. American Journal of Epidemiology 81(1): 2–22. doi: 10.1093/oxfordjournals.aje.a120493.

Sermage-Faure, C., D. Laurier, S. Goujon-Bellec, M. Chartier, A. Guyot-Goubin, J. Rudant, D. Hémon, and J. Clavel. (2012). "Childhood leukemia around French nuclear power plants—The geocap study, 2002–2007." International Journal of Cancer 131(5): E769–E780. doi: 10.1002/ijc.27425.

Shakhov, A. N., V. K. Singh, F. Bone, A. Cheney, Y. Kononov, P. B.-T. Krasnov, T. K. Bratanova-Toshkova, V. V. Shakhova, J. Young, M. M. Weil, A. Panoskaltsis-Mortari, C. M. Orschell, P. S. Baker, A. Gudkov, and E. Feinstein. (2012). "Prevention and mitigation of acute radiation syndrome in mice by synthetic lipopeptide agonists of Toll-like receptor 2 (TLR2)." PLoS ONE 7(3): e33044. doi: 10.1371/journal.pone.0033044.

Shaw, P. A., P. Gustafson, R. J. Carroll, V. Deffner, K. W Dodd., R. H. Keogh, V. Kipnis, J. A. Tooze, M. P. Wallace, H. Küchenhoff, and L. S. Freedman. (2020). "STRATOS guidance document on measurement error and misclassification of variables in observational epidemiology: Part 2—More complex methods of adjustment and advanced topics." Statistics in Medicine 39(16): 2232–2263. doi: 10.1002/sim.8531.

Shaw, P. A., J. He, and B. E. Shepherd. (2021). "Regression calibration to correct correlated errors in outcome and exposure." Statistic in Medicine 40(2): 271–286. doi: 10.1002/sim.8773.

Shimura, T., J. Kobayashi, K. Komatsu, and N. Kunugita. (2016). "Severe mitochondrial damage associated with low-dose radiation sensitivity in ATM- and NBS1-deficient cells." Cell Cycle 15(8): 1099–1107. doi: 10.1080/15384101.2016.1156276.

Shore, R. E. (2016). "Radiation and cataract risk: Impact of recent epidemiologic studies on ICRP judgments." Mutation Research—Reviews in Mutation Research 770(Pt. B): 231–237. doi: 10.1016/j.mrrev.2016.06.006.

Signorello, L. B., H. M. Munro, J. D. Boice, Jr., J. J. Mulvihill, D. M. Green, L. L. Robison, M. Stovall, R. E. Weathers, A. C. Mertens, and J. A. Whitton. (2010). "Stillbirth and neonatal death in relation to radiation exposure before conception: A retrospective cohort study." The Lancet 376(9741): 624–630. doi: 10.1016/S0140-6736(10)60752-0.

Signorello, L. B., J. J. Mulvihill, D. M. Green, H. M. Munro, M. Stovall, R. E. Weathers, A. C. Mertens, J. A. Whitton, L. L. Robison, and J. D. Boice, Jr. (2012). "Congenital anomalies in the children of cancer survivors: A report from the childhood cancer survivor study." Journal of Clinical Oncology 30(3): 239–245. doi: 10.1200/JCO.2011.37.2938.

Sigurdson, A. J., and E. Ron. (2004). "Cosmic radiation exposure and cancer risk among flight crew." Cancer Investigation 22(5): 743–761. doi: 10.1081/cnv-200032767.

Simon, S. L., and M. S. Linet. (2014). "Radiation-exposed populations: Who, why, and how to study." Health Physics 106(2): 182–195. doi: 10.1097/HP.0000000000000006.

Simon, S. L., F. O. Hoffman, and E. Hofer. (2015). "The two-dimensional Monte Carlo: A new methodologic paradigm for dose reconstruction for epidemiological studies." Radiation Research 183(1): 27–41. doi: 10.1667/RR13729.1.

Simon, S. L., A. Bouville, H. L. Beck, and D. R. Melo. (2020). "Estimated radiation doses received by New Mexico residents from the 1945 Trinity Nuclear Test." Health Physics 119(4): 428–477. doi: 10.1097/HP.0000000000001328.

Simonsen, L. C., T. C. Slaba, P. Guida, and A. Rusek. (2020). "NASA's first ground-based Galactic Cosmic Ray Simulator: Enabling a new era in space radiobiology research." PLoS Biology 18: e3000669. doi: 10.1371/journal.pbio.3000669.

Slovic, P. (2012). "The perception gap: Radiation and risk." Bulletin of the Atomic Scientists 68(3): 67–75. https://doi.org/10.1177/0096340212444870.

Smith, C., K. Shirvan, J. Christensen, and K. Vedros. (2021). "Making emergency planning zones smarter: A risk-informed approach for new reactors." Nuclear Newswire, April 16.

Smith, T. C., D. J. Spiegelhalter, and A. Thomas. (1995). "Bayesian approaches to random-effects meta-analysis: A comparative study." Statistics in Medicine 14(24): 2685–2699. doi: 10.1002/sim.4780142408.

Smith-Bindman, R., C. Aubin, J. Bailitz, R. N. Bengiamin, C. A. Camargo, J. Corbo, A. J. Dean, R. B. Goldstein, R. T. Griffey, G. D. Jay, T. L. Kang, D. R. Kriesel, O. J. Ma, M. Mallin, W. Manson, J. Melnikow, D. L. Miglioretti, S. K. Miller, L. D. Mills, J. R. Miner, M. Moghadassi, V. E. Noble, G. M. Press, M. L. Stoller, V. E. Valencia, J. Wang, R. C. Wang, and S. R. Cummings. (2014). "Ultrasonography versus computed tomography for suspected nephrolithiasis." New England Journal of Medicine 371: 1100–1110. doi: 10.1056/NEJMoa1404446.

Smith-Bindman, R., M. Moghadassi, R. T. Griffey, C. A. Camargo, Jr., J. Bailitz, M. Beland, and D. L. Miglioretti. (2015). "Computed tomography radiation dose in patients with suspected urolithiasis." JAMA Internal Medicine 175(8): 1413–1416. doi: 10.1001/jamainternmed.2015.2697.

Snijders, A. M., F. Marchetti, S. Bhatnagar, N. Duru, J. Han, Z. Hu, J.-H. Mao, J. W. Gray, and A. J. Wyrobek. (2012). "Genetic differences in transcript responses to low-dose ionizing radiation identify tissue functions associated with breast cancer susceptibility." PLoS ONE 7: e45394. doi: 10.1371/journal.pone.0045394.

Soares, S., S. G. Guerreiro, N. Cruz-Martins, I. Faria, P. Baylina, M. G. Sales, M. A. Correa-Duarte, and R. Fernandes. (2021). "The influence of miRNAs on radiotherapy treatment in prostate cancer—A systematic review." Frontiers in Oncology 11: 704664. doi: 10.3389/fonc.2021.704664.

SPEERA (Secretarial Panel for the Evaluation of Epidemiological Research Activities for the Department of Energy). (1990). Report to the Secretary: Secretarial Panel for the Evaluation of Epidemiological Research Activities for the Department of Energy. Washington, DC, Department of Energy.

Spix, C., S. Schmiedel, P. Kaatsch, R. Schulze-Rath, and M. Blettner. (2008). "Case-control study on childhood cancer in the vicinity of nuclear power plants in Germany 1980–2003." European Journal of Cancer 44(2): 275–284. doi: 10.1016/j.ejca.2007.10.024.

Spix, C., B. Grosche, M. Bleher, P. Kaatsch, P. Scholz-Kreisel, and M. Blettner. (2017). "Background gamma radiation and childhood cancer in Germany: An ecological study." Radiation and Environmental Biophysics 56(2): 127–138. doi: 10.1007/s00411-017-0689-2.

Sprung, C. N., A. Ivashkevich, H. B. Forrester, C. E. Redon, A. Georgakilas, and O. A. Martin. (2015). Oxidative DNA damage caused by inflammation may link to stress-induced non-targeted effects." Cancer Letters 356(1): 72–81. doi: 10.1016/j.canlet.2013.09.008.

SSFL (Santa Susana Field Laboratory) Advisory Panel. (2006). Report of the Santa Susana Field Laboratory Advisory Panel. https://www.ssflpanel.org/files/SSFLPanelReport.pdf.

Stadtmann, H., A. F. McWhan, T. W. M. Grimbergen, M. Figel, A. M. Romero, C. Gärtner, and C. Hranitzky. (2018). EURADOS Intercomparison 2014 for Whole Body Dosemeters in Photon Fields. Neuherberg, European Radiation Dosimetry Group. doi: 10.12768/fkb8-5798.

Stap, J., P. M. Krawczyk, C. H. Van Oven, G. W. Barendsen, J. Essers, R. Kanaar, and J. A. Aten. (2008). "Induction of linear tracks of DNA double-strand breaks by alpha-particle irradiation of cells." Nature Methods 5(3): 261–266. doi: 10.1038/nmeth.f.206.

Stram, D. O., D. L. Preston, M. Sokolnikov, B. Napier, K. J. Kopecky, J. Boice, H. Beck, J. Till, and A. Bouville. (2015). Shared dosimetry error in epidemiological dose-response analyses. PLoS ONE 10(3): e0119418. doi: 10.1371/journal.pone.0119418. Erratum, PLoS ONE 10(5): e0126041 (2015).

Stram, D. O., M. Sokolnikov, B. A. Napier, V. V. Vostrotin, A. Efimov, and D. L. Preston. (2021). "Lung cancer in the Mayak workers cohort: Risk estimation and uncertainty analysis." Radiation Research 195(4): 334–346. doi: 10.1667/RADE-20-00094.1.

Stricklin, D. L., J. VanHorne-Sealy, C. I. Rios, L. A. Scott Carnell, and L. P. Taliaferro. (2021). "Neutron radiobiology and dosimetry." Radiation Research 195(5): 480–496. doi: 10.1667/RADE-20-00213.1.

Stuart, T., A. Butler, P. Hoffman, C. Hafemeister, E. Papalexi, W. M. Mauck, III, Y. Hao, M. Stoeckius, P. Smibert, and R. Satija. (2019). "Comprehensive integration of single-cell data. Cell 177(7): 1888–1902. doi: 10.1016/j.cell.2019.05.031.

Suckert, T., S. Nexhipi, A. Dietrich, R. Koch, L.A. Kunz-Schughart, E. Bahn, and E. Beyreuther. (2021). "Models for translational proton radiobiology—From bench to bedside and back." Cancers (Basel) 13(16): 4216. doi: 10.3390/cancers13164216.

Sugiyama, H., M. Misumi, R. Sakata, A. V. Brenner, M. Utada, and K. Ozasa. (2021). "Mortality among individuals exposed to atomic bomb radiation in utero: 1950–2012." European Journal of Epidemiology 36(4): 415–428. doi: 10.1007/s10654-020-00713-5.

Sugiyama, T., M. Iwaizumi, M. Kaneko, S. Tani, M. Yamade, Y. Hamaya, T. Furuta, H. Miyajima, S. Osawa, S. Baba, M. Maekawa, and K. Sugimoto. (2020). "DNA mismatch repair is not disrupted in stage 0 colorectal cancer resected using endoscopic submucosal dissection." Oncology Letters 20(3): 2435–2441. doi: 10.3892/ol.2020.11799.

Sun, H., S. Cao, R. J. Mashl, C. K. Mo, S. Zaccaria, M. C. Wendl, S. R. Davies, M. H. Bailey, T. M. Primeau, J. Hoog, J. L. Mudd, D. A. Dean II, R. Patidar, L. Chen, M. A. Wyczalkowski, R. G. Jayasinghe, F. M. Rodrigues, N. V. Terekhanova, Y. Li, K. H. Lim, A. Wang-Gillam, B. A. Van Tine, C. X. Ma, R. Aft, K. C. Fuh, J. K. Schwarz, J. P. Zevallos, S. V. Puram, J. F. Dipersio, NCI PDXNet Consortium; B. Davis-Dusenbery, M. J. Ellis, M. T. Lewis, M. A. Davies, M. Herlyn, B. Fang, J. A. Roth, A. L. Welm, B. E. Welm, F. Meric-Bernstam, F. Chen, R. C. Fields, S. Li, R. Govindan, J. H. Doroshow, J. A. Moscow, Y. A. Evrard, J. H. Chuang, B. J. Raphael, and L. Ding. (2021). "Comprehensive characterization of 536 patient-derived xenograft models prioritizes candidates for targeted treatment." Nature Communications 12(1): 5086. doi: 10.1038/s41467-021-25177-3. Erratum, Nature Communications 13(1): 294 (2022).

Sunstein, C. R. (2002). Risk and Reason: Safety, Law, and the Environment. Cambridge, UK, Cambridge University Press.

Sunstein, C. R. (2017). "Cost-benefit analysis and arbitrariness review." Harvard Environmental Law Review 41(1): 1–41.

Suzuki, Y., H. Yabe, S. Yasumura, T. Ohira, S.-I. Niwa, A. Ohtsuru, H. Mashiko, M. Maeda, and M. Abe. (2015). "Psychological distress and the perception of radiation risks: The Fukushima Health Management Survey." Bulletin of the World Health Organization 93(9): 598–605. doi: 10.2471/BLT.14.146498.

Suzuki, Y., Y. Takebayashi, M. Murakami, S. Yasumura, M. Harigane, H. Yabe, T. Ohira, A. Ohtsuru, S. Nakajima, and M. Maeda. (2018). "Changes in risk perception of the health effects of radiation and mental health status: The Fukushima Health Management Survey." International Journal of Environmental Research and Public Health 15(6): 1219. doi: 10.3390/ijerph15061219.

Svingen, T., D. L. Villeneuve, D. Knapen, E. M. Panagiotou, M. K. Draskau, P. Damdimopoulou, and J. M. O'Brien. (2021). "A pragmatic approach to adverse outcome pathway development and evaluation." Toxicological Sciences 184(2): 183–190. doi: 10.1093/toxsci/kfab113.

Sykes, A. J., P. D. Larsen, R. F. Griffiths, and S. Aldington. (2012). "A study of airline pilot morbidity." Aviation, Space, and Environmental Medicine 83(10): 1001–1006.

Tabachnik, S. (2019). "Recent soil samples suggest Rocky Flats still unsafe, environmental groups contend." Denver Post, September 3. https://www.denverpost.com/2019/09/03/rocky-flats-lawsuit-safety.

Taliaferro, L. P., D. R. Cassatt, Z. P. Horta, and M. M. Satyamitra. (2021). "Meeting report: A poly-pharmacy approach to mitigate acute radiation syndrome." Radiation Research 196(4): 436–446. doi: 10.1667/RADE-21-00048.1.

Tallarita, R. (2020). "The tragedy of costs and benefits." Boston Review. https://bostonreview.net/articles/roberto-tallarita-tragedy-costs-and-benefits.

Tao, R., D. Zeng, and D. Y. Lin. (2020). "Optimal designs of two-phase studies." Journal of the American Statistical Association 115(532): 1946–1959. doi: 10.1080/01621459.2019.1671200.

Tao, Z., S. Akiba, Y. Zha, Q. Sun, J. Zou, J. Li, Y. Liu, Y. Yuan, S. Tokonami, H. Morishoma, T. Koga, S. Nakamura, T. Sugahara, and L. Wei. (2012). "Cancer and non-cancer mortality among inhabitants in the high background radiation area of Yangjiang, China (1979–1998). Health Physics 102(2): 173–181. doi: 10.1097/HP.0b013e31822c7f1e.

Tapio, S., M. P. Little, J. C. Kaiser, N. Impens, N. Hamada, A. G. Georgakilas, D. Simar, and S. Salomaa. (2021). "Ionizing radiation-induced circulatory and metabolic diseases." Environment International 146: 106235. doi: 10.1016/j.envint.2020.106235.

Tawn, E. J., G. S. Rees, C. Leith, J. F. Winther, G. B. Curwen, M. Stovall, J. H. Olsen, C. Rechnitzer, H. Schroeder, P. Guldberg, and J. D. Boice, Jr. (2011). "Germline minisatellite mutations in survivors of childhood and young adult cancer treated with radiation." International Journal of Radiation Biology 87: 330–340. doi: 10.3109/09553002.2011.530338.

Teschendorff, A. E, and A. P. Feinberg. (2021). "Statistical mechanics meets single-cell biology." Nature Reviews Genetics 22(7): 459–476. doi: 10.1038/s41576-021-00341-z.

Tharmalingam, S., S. Sreetharan, A. V. Kulesza, D. R. Boreham, and T. C. Tai. (2017). "Low-dose ionizing radiation exposure, oxidative stress and epigenetic programing of health and disease." Radiation Research 188(4.2): 525–538. doi: 10.1667/RR14587.1.

Thierry-Chef, I., G. Ferro, L. Le Cornet, J. Dabin, T. S. Istad, A. Jahnen, C. Lee, C. Maccia, F. Malchair, H. M. Olerud, R. W. Harbron, J. Figuerola, J. Hermen, M. Moissonnier, M. O. Bernier, M. B. Bosch de Basea, G. Byrnes, E. Cardis, M. Hauptmann, N. Journy, A. Kesminiene, J. M. Meulepas, R. Pokora, and S. L. Simon. (2021). "Dose estimation for the European Epidemiological Study on Pediatric Computed Tomography (EPI-CT)." Radiation Research 196(1): 74–99. doi: 10.1667/RADE-20-00231.1.

Thome, C., D. B. Chambers, A. M. Hooker, J. W. Thompson, and D. R. Boreham. (2018). "Deterministic effects to the lens of the eye following ionizing radiation exposure: Is there evidence to support a reduction in threshold dose?" Health Physics 114(3): 328–343. doi: 10.1097/HP.0000000000000810.

Tognon, C. E., R. C. Sears, G. B. Mills, J. W. Gray, and J. W. Tyner. (2021). "*Ex vivo* analysis of primary tumor specimens for evaluation of cancer therapeutics." Annual Review of Cancer Biology 5: 39–57. doi: 10.1146/annurev-cancerbio-043020-125955.

Tomasek, L. (2012). "Lung cancer mortality among Czech uranium miners—60 years since exposure." Journal of Radiological Protection 32(3): 301–314. doi: 10.1088/0952-4746/32/3/301.

Tomasek, L. (2013). "Lung cancer risk from occupational and environmental radon and role of smoking in two Czech nested case-control studies." International Journal of Environmental Research and Public Health 10(3): 963–979. doi: 10.3390/ijerph10030963.

Tomita, M., and M. Maeda. (2015). "Mechanisms and biological importance of photon-induced bystander responses: Do they have an impact on low-dose radiation responses." Journal of Radiation Research 56(2): 205–219. doi: 10.1093/jrr/rru099.

Topol, E. J. (2019). "High-performance medicine: The convergence of human and artificial intelligence." Nature Medicine 25(1): 44–56. doi: 10.1038/s41591-018-0300-7.

Tracy, B. S. (2020). An Overview of Rare Earth Elements and Related Issues for Congress. Washington, DC, Congressional Research Service. https://crsreports.congress.gov/product/pdf/R/R46618.

Tran, V., L. B. Zablotska, A. V. Brenner, and M. P. Little. (2017). "Radiation-associated circulatory disease mortality in a pooled analysis of 77,275 patients from the Massachusetts and Canadian tuberculosis fluoroscopy cohorts." Scientific Reports 7(1): 44147. doi: 10.1038/srep44147.

Trichopoulos, D., X. Zavitsanos, C. Koutis, P. Drogari, C. Proukakis, and E. Petridou. (1987). "The victims of Chernobyl in Greece: Induced abortions after the accident." British Medical Journal 295(6606): 1100. doi: 10.1136/bmj.295.6606.1100.

Trott, K. R., and F. Kamprad. (1999). "Radiobiological mechanisms of anti-inflammatory radiotherapy. Radiotherapy and Oncology 51(3): 197–203. doi: 10.1016/s0167-8140(99)00066-3.

Tsuruoka, C., M. Kaminishi, M. Shinagawa, Y. Shang, Y. Amasaki, Y. Shimada, and S. Kakinuma. (2021). "High relative biological effectiveness of 2 MeV fast neutrons for induction of medulloblastoma in Ptch1+/- mice with radiation-specific deletion on chromosome 13." Radiation Research 196(2): 225–234. doi: 10.1667/RADE-20-00025.1.

Turner, M. C., D. Krewski, Y. Chen, C. A. Pope, III, S. Gapstur, and M. J. Thun. (2011). "Radon and lung cancer in the American Cancer Society cohort." Cancer Epidemiology, Biomarkers and Prevention 20(3): 438–448. https://doi.org/10.1158/1055-9965.EPI-10-1153.

Tyldesley, S., G. Delaney, F. Foroudi, L. Barbera, M. Kerba, and W. Mackillop. (2011). "Estimating the need for radiotherapy for patients with prostate, breast, and lung cancers: Verification of model estimates of need with radiotherapy utilization data from British Columbia." International Journal of Radiation Oncology, Biology and Physics 79(5): 1507–1515. doi: 10.1016/j.ijrobp.2009.12.070.

Ulsh, B. A., F. W. Whicker, T. G. Hinton, J. D. Congdon, and J. S. Bedford. (2001). "Chromosome translocations in *T. scripta*: The dose-rate effect and in vivo lymphocyte radiation response." Radiation Research 155(1): 63–73. doi: 10.1667/0033-7587(2001)155[0063:ctitst]2.0.co;2.

UN (United Nations). (2021). 2021 Universal Declaration of Human Rights. https://www.un.org/en/about-us/universal-declaration-of-human-rights.

UNSCEAR (United Nations Scientific Committee on the Effects of Atomic Radiation). (2000). UNSCEAR 2000 Report. Vol. II: Sources and Effects of Ionizing Radiation, Annex H: Combined effects of radiation and other agents. New York, United Nations.

UNSCEAR. (2006a). Effects of Ionizing Radiation, Annex A: Epidemiological studies of radiation and cancer. New York, United Nations. https://www.unscear.org/docs/publications/2006/UNSCEAR_2006_Annex-A-CORR.pdf.

UNSCEAR. (2006b). Effects of Ionizing Radiation, Annex D: Effects of Ionizing Radiation on the Immune System. New York, United Nations. https://www.unscear.org/docs/publications/2006/UNSCEAR_2006_Annex-D.pdf.

UNSCEAR. (2008). Sources and Effects of Ionizing Radiation, Annex B: Exposures of the public and workers from various sources of radiation. https://www.unscear.org/docs/publications/2008/UNSCEAR_2008_Annex-B-CORR2.pdf.

UNSCEAR. (2016). Sources, Effects, and Risks of Ionizing Radiation, Annex B: Radiation exposures from electricity generation. https://www.unscear.org/docs/publications/2016/UNSCEAR_2016_Annex-B-CORR2.pdf.

UNSCEAR. (2020a). Report of the United Nations Scientific Committee on the Effects of Atomic Radiation. Sixty-seventh session (2-6 November 2020). Report A/76/46 Part 1, pp. 1–22. New York, United Nations. https://www.unscear.org/docs/GAreports/2020/UNSCEAR_Report_General_Assembly_A_76_46_Part1.pdf.

UNSCEAR. (2020b). Sources, Effects and Risks of Ionizing Radiation: UNSCEAR 2020 Report, Scientific Annex B: Levels and effects of radiation exposure due to the accident at the Fukushima Daiichi Nuclear Power Station: Implications of information published since the UNSCEAR 2013 Report. https://www.unscear.org/docs/publications/2020/UNSCEAR_2020_AnnexB_AdvanceCopy.pdf.

UNSCEAR. (2021). Sources, Effects and Risks of Ionizing Radiation: UNSCEAR 2020/2021, Report to the General Assembly, with Scientific Annexes, Volume III, Scientific Annex C: Biological mechanisms relevant for the inference of cancer risks from low-dose and low-dose-rate radiation. New York, United Nations. https://www.unscear.org/docs/publications/2020/UNSCEAR_2020_21_Annex-C.pdf.

Unternaehrer-Hamm, J., E. Chirshev, N. Hojo; A. Bertucci, L. Sanderman, N. Nguyen, H. Wang, T. Suzuki, E. Brito, S. Martinez, C. Castañón, S. Mirshahidi, M. E. Vazquez, K. Oberg, and Y. Ioffe. (2020). "Epithelial/mesenchymal heterogeneity of high-grade serous ovarian carcinoma samples correlates with let-7 levels and predicts tumor growth and metastasis." Molecular Oncology 14(11): 2796–2813. doi: 10.1002/1878-0261.12762.

U.S. Congress, House. (2021). Examining the Need to Expand Eligibility Under the Radiation Exposure Compensation Act. Hearing Before the Committee on the Judiciary Subcommittee on the Constitution, Civil Rights, and Civil Liberties (statement of Scott D. Szymendera, Analyst in Disability Policy, March 24). Washington, DC, Congressional Research Service.

U.S. Congress, Senate. (1998). Radioactive Fallout from Nuclear Testing at Nevada Test Site, 1950-60. Hearing before a Subcommittee of the Committee on Appropriations, 105th Congress, 1st Session. Washington, DC, U.S. Government Printing Office. https://www.govinfo.gov/content/pkg/CHRG-105shrg44045/html/CHRG-105shrg44045.htm.

U.S. NRC (United States Nuclear Regulatory Commission). (1986). "Safety goals for the operation of nuclear power plants (51 FR 28044; August 4, 1986 as corrected and re-published at 51 FR 30028; August 21, 1986)." Federal Register 51: 30028.

U.S. NRC. (1995). Reassessment of NRC's Dollar per Person-rem Conversion Factor Policy. Washington, DC, Office of Nuclear Regulatory Research, Division of Regulatory Applications, U.S. Nuclear Regulatory Commission.

U.S. NRC. (2012). Technical Evaluation Report: For the U.S. Department of Energy West Valley Draft Waste Incidental to Reprocessing Evaluation for the Concentrator Feed Makeup Tank and the Melter Feed Hold Tank Final Report. Washington, DC, Office of Federal and State Materials and Environmental Management Programs, U.S. Nuclear Regulatory Commission. https://www.nrc.gov/docs/ML1227/ML12270A279.pdf.

U.S. NRC. (2015a). 10 CFR Part 20 [Docket Nos. PRM-20-28, PRM-20-29, and PRM-20-30; NRC-2015-0057], Linear No-Threshold Model and Standards for Protection Against Radiation. Rockville, MD, U.S. Nuclear Regulatory Commission.

U.S. NRC. (2015b). Examining the Reasons for Ending the Cancer Risk Study. https://public-blog.nrc-gateway.gov/2015/10/06/examining-the-reasons-for-ending-the-cancer-risk-study.

U.S. NRC. (2017). Regulatory Analysis Guidelines of the U.S. Nuclear Regulatory Commission, Draft Report for Comment. Washington, DC, Office of Nuclear Regulatory Research, U.S. Nuclear Regulatory Commission.

U.S. NRC. (2020a). NRC Non-Light Water Reactor (Non-LWR) Vision and Strategy, Volume 4: Licensing and Siting Dose Assessment Codes [DRAFT]. Washington, DC, U.S. Nuclear Regulatory Commission.

U.S. NRC. (2020b). Valuing Nonfatal Cancer Risks in Cost-Benefit Analysis. https://www.nrc.gov/docs/ML2005/ML20058C222.pdf.

U.S. NRC. (2021). "Linear no-threshold model and standards for protection against radiation: A proposed rule by the Nuclear Regulatory Commission on 08/17/2021." Federal Register 86: 45923–45936.

U.S. NRC. (2022). Reassessment of NRC's Dollar per Person-rem Conversion Factor Policy, Revision 1. Washington, DC, Office of Nuclear Material Safety and Safeguards, U.S. Nuclear Regulatory Commission. https://www.nrc.gov/docs/ML2205/ML22053A025.pdf.

Utada, M., A. V. Brenner, D. L. Preston, J. B. Cologne, R. Sakata, H. Sugiyama, A. Sadakane, E. J. Grant, E. K. Cahoon, K. Ozasa, and K. Mabuchi. (2018). "Radiation risks of uterine cancer in atomic bomb survivors: 1958–2009." JNCI Cancer Spectrum 2(4): pky081. doi: 10.1093/jncics/pky081.

Utada, M., A. V. Brenner, D. L. Preston, J. B. Cologne, R. Sakata, H. Sugiyama, N. Kato, E. J. Grant, E. J. Cahoon, K. Mabuchi, and K. Ozasa. (2020). "Radiation risk of ovarian cancer in atomic bomb survivors: 1958–2009." Radiation Research 195(1): 60–65.

Van Dilla, M. A., T. T. Trujillo, P. F. Mullaney, and J. R. Coulter. (1969). "Cell microfluorometry: A method for rapid fluorescence measurement." Science 163(3872): 1213–1214. doi: 10.1126/science.163.3872.1213.

Van Voorhies, W. A., H. A. Castillo, C. N. Thawng, and G. B. Smith. (2020). "The phenotypic and transcriptomic response of the *Caenorhabditis elegans* nematode to background and below-background radiation levels." Frontiers in Public Health 8: 581796. doi: 10.3389/fpubh.2020.581796.

Vandiver, A. R., R. A. Irizarry, K. D. Hansen, L. A. Garza, A. Runarsson, X. Li, A. L. Chien, T. S. Wang, S. G. Leung, S. Kang, and A. P. Feinberg. (2015). "Age and sun exposure-related widespread genomic blocks of hypomethylation in nonmalignant skin." Genome Biology 16(1): 1–15. doi: 10.1186/s13059-015-0644-y.

Velazquez-Kronen, R., E. S. Gilbert, M. S. Linet, K. B. Moysich, J. L. Freudenheim, J. Wactawski-Wende, S. L. Simon, E. K. Cahoon, B. H. Alexander, M. M. Doody, and C. M. Kitahara. (2020). "Lung cancer mortality associated with protracted low-dose occupational radiation exposures and smoking behaviors in U.S. radiologic technologists, 1983–2012." International Journal of Cancer 147(11): 3130–3138. doi: 10.1002/ijc.33141.

Viscusi, W. K. (2018). Pricing Lives: Guideposts for a Safer Society. Princeton, NJ, Princeton University Press.

Wakeford, R. (2019). "Does low-level exposure to ionizing radiation increase the risk of cardiovascular disease?" Hypertension 73: 1170–1171. doi: 10.1161/HYPERTENSIONAHA.119.11892.

Wakeford, R., and J. F. Bithell. (2021). "A review of the types of childhood cancer associated with a medical X-ray examination of the pregnant mother." International Journal of Radiation Biology 97(5): 571–592. doi: 10.1080/09553002.2021.1906463.

Wakeford, R., and M. P. Little. (2003). "Risk coefficients for childhood cancer after intrauterine irradiation: A review." International Journal of Radiation Biology 79(5): 293–309. doi: 10.1080/0955300031000114729.

Wasserstein, D. L., and N. A. Lazar. (2016). "The ASA statement on *p*-values: Context, process, and purpose." American Statistician 70(2): 129–133. doi: 10.1080/00031305.2016.1154108.

Weinstein, N. D., K. Kolb, and B. D. Goldstein. (1996). "Using time intervals between expected events to communicate risk magnitudes." Risk Analysis 16(3): 305–308. doi: 10.1111/j.1539-6924.1996.tb01464.x.

Whipple, C. (1987). De Minimis Risk. Boston, MA, Springer-Verlag.

White-Koning, M. L., D. Hémon, D. Laurier, M. Tirmarche, E. Jougla, A. Goubin, and J. Clavel. (2004). "Incidence of childhood leukaemia in the vicinity of nuclear sites in France, 1990–1998." British Journal of Cancer 91(5): 916–922. doi: 10.1038/sj.bjc.6602068.

Wieselquist, W. A., R. A. Lefebvre, and M. A. Jessee (eds.). (2020). SCALE Code System, ORNL/TM-2005/39, Version 6.2.4. Oak Ridge, TN, Oak Ridge National Laboratory.

Wilkinson, M. D., M. Dumontier, I. J. Aalbersberg, G. Appleton, M. Axton, A. Baak, N. Blomberg, J.-W. Boiten, L. B. Da Silva Santos, P. E. Bourne, J. Bouwman, A. J. Brookes, T. Clark, M. Crosas, I. Dillo, O. Dumon, S. Edmunds, C. T. Evelo, R. Finkers, A. Gonzalez-Beltran, A. J. Gray, P. Groth, C. Goble, J. S. Grethe, J. Heringa, P. A. Hoen, R. Hooft, T. Kuhn, R. Kok, J. Kok, S. J. Lusher, M. E. Martone, A. Mons, A. L. Packer, B. Persson, P. Rocca-Serra, M. Roos, R. Van Schaik, S.-A. Sansone, E. Schultes, T. Sengstag, T. Slater, G. Strawn, M. A. Swertz, M. Thompson, J. Van Der Lei, E. Van Mulligen, J. Velterop, A. Waagmeester, P. Wittenburg, K. Wolstencroft, J. Zhao, and B. Mons. (2016). "The FAIR guiding principles for scientific data management and stewardship." Scientific Data 3: 160018. doi: 10.1038/sdata.2016.18.

Wilson, P. F., H. Nagasawa, C. L. Warner, M. M. Fitzek, J. B. Little, and J. S. Bedford. (2008). "Radiation sensitivity of primary fibroblasts from hereditary retinoblastoma family members and some apparently normal controls: Colony formation ability during continuous low-dose-rate gamma irradiation." Radiation Research 169(5): 483–494. doi: 10.1667/RR1333.1.

Wilson, R. H., K. Vishwanath, and M. A. Mycek. (2016). "Optical methods for quantitative and label-free sensing in living human tissues: Principles, techniques, and applications." Advances in Physics 1(4): 523–543. doi: 10.1080/23746149.2016.1221739.

WNN. (2021). "Fukushima water release will have minimal impact, Tepco says." World Nuclear News, November 17.

Wojcik, A., S. Bouffler, M. Hauptmann, and P. Rajaraman. (2018). "Considerations on the use of the terms radiosensitivity and radiosusceptibility." Journal of Radiological Protection 38(3): N25–N29.

Wu, Y., F. O. Hoffman, A. I. Apostoaei, D. Kwon, B. A. Thomas, R. Glass, and L. B. Zablotska. (2019). "Methods to account for uncertainties in exposure assessment in studies of environmental exposures." Environmental Health 18(1): 31. doi: 10.1186/s12940-019-0468-4.

Xu, Y., G. Randers-Pehrson, H. C. Turner, S. A. Marino, C. R. Geard, D. J. Brenner, and G. Garty. (2015). "Accelerator-based biological irradiation facility simulating neutron exposure from an improvised nuclear device. Radiation Research 184(4): 404–410. doi: 10.1667/RR14036.1.

Yamada, M., K. Furukawa, Y. Tatsukawa, K. Marumo, S. Funamoto, R. Sakata, K. Ozasa, H. M. Cullings, D. L. Preston, and P. Kurttio. (2021). "Congenital malformations and perinatal deaths among the children of atomic bomb survivors: A reappraisal." American Journal of Epidemiology 190(11): 2323–2333. doi: 10.1093/aje/kwab099.

Yeager, M., M. J. Machiela, P. Kothiyal, M. Dean, C. Bodelon, S. Suman, M. Wang, L. Mirabello, C. W. Nelson, W. Zhou, C. Palmer, B. Ballew, L. M. Colli, N. D. Freedman, C. Dagnall, A. Hutchinson, V. Vij, Y. Maruvka, M. Hatch, I. Illienko, Y. Belayev, N. Nakamura, V. Chumak, E. Bakhanova, D. Belyi, V. Kryuchkov, I. Golovanov, N. Gudzenko, E. K. Cahoon, P. Albert, V. Drozdovitch, M. P. Little, K. Mabuchi, C. Stewart, G. Getz, D. Bazyka, A. Berrington de Gonzalez, and S. J. Chanock. (2021). "Lack of transgenerational effects of ionizing radiation exposure from the Chernobyl accident." Science 372(6543): 725–729. doi: 10.1126/science.abg2365.

Yeom, Y. S., H. Han, C. Choi, T. T. Nguyen, B. Shin, C. Lee, and C. H. Kim. (2019). "Posture-dependent dose coefficients of mesh-type ICRP reference computational phantoms for photon external exposures." Physics in Medicine and Biology 64(7): 075018. doi: 10.1088/1361-6560/ab0917.

Yeom, Y. S., K. Griffin, H. Han, C. Choi, B. Shin, T. T. Nguyen, C. H. Kim, and C. Lee. (2021). "Dose conversion coefficients for neutron external exposures with five postures: Walking, sitting, bending, kneeling, and squatting." Radiation and Environmental Biophysics 60(2): 317–328. doi: 10.1007/s00411-021-00900-2.

Yong, L. C., L. E. Pinkerton, J. H. Yiin, J. L. Anderson, and J. A. Deddens. (2014). "Mortality among a cohort of U.S. commercial airline cockpit crew." American Journal of Industrial Medicine 57(8): 906–914. doi: 10.1002/ajim.22318.

Yoshida, K., B. French, N. Yoshida, A. Hida, W. Ohishi, and Y. Kusunoki. (2019). "Radiation exposure and longitudinal changes in peripheral monocytes over 50 years: The Adult Health Study of atomic-bomb survivors." British Journal of Haematology 185(1): 107–115. doi: 10.1111/bjh.15750.

Young, A. L. (2020). "Radiation research and policy coordination: A successful model." Urban Studies and Public Administration 3(3): 183–193. doi: 10.22158/uspa.v3n3p183.

Zablotska, L. B., R. S. D. Lane, and P. A. Thompson. (2014a). "A reanalysis of cancer mortality in Canadian nuclear workers (1956–1994) based on revised exposure and cohort data." British Journal of Cancer 110(1): 214–223. doi: 10.1038/bjc.2013.592.

Zablotska, L. B., M. P. Little, and R. J. Cornett (2014b). Potential increased risk of ischemic heart disease mortality with significant dose fractionation in the Canadian Fluoroscopy Cohort Study. American Journal of Epidemiology 179(1): 120–131. doi: 10.1093/aje/kwt244.

Zander, A., T. Paunesku, and G. Woloschak. (2019). "Radiation databases and archives—examples and comparisons." International Journal of Radiation Biology 95(10): 1378–1389. doi: 10.1080/09553002.2019.1572249.

Zeeb, H., G. P. Hammer, I. Langner, T. Schafft, S. Bennack, and M. Blettner. (2010). "Cancer mortality among German aircrew: Second follow-up." Radiation and Environmental Biophysics 49(2): 187–194. doi: 10.1007/s00411-009-0248-6.

Zeeb, H., G. P. Hammer, and M. Blettner. (2012). "Epidemiological investigations of aircrew: An occupational group with low-level cosmic radiation exposure." Journal of Radiological Protection 32(1): N15–N19. doi: 10.1088/0952-4746/32/1/N15.

Zhang, W., R. G. E. Haylock, M. Gillies, and N. Hunter. (2019). "Mortality from heart diseases following occupational radiation exposure: Analysis of the National Registry for Radiation Workers (NRRW) in the United Kingdom." Journal of Radiological Protection 39(2): 327–353. doi: 10.1088/1361-6498/ab02b2.

Zhang, Y. S., G. T. Santiago, M. M. Alvarez, S. J. Schiff, E. S. Boyden, and A. Khademhosseini. (2017). "Expansion mini-microscopy: An enabling alternative in point-of-care diagnostics." Current Opinion in Biomedical Engineering 1: 45–53. doi: 10.1016/j.cobme.2017.03.001.

Zhao, T., Z. D. Chiang, J. W. Morriss, L. M. LaFave, E. M. Murray, I. Del Priore, K. Meli, C. A. Lareau, N. M. Nadaf, J. Li, A. S. Earl, E. Z. Macosko, T. Jacks, J. D. Buenrostro, and F. Chen. (2022). "Spatial genomics enables multi-modal study of clonal heterogeneity in tissues." Nature 601(7891): 85–91. doi: 10.1038/s41586-021-04217-4.

Appendix A

Consolidated Appropriations Act, 2021

SEC. 11001. LOW-DOSE RADIATION RESEARCH

(a) LOW-DOSE RADIATION RESEARCH PROGRAM.—Section 306(c) of the Department of Energy Research and Innovation Act (42 U.S.C. 18644(c)) is amended to read as follows:
"(c) LOW-DOSE RADIATION RESEARCH PROGRAM.—
"(1) IN GENERAL.—The Secretary shall carry out a research program on low-dose and low-dose-rate radiation to—
"(A) enhance the scientific understanding of, and reduce uncertainties associated with, the effects of exposure to low-dose and low-dose-rate radiation; and
"(B) inform improved risk-assessment and risk-management methods with respect to such radiation.
"(2) PROGRAM COMPONENTS.—In carrying out the program required under paragraph (1), the Secretary shall—
"(A) support and carry out the directives under section 106(b) of the American Innovation and Competitiveness Act (42 U.S.C. 6601 note), except that such section shall be treated for purposes of this subsection as applying to low-dose and low-dose rate radiation research, in coordination with the Physical Science Subcommittee of the National Science and Technology Council;
"(B) identify and, to the extent possible, quantify, potential monetary and health-related impacts to Federal agencies, the general public, industry,

research communities, and other users of information produced by such research program;

"(C) leverage the collective body of knowledge from existing low-dose and low-dose-rate radiation research;

"(D) engage with other Federal agencies, research communities, and potential users of information produced under this section, including institutions performing or utilizing radiation research, medical physics, radiology, health physics, and emergency response measures; and

"(E) support education and outreach activities to disseminate information and promote public understanding of low-dose radiation, with a focus on non-emergency situations such as medical physics, space exploration, and naturally occurring radiation.

"(3) RESEARCH PLAN.—

"(A) Not later than 90 days after the date of enactment of the Energy Act of 2020, the Secretary shall enter into an agreement with the National Academy of Sciences to develop a long-term strategic and prioritized research agenda for the program described in paragraph (2);

"(B) Not later than one year after the date of enactment of the Energy Act of 2020, the Secretary shall transmit this research plan developed in subparagraph (A) to the Committee on Science, Space, and Technology of the House of Representatives and the Committee on Energy and Natural Resources of the Senate.

"(4) GAO STUDY.—Not later than 3 years after the date of enactment of the Energy Act of 2020, the Comptroller General shall transmit to the Committee on Science, Space, and Technology of the House of Representatives and the Committee on Energy and Natural Resources of the Senate, a report on:

"(A) an evaluation of the program activities carried out under this section;

"(B) the effectiveness of the coordination and management of the program; and

"(C) the implementation of the research plan outlined in paragraph (3).

"(6) DEFINITIONS.—In this subsection:

"(A) LOW-DOSE RADIATION.—The term 'low-dose radiation' means a radiation dose of less than 100 millisieverts.

"(B) LOW-DOSE-RATE RADIATION.—The term 'low-dose-rate radiation' means a radiation dose rate of less than 5 millisieverts per hour.

"(7) RULE OF CONSTRUCTION.—Nothing in this subsection shall be construed to subject any research carried out by the Secretary for the program under this subsection to any limitations described in section 977(e) of the Energy Policy Act of 2005 (42 U.S.C. 16317(e)).

"(8) FUNDING.—For purposes of carrying out this subsection, the Secretary is authorized to make available from funds provided to the Biological and Environmental Research Program—

"(A) $20,000,000 for fiscal year 2021;
"(B) $20,000,000 for fiscal year 2022;
"(C) $30,000,000 for fiscal year 2023; and
"(D) $40,000,000 for fiscal year 2024."
(b) SPACE RADIATION RESEARCH.—Section 306 of the Department of Energy Research and Innovation Act (42 U.S.C. 18644) is amended by adding at the end the following:
"(d) SPACE RADIATION RESEARCH.—The Secretary of Energy shall continue and strengthen collaboration with the Administrator of the National Aeronautics and Space Administration on basic research to understand the effects and risks of human exposure to ionizing radiation in low Earth orbit, and in the space environment."

Appendix B

Committee and Staff Biographies

CHAIR

Joe W. Gray is a physicist and an engineer by training and is currently a professor emeritus of laboratory medicine at the University of California, San Francisco, and biomedical engineering at Oregon Health & Science University (OHSU). His laboratory developed and applied advanced measurement technologies to elucidate mechanisms involved in cancer genesis, progression, and response to therapy, and he applied systems control strategies to develop more durable and tolerable cancer treatments. His work is described in more than 550 publications and 90 U.S. patents. Prior to joining OHSU, Dr. Gray was a staff scientist in the biomedical sciences division of the Lawrence Livermore National Laboratory (1972–1991); a professor of laboratory medicine at the University of California, San Francisco (1991–2011); and an associate laboratory director for biosciences and the director of life sciences at the Lawrence Berkeley National Laboratory (2003–2011). He is a fellow of the American Association for the Advancement of Science, the American Institute for Medical and Biological Engineering, and the American Association of Cancer Research Academy, and a member of the National Academy of Medicine. He also serves on the Board of Counselors for the Radiation Effects Research Foundation. Dr. Gray has a B.S. in engineering physics from the Colorado School of Mines (1968) and a Ph.D. in physics from Kansas State University (1972).

MEMBERS

Simon D. Bouffler is the head of the Radiation Effects Department at Public Health England's (PHE's) Centre for Radiation, Chemical and Environmental Hazards in the United Kingdom (note that PHE became part of the UK Health Security Agency as of October 1, 2021). He has more than 30 years of experience in radiation protection research and has responsibility for epidemiological and experimental research related to radiation risk; this includes both ionizing and non-ionizing radiation and ultraviolet light. He has wide-ranging research interests on the mechanisms of radiogenic diseases, particularly at low doses and low dose rates of exposure, with more than 120 relevant peer-reviewed publications. He was awarded a B.Sc. (1981) and a Ph.D. (1984) in biology from the University of Southampton, United Kingdom. He has been involved in many radiation protection research projects and provided leadership on stakeholder engagement for the EU CONCERT project. He is the chair of the MELODI Strategic Research Agenda working group and coordinated the RISK-IR project that investigated the effects of ionizing radiation, particularly at low doses, on stem cell function. He has served as the UK representative to the United Nations Scientific Committee on the Effects of Atomic Radiation since 2015, having worked for the Committee since 2008; additionally since 2017, he has served on the Main Commission of the International Commission on Radiological Protection. In 2018, he was awarded the Weiss Medal by the UK Association for Radiation Research.

Shaheen A. Dewji is an assistant professor in the Nuclear and Radiological Engineering and Medical Physics Programs in the George W. Woodruff School of Mechanical Engineering at the Georgia Institute of Technology. Previously, Dr. Dewji was a faculty member in the Department of Nuclear Engineering at Texas A&M University and a Faculty Fellow of the Center for Nuclear Security Science and Policy Initiatives. In her preceding role at Oak Ridge National Laboratory, Dr. Dewji was a radiological scientist in the Center for Radiation Protection Knowledge, where her recent work has included assessment of patient release criteria for nuclear medicine patients and development of dose coefficients associated with the external exposure and internal uptake of radionuclides due to environmental or nuclear security exposures. Dr. Dewji completed her M.S. (2009) and Ph.D. (2014) in nuclear and radiological engineering at the Georgia Institute of Technology in Atlanta, and is an alumna of the Sam Nunn Security Program. As a native of Vancouver, Canada, she received her B.S. in physics from The University of British Columbia (2006). Since 2020, Dr. Dewji has served as a member of the National Academies of Sciences, Engineering, and Medicine's Nuclear and Radiation Studies Board and was a member of the 2021

Panel on Review of Selected Research Areas at the Physical Measurement Laboratory of the National Institute of Standards and Technology.

Andrew P. Feinberg studied mathematics and humanities at Yale University in the Directed Studies honors program, and he received his B.A. (1973) and M.D. (1976) from the accelerated medical program at Johns Hopkins University, as well as an M.P.H. from Johns Hopkins (1981). He performed a postdoctoral fellowship in developmental biology at the University of California, San Diego; clinical training in medicine at the University of Pennsylvania; and genetics research and clinical training at Johns Hopkins. Dr. Feinberg is considered the founder of the field of cancer epigenetics, having discovered altered DNA methylation in cancer in the early 1980s with Bert Vogelstein. Over the decades since, Dr. Feinberg and his colleagues have shaped the landscape of understanding of DNA methylation and other epigenetic changes, and their applications to epidemiology and medicine, and introduced groundbreaking statistical and laboratory methods to the study of the epigenome. He and his colleagues discovered human imprinted genes and loss of imprinting in cancer, and they proved the epigenetic hypothesis of cancer through their work on Beckwith-Wiedemann syndrome. Most recently, they pioneered genome-scale epigenetics (epigenomics), with the first National Institutes of Health (NIH)-funded Epigenome Center, pioneering methods including the first comprehensive genome-scale methylation discovering the major target for epigenetic variation in humans, CpG island shores. He led the first whole genome bisulfite sequencing analysis of human cancer, discovering large hypomethylated blocks that correspond to nuclear lamina-associated heterochromatin, as well as a mechanism for disruption of these blocks in epithelial-mesenchymal transition. He has also helped to create the field of epigenetic epidemiology, discovering epigenetic mediation of genetic variants in disease. He has made several important theoretical contributions as well, including the epigenetic progenitor hypothesis of cancer and the role of entropy in epigenetic development and disease. He is a Bloomberg Distinguished Professor in the Johns Hopkins University Schools of Medicine, Engineering, and Public Health, where he is the director of the Center for Epigenetics. He is a recipient of an NIH Director's Pioneer Award; a member of the National Academy of Medicine, the American Academy of Arts and Sciences, and the NIH Council of Councils; and received honorary doctorates from the University of Uppsala, the Karolinska Institute, and the University of Amsterdam.

Benjamin French is an associate professor of biostatistics in the Department of Biostatistics at Vanderbilt University and an expert advisor to the Department of Statistics at the Radiation Effects Research Foundation (RERF), where he previously served as a senior scientist and the interim department chief. He received his undergraduate degree in mathematics and Norwegian from St. Olaf College and a Ph.D. in biostatistics from the University of Washington. His methodological research focuses on analysis methods for longitudinal (or correlated) and survival (or event-time) data. At RERF, he developed novel analysis approaches for radiation risk estimation for cancer mortality and incidence, while accounting for potential sources of unmeasured confounding and outcome misclassification. As a collaborative biostatistician, he has led or participated in a wide range of biomedical research projects, most recently as the director of the biostatistics core for an international consortium studying outcomes among cancer patients diagnosed with COVID-19. He has taught short courses on longitudinal data analysis and joint modeling of longitudinal and survival outcomes in the United States and abroad.

Bernard D. Goldstein, University of Pittsburgh (retired), is an emeritus dean and an emeritus professor of environmental and occupational health at the University of Pittsburgh School of Public Health. He is an elected member of the National Academy of Medicine (NAM), and has chaired more than a dozen NAM or National Research Council committees. He has also chaired committees related to environmental health for the World Health Organization and the United Nations Environment Programme. His past experience includes service as the assistant administrator for research and development of the Environmental Protection Agency, 1983–1985, and the president of the Society for Risk Analysis. Dr. Goldstein was the founding director of the Environmental and Occupational Health Sciences Institute (EOHSI) of Rutgers University. While at EOHSI, he was the initial principal investigator of the Consortium for Risk Evaluation with Stakeholder Participation (CRESP), a multi-university program responsive to the Department of Energy's research needs related to the cleanup of nuclear weapon sites, a position he held from 1995 to 2001. Since then, he has continued occasional involvement in CRESP and in other nuclear-related activities, including participating in a congressionally mandated committee to review risk-based approaches to cleanup of aspects of the Hanford Site and authoring a recent op-ed related to the risk of nuclear waste. He also has been significantly involved in other energy issues including the use of methyl tert-butyl ether as a gasoline additive, the risk of unconventional national gas drilling, and the health impact of the *Deepwater Horizon* oil spill. Dr. Goldstein holds a B.S. in psychology from University of Wisconsin–Madison (1958) and an M.D. from the New York University School of Medicine (1962).

John D. Graham is the dean of the Indiana University School of Public and Environmental Affairs (SPEA). Dr. Graham's research interests include government reform, energy and the environment, and the future of the automobile in both developed and developing countries. He came to SPEA after serving as the dean of the Frederick Pardee RAND Graduate School at the RAND Corporation in California. Prior to joining RAND, Dr. Graham served in the White House Office of Management and Budget (OMB) from 2001 to 2006. As the Senate-confirmed administrator of the Office of Information and Regulatory Affairs, he led a staff of 50 career policy analysts who reviewed major regulatory proposals from Cabinet agencies. Prior to his role at OMB, Dr. Graham was a professor of policy and decision sciences at the Harvard T.H. Chan School of Public Health. From 1990 to 2001, Dr. Graham founded and led the Harvard Center for Risk Analysis. In 1995, he was elected the president of the Society for Risk Analysis, an international membership organization of 2,400 scientists and engineers. Dr. Graham holds a B.A. (with honors) in economics and politics from Wake Forest University (1978), an M.A. in public affairs from Duke University (1980), and a Ph.D. in urban and public affairs from Carnegie Mellon University (1983).

Elizabeth M. Jaffee is an internationally recognized expert in cancer immunology and pancreatic cancer. She is the deputy director of the Sidney Kimmel Comprehensive Cancer Center at Johns Hopkins, the co-director of the Skip Viragh Pancreatic Cancer Center, and the associate director of the Bloomberg Kimmel Institute for Cancer Immunotherapy. Her research focus is on developing novel immunotherapies for the treatment and prevention of pancreatic cancer. Dr. Jaffee is a past president of the American Association for Cancer Research. She has served on a number of committees at the National Cancer Institute including as the co-chair of the Blue Ribbon Panel that provided scientific advice to Vice President Biden's Moonshot Initiative. She currently serves as the chair of the National Cancer Advisory Board and the chief medical advisor to the Lustgarten Foundation for Pancreatic Cancer Research. She is the inaugural director of the new Convergence Institute at Johns Hopkins. She was recently elected to the National Academy of Medicine and is a fellow of the American College of Physicians. Dr. Jaffee graduated magna cum laude from Brandeis University (1981) before receiving her M.D. from New York Medical College.

Evagelia C. Laiakis received her Ph.D. in human genetics from the University of Maryland, Baltimore (2006), studying radiation-induced genomic instability and the contribution of pro-inflammatory processes. She subsequently completed her postdoctoral fellowship at Georgetown University (2012) in the field of radiation biodosimetry through metabolomics. She is currently an associate professor in the Department of Oncology at the Lombardi Comprehensive Cancer Center with a secondary appointment in the Department of Biochemistry and Molecular and Cellular Biology. Dr.

Laiakis is an elected council member to the National Council on Radiation Protection and Measurements (NCRP) and has been serving as a member of PAC-1 of NCRP (Basic Criteria, Epidemiology, Radiobiology, and Risk) since 2016. She served as a program committee member for the 2021 Annual NCRP meeting and is a co-chair for the 2022 annual NCRP meeting. Dr. Laiakis's laboratory aims to expand the field of radiation metabolomics and lipidomics through mass spectrometry with untargeted and targeted approaches. Her research focus includes understanding metabolic responses to scenarios involving a wide range of doses (low dose to acute radiation syndrome–associated doses), dose rates, normal tissue responses, and radiation quality effects (photons, neutrons, high-energy particles), utilizing biofluids and tissues from rodents to humans. Her work has also expanded to space radiation effects, in combination with stressors such as microgravity, with emphasis on skeletal muscle metabolism–related changes. Finally, she is an associate editor for the *International Journal of Radiation Biology* and *Radiation Research*, and the 2019 recipient of the Jack Fowler award from the Radiation Research Society.

Lindsay M. Morton is currently a senior investigator and the deputy chief of the Radiation Epidemiology Branch, Division of Cancer Epidemiology and Genetics, National Cancer Institute (NCI). She trained in molecular epidemiology as a postdoctoral fellow at NCI after earning a Ph.D. in epidemiology with a focus on cancer from Yale University and an A.B. from Dartmouth College. Dr. Morton's research focuses on quantifying risks of subsequent malignancies among cancer survivors, particularly following treatment with radiotherapy and/or systemic therapies (chemotherapy, immunotherapy) and also incorporating research on germline genetic susceptibility. Much of her research is focused on high-risk populations such as childhood cancer survivors, individuals with inherited cancer predisposition syndromes, and stem cell transplant recipients. She also has a long-term interest in the etiology and survivorship of hematologic malignancies and has led research on the somatic changes in tumors that arise following radiation exposure, particularly thyroid cancer following the Chernobyl nuclear power plant accident. Based on 200 peer-reviewed publications, findings from Dr. Morton's studies have contributed to assessments of the risks and benefits of cancer treatments, guidelines for long-term surveillance of cancer survivors, methodological improvements in data collection for cancer survivors, and understanding of the biological basis of radiation carcinogenesis. She has served as the co-chair of the Late Effects Task Force of the Center for International Blood and Marrow Transplant Research; as an associate editor for the *Journal of the National Cancer Institute*; on the editorial boards of *Cancer Research*, *British Journal of Cancer*, and *Leukemia and Lymphoma*; and as a member of the Radiogenomics Consortium

Steering Committee. Dr. Morton is an elected member of the American Epidemiological Society.

David B. Richardson is the associate dean for research in public health and a professor in environmental and occupational health at the University of California, Irvine. Prior to this position he was a professor in the Department of Epidemiology in the School of Public Health at the University of North Carolina at Chapel Hill; and the deputy director of the North Carolina Occupational Safety and Health Education and Research Center and the director of the center's Program in Occupational Epidemiology. His research focuses on the health effects of occupational and environmental exposures, particularly with regard to carcinogens. He has conducted studies of cancer among workers in the United States and abroad. Dr. Richardson's current research includes studies of mortality among nuclear industry workers and uranium miners, and development of new methods for occupational cohort studies. He is a member of Committee 1 (Radiation Effects) of the International Commission on Radiological Protection; serves as a lead coordinating writer for the United Nations Committee on Epidemiological Studies of Radiation and Cancer, Scientific Committee on the Effects of Atomic Radiation; and serves as the associate editor of the journals *Occupational and Environmental Medicine* and *American Journal of Epidemiology*. His service on National Academies' committees includes the Committee to Review the Health Effects in Vietnam Veterans of Exposure to Herbicides—Tenth Biennial Update and the Committee on the Review of the Department of Labor's Site Exposure Matrix (SEM) Database. Dr. Richardson received a Ph.D. and an M.S.P.H., both in epidemiology, from the University of North Carolina at Chapel Hill.

Dörthe Schaue is an associate professor of radiation oncology at the University of California, Los Angeles (UCLA). For two decades her work has focused on the effects of ionizing radiation on the immune system, on tumor immunity, and on radiation mitigation. Originally trained at radiation research institutions in the United Kingdom and Germany, including the Gray Lab in London and the Paterson Institute in Manchester, Dr. Schaue developed an interest in the immunological aspects of low-dose radiation exposures and was able to build on this knowledge since joining UCLA in 2004. Her current National Institutes of Health–funded research efforts focus on understanding the complex interaction at the irradiated immune-tumor-host interface, and the development of immunoPET for monitoring these interactions in vivo. Her interests in radiation-induced immune imbalances and the role of chronic inflammation, fibrosis, and tissue remodeling in late effects of radiation damage and life shortening grew through her involvement in extensive radiation mitigation studies. She has mentored numerous students, residents, and postgraduate researchers, and she is a member of the Physics and Biology in Medicine Graduate program at UCLA where she teaches radiation biology and immunity in addition to basic and translational radiobiology to UCLA Radiation Oncology residents. She is an associate editor for the *International Journal of Radiation Biology* and a reviewer for the National Cancer Institute's Clinical and Translational Exploratory/Developmental Studies as well as other study sections. She currently serves on multiple national radiation interest committees, including the National Council on Radiation Protection and Measurements' PAC1, ASTRO's Radiobiology Task Force, and the Radiation Research Society.

Rashid A. Shaikh is the director of science (emeritus) at the Health Effects Institute (HEI), a nonprofit, independent research organization. He led scientific strategic planning for HEI, and he was responsible for the management and oversight of HEI's diverse research portfolio and review activities. Working closely with multidisciplinary expert committees and paying close attention to policy and regulatory needs, he directed the planning and execution of HEI's research on particulate matter, exposure assessment, accountability, ozone, diesel emissions, and other air pollutants; many of HEI's studies have provided important information for regulatory policy. His responsibilities included the rigorous, independent peer review and preparation of commentary on all completed HEI-sponsored research. Additionally, he convened and managed several comprehensive and state-of-the-science reviews of research on air pollution and its health effects prepared by scientific panels. He also worked on science policy issues, including the use of human subjects, conflict of interest, data confidentiality and data access, and publication policy. Dr. Shaikh has served on several national scientific committees, including those at the Environmental Protection Agency and the California Air Resources Board, and he has served on the Board of Advisors at the Center for Environmental Research and Technology, University of California, Irvine. He has a special interest in air quality and health issues, the use of new fuels and technologies for automobiles, air pollution, and strategic research planning the use of scientific information for policy making. Dr. Shaikh received his bachelor's degree from St. Xavier's College in Bombay, India, and his master's degree from the Indian Institute of Technology in Kanpur, India. He received his doctorate in biology from the Massachusetts Institute of Technology, Cambridge.

Richard L. Wahl is the Elizabeth E. Mallinckrodt Professor and the head of the Department of Radiology at the Washington University School of Medicine in St. Louis. Dr. Wahl is also the director of the university's Mallinckrodt Institute of Radiology and a professor of radiation oncology. He has been at the forefront of efforts to combine quantitative data from multiple kinds of scans to form so-called fusion images that can help physicians more precisely diagnose and characterize cancers. He was also among the first to harness the power of the immune system to precisely target radiation therapy to cancers, a technique that has become known as radioimmunotherapy. His clinical and research interests include radiopharmaceutical therapies, radioimmunotherapies, quantitative imaging, and imaging of the immune system. Dr. Wahl is an elected member of the American Society for Clinical Investigation, the American Association of Physicians, and the National Academy of Medicine. He serves as the chair of the Research and Discovery domain for the Society of Nuclear Medicine and Molecular Imaging's (SNMMI's) Value Initiative. He was also elected president of SNMMI. Dr. Wahl has a B.A. in chemistry and an Sc.D. from Wartburg College and an M.D. from the Washington University School of Medicine in St. Louis.

Gayle E. Woloschak is currently a professor of radiation oncology at Northwestern University in Chicago and an adjunct professor of religion and science at the Lutheran School of Theology Chicago and at the Pittsburgh Theological Seminary. She holds a Ph.D. in biomedical sciences from the University of Toledo (Medical College of Ohio) and a D.M. in Eastern Christian studies from the Pittsburgh Theological Seminary. Her laboratory interests include molecular biology, radiation biology, and nano-biotechnology, and her science-religion fields include biological evolution, stem cell research, and ecology.

STAFF

Ourania "Rania" Kosti is a senior program officer at the Nuclear and Radiation Studies Board (NRSB) of the National Academies of Sciences, Engineering, and Medicine and the acting executive director of the InterAcademy Partnership, DC, office. Dr. Kosti's interests within NRSB focus on radiation health effects, and she is the principal investigator for the National Academies' Radiation Effects Research Foundation Program that supports studies of the atomic bombing survivors in Japan. Prior to her current appointment, she was a postdoctoral fellow at the Lombardi Comprehensive Cancer Center at Georgetown University Hospital in Washington, DC, where she conducted research on biomarker development for early cancer detection using case-control epidemiological study designs. Dr. Kosti also trained at the National Cancer Institute (2005–2007). She received a B.S. in biochemistry from the University of Surrey, United Kingdom; an M.S. in molecular medicine from the University College London; and a Ph.D. in molecular endocrinology from St. Bartholomew's Hospital in London, United Kingdom.

Appendix C

Information-Gathering Meetings

JULY 21, 2021, ONLINE MEETING ONLY

Views and Perspectives from the Department of Energy (DOE)

    Todd Anderson, Director, Biological Systems Science Division, Office of Biological and Environmental Research, DOE Office of Science

AUGUST 26, 2021, ONLINE MEETING ONLY

Comments from Congress on the Request for the Study

    Alyse Huffman and Adam Rosenberg, Committee on Science, Space, and Technology, Energy Subcommittee, U.S. House of Representatives

Perspectives from the Interagency Steering Committee on Radiation Standards (ISCORS)

    Mike Boyd, Environmental Protection Agency
    Vince Holahan, U.S. Nuclear Regulatory Commission

DOE Office of Domestic and International Health Studies Radiation Health Studies Programs

    Anthony Pierpoint, Director, Office of Domestic and International Health Studies

Perspectives from the Previous DOE Low-Dose Program

Tony Brooks, Washington State University Tri-Cities (emeritus)

Cooperation and Coordination of the Previous DOE Low-Dose Program and Research at NASA

Francis Cucinotta, University of Nevada, Las Vegas

Panel Discussion

Edouard Azzam, Canadian Nuclear Laboratories
David Brenner, Columbia University
Amy Kronenberg, Lawrence Berkeley National Laboratory
Albert Fornace, Jr., Georgetown University
Zhi-Min Yuan, Harvard T.H. Chan School of Public Health

SEPTEMBER 24, 2021, ONLINE MEETING ONLY

Coordination of Low-Dose Radiation Research with the National Cancer Institute (NCI)

Amy Berrington de González, Division of Cancer Epidemiology and Genetics, NCI
C. Norman Coleman, Center for Cancer Research, NCI

Coordination of Low-Dose Radiation Research with the Nuclear Energy Agency/Organisation for Economic Co-operation and Development (NEA/OECD)

Jacqueline Garnier-Laplace, Division of Radiological Protection and Human Aspects of Nuclear Safety, Nuclear Energy Agency, OECD
Dominique Laurier, French Institute for Radiological Protection and Nuclear Safety (IRSN) and Chair of NEA's High-Level Group on Low-Dose Research

Coordination of Low-Dose Radiation Research with the National Institute of Allergy and Infectious Diseases (NIAID)

Andrea L. DiCarlo-Cohen, Radiation and Nuclear Countermeasures Program, NIAID

APPENDIX C   283

Coordination of Low-Dose Radiation Research with the National Institute for Occupational Safety and Health (NIOSH)

    Kaitlin Kelly-Reif, Division of Field Studies and Engineering, NIOSH

Coordination of Low-Dose Radiation Research with the Armed Forces Radiobiology Research Institute (AFRRI)

    Alexandra C. Miller, PhD, Uniformed Services University of the Health Sciences (USUHS) Institutional Animal Care and Use Committee Chair and Senior Scientist, Science Research Department, AFRRI, USUHS

Coordination of Low-Dose Radiation Research with the Centers for Disease Control and Prevention (CDC)

    Armin Ansari, Radiological Assessment Team, CDC

Coordination of Low-Dose Radiation Research with the Electric Power Research Institute (EPRI)

    Don Cool, Radiation Safety, EPRI

Space Radiation: Opportunities for Tactical Collaboration

    S. Robin Elgart, Human Research Program, National Aeronautics and Space Administration (NASA)

NASA Division of Biological and Physical SciencesOpen Science Data Systems for Low-Dose Data

    Sylvain Costes, Radiation Biophysics Laboratory, NASA

Perspectives from DOE Management of the Previous DOE Low-Dose Radiation Research Program

    Arthur Katz, Biological and Environmental Research, DOE (retired)

OCTOBER 27–28, 2021, ONLINE MEETING ONLY

The Science of Risk Communication

    Baruch Fischhoff, Carnegie Mellon University

Government Perspectives on Communication of Low-Dose Radiation Risks

    Kristen Ellis, Department of Energy-Environmental Management
    Jonathan Gill, Department of Homeland Security
    Angela Leek, Iowa Department of Public Health
    Trish Milligan, U.S. Nuclear Regulatory Commission (retired)
    Jessica Wieder, Environmental Protection Agency

Perspectives from Nongovernmental Organizations on Communication of Low-Dose Radiation Risks

    Bemnet Alemayehu, Natural Resources Defense Council
    Terrie Barrie, Alliance of Nuclear Worker Advocacy Groups
    Dan Hirsch, Committee to Bridge the Gap

Medical, Research, and Industry Perspectives

    Gerry Thomas, Imperial College London
    Aditi Verma, Harvard Kennedy School
    Nima Ashkeboussi, Nuclear Energy Institute
    Nick Priest, CANDU Owners Group (COG) Expert Advisor for the Low-Dose Strategic Program
    Rebecca Smith-Bindman, University of California, San Francisco

Risk Management, Safety Policies, and Economics

    Robin Cantor, Berkeley Research Group LLC
    Lisa Robinson, Harvard T.H. Chan School of Public Health

Risk Perception and Public Policy

    Hank Jenkins-Smith, University of Oklahoma

Stakeholder Engagement

    Moderator: Lilly Adams, Union of Concerned Scientists
    President Jonathan Nez, Navajo Nation
    Jill Jim, Navajo Nation Department of Health
    Mary Dickson, representative of downwinders of U.S. nuclear tests
    Keith Kiefer, National Commander of the National Association of Atomic Veterans
    Benetick Maddison, Marshallese Educational Initiative (prerecorded presentation)

Arjun Makhijani, Institute for Energy and Environmental Research
Trisha Pritikin, Hanford Downwinder, author of *The Hanford Plaintiffs: Voices from the Fight for Atomic Justice*
Beata Tsosie-Peña, Environmental Health and Justice Program at Tewa Women United in New Mexico (prerecorded presentation)

Research Needs in Radiation Risk Communication

Randall Hyer, Center for Risk Communication

NOVEMBER 16–17, 2021, ONLINE MEETING ONLY

Setting the Stage: New Directions for Low-Dose Radiation Research

Jonine Bernstein, Memorial Sloan Kettering

Genetics, Epigenetics, and the Microbiome

Dale Ramsden, University of North Carolina at Chapel Hill
Chris Mason, Weill Cornell Medicine

In Utero Exposure

Richard Wakeford, University of Manchester

The Future of Low-Dose Radiation Risk Modeling

Dale Preston, Hirosoft International
Igor Shuryak, Columbia University

The Future of Low-Dose Radiation Dosimetry

Wes Bolch, University of Florida
Choonsik Lee, NCI

Modern Tools in Neuroscience and Tumor Immunogenicity Research

Ruben Gur, University of Pennsylvania
Daniel Marks, Oregon Health & Science University
Sandra Demaria, Weill Cornell

Social Disparities and Environmental Exposures

Johnnye Lewis, University of New Mexico

Low-Dose Radiation Research in Japan

Tatsuhiko Imaoka, Quantum and Radiological Science and Technology (QST), Japan
Shizuko Kakinuma, QST
Yoshiya Shimada, Institute for Environmental Sciences

Advances in Understanding Cancer Evolution and Cellular Response to Radiation

Stephen Chanock, NCI
Phil Jones, Sanger Institute
Serge Candéias, CEA, France
Ed Harlow, Harvard Medical School
Mike Snyder, Stanford
Cheryl Walker, Baylor College of Medicine

DECEMBER 9, 2021, ONLINE MEETING ONLY

Lessons Learned from Research in Air Pollution

Daniel Krewski, University of Ottawa
Jonathan Samet, Colorado School of Public Health
Francesca Dominici, Harvard T.H. Chan School of Public Health

Consortium for Risk Evaluation with Stakeholder Participation (CRESP): Lessons Learned in Community Outreach and Communications

David Kosson, Vanderbilt University
Michael R. Greenberg, Rutgers University
Steve Krahn, Vanderbilt University

JANUARY 24, 2022, ONLINE MEETING ONLY

Opportunities in Low-Dose Radiation Research

Andrew Wyrobek, Lawrence Berkeley National Laboratory (LBNL)
Antoine Snijders, LBNL

Radiation Biology: A Response to the American Innovation and Competitiveness Act

Kartik Sheth, White House Office of Science and Technology Policy

Challenges and Opportunities for Dosimetry in Low-dose Radiation Research

    Derek Jokisch, Francis Marion University and Oak Ridge National Laboratory
    John Klumpp, Los Alamos National Laboratory

Updates and Final Remarks from DOE on the Study Task

    Todd Anderson, DOE Office of Science

Current Research and Future Directions at the Radiation Effects Research Foundation (RERF), Japan

    Bob Ullrich, RERF

Appendix D

Projects Designated by the Department of Energy as "Low-Dose Radiation Projects" Carried Out at National Laboratories (2016–2021)

DOE Laboratory	Funding Year	Amount	Source
ANL	2020[a]	$2,200,000	BER
ANL	2021[a]	$2,528,000	BER
BNL	2020[a]	$1,400,000	BER
BNL	2021[a]	$1,000,000	BER
LANL	2017–2021	$1,950,000	DOE-NNSA
LANL	2020–2022	$245,000	DTRA
LANL	2021–2023	$5,100,000	LDRD
LBNL	2006–2017	$500,000 in 2016b	DOE-BER
LBNL	2011–2016	N/A (JGI user facility provided at no cost to users)	DOE JGI
LBNL	2011–2016	$3,600,531	NASA
LBNL	2012–2016	$1,654,643	NASA
LBNL	2012–2017	$990,770	NASA
LBNL	2012–2017	$2,025,709	NIH
LBNL	2013–2016	$70,195	NASA
LBNL	2013–2017	$1,154,600	NASA
LBNL	2014–2017	$421,707	NASA (prime sponsor); Oregon Health & Science University (direct sponsor)
LBNL	2014–2019	$1,583,882	NASA
LBNL	2015–2016	$199,929	NASA
LBNL	2015–2017	$200,474	NASA
LBNL	2015–2019	$297,416	NASA (prime sponsor); Medical College of Wisconsin (direct sponsor)
LBNL	2016–2019	$1,741,387	NASA
LBNL	2016–2019	$492,041	NASA
LBNL	2016–2021	$3,959,623	NASA
LBNL	2019–2022	$215,999	NASA
LBNL	2019–2021	$504,391	NASA
LBNL	2019–2022	$216,118	NASA

Title
Exploration of the Potential for Artificial Intelligence and Machine Learning to Advance Low-Dose Radiation Biology Research (RadBio-AI)
AI-driven data integration and multiscale modeling approaches to low-dose radiation effects understanding
Exploration of the Potential for Artificial Intelligence and Machine Learning to Advance Low-Dose Radiation Biology Research (RadBio-AI)
AI-driven data integration and multiscale modeling approaches to low-dose radiation effects understanding
Leaf microbiome as a monitoring tool for nuclear activities
Understanding the impact of space radiation on human gut microbiome
Human Exposure of Radiation using Organ Systems (HEROS)
Low-dose scientific focus area
The identification of specific genetic and molecular profiles induced by low-dose radiation that lead to loss of mammary tissue architecture and tumor progression
Harderian gland tumorigenesis low-dose, low-dose-rate, and LET response
Comparative analysis of charged particle–induced autosomal mutagenesis in murine tissue and cells
Space radiation risk assessment project
Novel interactions of DNA repair processes in replication fork maintenance
Effects of low-dose radiation on long-term synaptic plasticity and neurogenesis in normal and Alzheimer's disease transgenic mice
Impact of age, genetic variants, and high-LET track structure on mammary cancer risk estimates
The relation between mutagenesis and genomic instability after particle exposure in vivo
Molecular characterization of choroid plexus and hippocampal damage and degenerative CNS risks from space radiation
Integrating LBNL DSB clustering model with NASA modeling tool to predict cell death and chromosomal aberration in human cells exposed to galactic cosmic ray
Space adaptation effects on immune system impacts reproductive function and mammary gland development across generations
Measurement of and countermeasures against, degenerative heart disease from space radiation
GCR simulator studies with human and mouse models
Blood-based multiscale model for cancer risk from galactic cosmic ray in genetically diverse populations
Simulation of GCR-induced Harderian gland and lung tumorigenesis
Defining the relationship between simulated weightlessness and space radiation on cardiovascular disease
Variation in CNS damage signaling and blood sentinels of neuropathology after exposure to space radiation
Molecular characterization of CNS tissue damage and neurocognitive risks from space radiation

continued

DOE Laboratory	Funding Year	Amount	Source
LBNL	2019–2025	$1,138,838	NIH (prime sponsor sponsor); Albert Einstein College of Medicine (direct sponsor)
LBNL	2020–2025	$1,200,000	NASA
LBNL	2020–2022	$497,795	NIH
LBNL	2021–2022	$784,812	NASA
LLNL	2011–2017	$1,925,000	NIH/NCI
LLNL	2013–2018	$1,650,000	NIH/NCI
LLNL	2016–2018	$200,000	NIH (prime); Columbia University (direct sponsor)
LLNL	2017–2021	$3,000,000	NASA (prime sponsor); Wake Forest University (direct sponsor)
LLNL	2017–2019	$700,000	LDRD
LLNL	2017–2022	$1,784,000	NIH/NCI (prime sponsor); UC Davis (direct sponsor)
LLNL	2018–2021	$6,000,000	LDRD
LLNL	2018–2023	$1,620,000	NIH/NCI (prime sponsor); Dana Farber Cancer Institute (direct sponsor)
LLNL	2020–2023	$2,250,000	LDRD
ORNL	2018	$180,000	LDRD
ORNL	2019	$1,000,000	LDRD
ORNL	2020	$130,000	Work for Others
ORNL	2020	$180,000	BER
ORNL	2020[a]	$1,400,000	BER
ORNL	2021[a]	$1,000,000	BER
ORNL	2021	N/A	Equipment
PNNL	2008–2016	$500,000 in 2016[b]	BER
PNNL	2020–2021	$330,000	NASA
PNNL	2020–2022	$485,000	NASA

[a] Appropriated by Congress to DOE as part of the new low-dose program.
[b] The last year of the previous low-dose radiation program.
NOTE: ANL = Argonne National Laboratory; BER = DOE-Biological and Environmental Research; BNL = Brookhaven National Laboratory; CNS = central nervous system; DOE = Department of Energy; DSB = double strand break; DTRA = Defense Threat Reduction Agency; GCR = galactic cosmic ray; JGI = Joint Genome Institute; LANL = Los Alamos National Laboratory; LBNL = Lawrence Berkeley National Laboratory; LDRD = Laboratory Directed

APPENDIX D *293*

Title
DNA repair, mutations, and cellular aging
Dose-rate effects and galactic cosmic ray simulation in cancer-relevant systems
Genetic determinants of radiation-induced hematologic toxicity
Simulation of GCR-induced Harderian gland and lung tumorigenesis
Characterization of HER2 family of proteins
Optimizing 131I-MIBG therapy for children with advanced neuroblastoma
Biodosimetry of exposure to internalized ^{131}Iodine in human relapsed or refractory cancer patients
Novel microfluidic biomarker detection platforms to monitor in vivo effects of solar particle events and galactic cosmic rays radiation, using mice with human hematopoietic systems
Diagnostic devices for detection in harsh environments
Mitochondrial bioenergetics in aggressive breast cancer growth
Instrumented tumor
Tumor and host markers of clinical outcomes after MIBG therapy in neuroblastoma
High-throughput protein biomanufacturing and in-situ assessment platform to enable rapid response capability
A microfluidic platform for identifying radiation/nuclear countermeasures for emergency situations
Next-generation radiotherapeutics and bioassessment platforms
Synthesis and evaluation of Z-glutamine analogs
Targeted delivery of radionuclides and chemotherapy to therapy-resistant cancer stem cells
Exploration of the Potential for Artificial Intelligence and Machine Learning to Advance Low-Dose Radiation Biology Research (RadBio-AI)
AI-driven data integration and multiscale modeling approaches to low-dose radiation effects understanding
Equipment to analyze trace materials
Linear and nonlinear tissue signaling mechanisms in response to low-dose and low-dose-rate radiation
C4 Photosynthesis in Space (C4Space)
Dynamics of Microbiomes in Space (DynaMoS)

Research and Development; LET = linear energy transfer; LLNL = Lawrence Livermore National Laboratory; MIPG = metaiodobenzylguanidine; NASA = National Aeronautics and Space Administration; NCI = National Cancer Institute; NIH = National Institutes of Health; NNSA = National Nuclear Security Administration; ORNL = Oak Ridge National Laboratory; PPNL = Pacific Northwest National Laboratory; UC = University of California.

Appendix E

Unedited Responses from Radiation Facilities

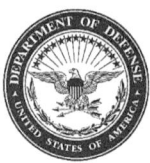 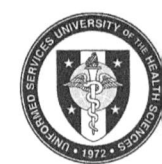

UNIFORMED SERVICES UNIVERSITY OF THE HEALTH SCIENCES

ARMED FORCES RADIOBIOLOGY RESEARCH INSTITUTE
4301 JONES BRIDGE ROAD, BUILDING 42
BETHESDA, MARYLAND 20889-5648
www.usuhs.edu/afrri

November 15, 2021

The National Academies of Sciences Engineering and Medicine
Nuclear and Radiation Studies Board
Washington, DC 20001
Attention: Study Director

Dear Dr. Kosti Ourania,

The Armed Forces Radiobiology Research Institute (AFRRI) is pleased to answer your list of questions related to our radiation sources and facilities that are currently used or could be used to support low-dose and low-dose rate radiation research.

Please see response to respective questions below:

1. Please provide a brief description of your radiation sources and facilities including location, type of source, first year of operation and expected date for removal/decommissioning, and types of activities these sources and facilities support (e.g., research, radiobiology experiments, radioisotope production, other).

TRIGA Reactor

AFRRI's TRIGA reactor is 1 of 66 worldwide. These types of reactors are used in university and government laboratories and medical centers for applications that include research, production of radio-isotopes for medicine and treating tumors, nondestructive testing, basic science research, education, and training. They operate at thermal power levels of <0.1–14 megawatts (MW) and may be pulsed up to 22,000 MW.

The reactor is licensed by the U.S. Nuclear Regulatory Commission (License R-84). As of 2005, it was one of 18 TRIGA reactors in the United States and the only one dedicated to applied medical radiobiology research. The AFRRI TRIGA Mark-F Nuclear Reactor Facility first went operational in 1962. It is a medium-sized unit that generates neutrons and gamma rays for radiation experiments. The reactor can produce a controlled, self-sustaining fission chain reaction in the reactor core. The core, in addition to the fuel elements and control rods (containing boron carbide), includes a neutron start-up source (americium/beryllium). It is suspended under 16 feet (~4.9 m) of water within a pool (an effective radiation shield) on a carriage assembly that allows movement of the core between two exposure rooms for experimental work with large animal or other studies (Dix, 2005). The advantages of such a movable reactor core are that the quantity and character of the radiation that reaches the exposure facilities can be controlled, and more than one exposure facility can be used during reactor operations. The reactor can operate in steady-state as well as pulse mode. It can operate from low power (100 watts) up to the maximum allowed steady-state power level of 1.0 MW. Its pulse mode can produce a short peak (from a prompt critical excursion) of up to 2,500 MW for brief periods (less than one second).

High-Level Cobalt-60 Facility

The High-Level Cobalt-60 facility at AFRRI first opened in 1969. The facility is located below ground in the AFRRI complex, with shielding provided by massive reinforced concrete and earth fill. Its panoramic irradiator is a wet-source storage unit consisting of a 450,000 Ci (at installation) Cobalt-60 source, water trench, source and storage racks, elevator mechanism, and associated equipment. The exposure room is 35ft ˜ 35ft and 25ft, 8in high (10.7m ˜ 10.7m ˜ 7.6m = 870 m3). The irradiator produces mono-energetic gamma rays at variable dose rates with flexible configurations in both unilateral and bilateral irradiation modes and may be used for acute and chronic studies of materials, biologic specimens, small and large. It has been employed in a variety of applications, including investigations of the effects of ionizing radiation exposure on cells, prognostic indicators of survival in a variety of mammals, the efficacy of radio-protective agents and the effects of radiation on unshielded electronics in space application. The facility source was replenished in 2013, and there is currently no plan to shut down the facility.

Low-Level Cobalt Facility

The Low-Level Cobalt Facility, formerly called the Chronic Irradiation Facility, is a second Cobalt-60 radiation source facility which provides low-dose-rate gamma radiation to simulate chronic exposure. The low-level cobalt facility consists of a dry, panoramic Cobalt-60 irradiator (1.17 MeV, 1.33 MeV gamma rays) capable of providing doses to samples over a long time frame. The source is located 1.5 meters from the floor in the center of a large 6 meter square room that can accommodate biological samples of all sizes. To meet various dose-rate requirements, attenuators (2x, 4x, 8x) are available. Additional attenuators can be procured as necessary. The room is climate controlled with the proper ventilation exchange rates along with a day/night lighting system to satisfy the most demanding animal care and use requirements. Video surveillance is also available for the monitoring of animals. Personnel are available to fully support all necessary experiment protocols. The facility is licensed for up to 100 Ci of Co-60.

Linear Accelerator (LINAC)

In August 2012, AFRRI retired its 47-year-old underground linear accelerator and replaced it with an Elektra Infinity clinical accelerator that is supported by a computed tomography (CT) unit. The purchased unit has received significant upgrades to hardware and software in 2021. It is capable of providing high-energy photons from 4 MeV up to 15 MeV with variable dose rates from 0.05 to 6 Gray per minute. Imaging capabilities are provided through a portal camera and cone-beam computed tomography.

Small Animal Radiation Research Platform (SARRP)

The institute commissioned the Small Animal Radiation Research Platform (SARRP) January 2015 which provides low-energy photons up to 220kVp to achieve 0.2 to 2.6 Gy/min dose rates to targets. Imaging is provided through portal camera and cone beam computed tomography.

2. What are the dose ranges, radiation qualities, energy, and dose-rates delivered in your facilities? Is operation pulsed or steady-state? Are the facilities suitable for inhalation experiments?

All radiation facilities at AFRRI are flexible to provide a variety of dose rates and total accumulated doses to experiments through manipulation of exposure time, distance, shielding, and strength of radiation source. The TRIGA reactor is unique in the ability to provide mixed-field (gamma and neutron) radiation to experiments of varying neutron energy levels.

In addition to the ability to provide a mixed field, the TRIGA also has an accompanying hot cell with a viewing port and robotic tele-operators. Our team has considered the question of inhalation experiments, and have promising ideas of how we can provide a space for dispersed irradiated particles inside a sealed space. Table 1 details the radiation quality, energy, operation type, possible dose rates and additional notes for each facility.

Table 1: An overview of available radiation qualities and rates possible at AFRRI facilities.

Facility	Radiation Quality	Energy	Operation	Dose Rates	NOTES
Reactor#	Mixed field, gamma/neutron	From thermal to fast	Pulse and Steady State	From less than 10 R/hr to more than 100 kR/hr	Target can be shielded for significantly lower dose
High Level Cobalt	Mono-energetic	1.33 and 1.17 MeV	Dose rate can be varied by source position adjustment	From less than 1 R/hr to more than 100 kR/hr	Target can be shielded for significantly lower dose

Low Level Cobalt#	Mono-energetic	1.33. and 1.17 MeV	Panoramic, with source in the middle of the room	From less than 1 mR/hr to more than 100 R/hr	Both source and target can be shielded for significantly lower dose. Dose rate also adjusted by target placement in exposure room
LINAC	Mono-energetic	4, 10, 15 MeV	Flexible platform that provides partial body irradiation for targets	From 0.05 to 6 Gy/min	
SARRP#	Mono-energetic	Up to 220kVp	Accurate and precise chamber for small animal with adjustable inserts	From 0.3 to 2.6 Gy/min	

\# Dose and dose rates reported will go into further validation upon return to operational status.

3. For radiobiology experiments, are your facilities mostly used for exposure of cells, tissues, or animals? Please describe and if possible provide publications that describe use of your radiation facilities to facilitate radiation research.

Irradiation facilities are configurable for live animals, cell cultures and tissues, and other inanimate projects/subjects. As an example, Table 2 below shows irradiation numbers in the HLCF from 2005 until now.

Table 2: History of Irradiation Sessions at HLCF.

	Irradiation sessions						Irradiation sessions			
year	total	animal	cells	spores	other	year	total	animal	cells	spores	Other
2005	131	67	30	21	13	2014	201	113	67		21
2006	163	67	35	43	18	2015	158	90	65		3
2007	208	113	26	38	31	2016	122	79	43		
2008	191	115	47	8	21	2017	163	86	77		
2009	208	108	70		30	2018	135	78	56		1
2010	212	113	86	3	10	2019	101	69	31		1
2011	206	123	81	2		2020	57	39	15		3
2012	170	117	49	4		2021	62	48	10		4
2013	151	108	37		6						

4. Are your facilities available for use to outside radiation researchers and other investigators?

Yes, our facilities are available to outside radiation researchers and other investigators. The proposed experiment will have to be coordinated with the Uniformed Services University of Health Sciences (USU) Vice President of Research's office, and approvals will be required by both our animal and safety committees. Interagency Agreement, Memoranda of Understanding or coordinated requirements definition could also provide access to external investigators. Naval Support Activity Bethesda (NSAB), COVID 19 Safety protocols, and USU/AFRRI security measures must be met but do not preclude profit or non-profit organizations from utilizing the AFRRI radiation sources. Foreign nationals may require special procedures for entry into NSAB and AFRRI.

5. Is there available adjacent infrastructure that facilitates radiation research such as tissue culture and animal facilities?

USU Department of Laboratory Animal Resources provides veterinary support for animal experiments. Also, the institute is expanding its animal facilities by constructing a new state of the art vivarium, expected to be complete by summer 2022. The vivarium is adjacent and connected to AFRRI, and will provide efficient and expedited handling of animals. Each of the facilities mentioned above also has co-located animal preparation areas next to the exposure rooms. These areas are used to hold and prep animals for experiments. The radiation facilities and tissue culture or animal facilities responsibilities are not integrated under a department, but all fall under AFRRI and or USU. Biological labs are located throughout the building for in-house Principal Investigators

AFRRI appreciates the great opportunity that the National Academy of Science Committee on Developing a Long-Term Strategy for Low-Dose Radiation Research in the United States is providing by inviting us to participate in the information gathering meeting last month and requesting additional information on radiation facilities. Should you need any further technical information, please contact Lieutenant Colonel Lu Makinde at (301) 295-9246.

_____   _____
Date   Mohammad Naeem, MD, FCCP, FACR
                                             Colonel, Medical Corps, US Army
                                             Director AFRRI

Colorado State University Radiation Facilities for Low-Dose Rate Radiation Research

Several facilities on the CSU campus are used for low dose rate radiation research.

Low dose rate γ-ray tissue culture facility (MRB 08). This facility is housed in a shielded vault in the Molecular and Radiological Biosciences (MRB) building on the Main CSU campus. It consists of a $_{137}$Cs γ-ray source mounted above a tissue culture incubator. The incubator sits on a hydraulic lift which allows it to be raised or lowered to adjust the dose rate to cell cultures inside. Attenuators provide additional dose rate control. The dose rate is currently set for 9.3 mGy/hr but can be increased to 60 mGy/hr at the current location and increased further to about 500 mGy/hr by adjusting the hydraulic lift. The dose rate can be decreased to near background by utilizing additional attenuators.

The facility is currently being used for radiobiology experiments, specifically continuous (weeks long) exposures of engineered human heart tissue.

Low dose rate γ-ray tissue culture facility (MRB 12). This facility is a 37° C warm room beneath which twelve $_{137}$Cs sources can be exposed. When MRB 12 was commissioned in 1997 the sources were each nominally 4 mCi (now about 2 mCi). Researchers can place their samples (typically cells in flasks) at various heights from the sources and irradiate at low dose rate for days. From a position of 56 cm to 180 cm above the sources, thirty-five stacks of T75 tissue culture flasks can be placed for different dose rates. A total 1190 T75 flasks can be irradiated simultaneously in this manner. The dose rates range from 1 mGy/h to 100 mGy/h depending on the number of sources used and the distance from sources.

Because the warm room is not a CO_2 incubator, culture media must be prepared by the addition of 10-25 mM HEPES buffer to ensure pH equilibration (pH 7.2-7.4).

Low dose rate neutron tissue culture facility (MRB 02). This facility is under construction and scheduled to be operational by the end of the 2021 calendar year. An Adelphi D-T neutron generator is being mounted above a tissue culture incubator. The generator will provide a maximum yield of $2 \cdot 10_9$ neutrons/s with an energy spectrum that is narrowly peaked at 14.1 MeV. Unscattered neutron fluences will correspond to a maximum dose rate of approximately 3.6 mGy/hr at a distance of 1 m. Neutrons will be scattered and neutron energies moderated by structural components and equipment in the room and most importantly by the shielding materials applied for radiation protection and field attenuation purposes. The neutron energies at the samples will present a spectrum and span a range of LET to be determined and can be modified further by the introduction of additional scattering material. Dose rates can be decreased by up to a factor of about 20 by reducing the generator current; additionally, the generator-incubator distance can be modified to increase or decrease the expected dose rate. The generator is expected to provide minimal background from photon radiation; photon contributions to the ambient dose rate from neutron capture reactions will be determined during the commissioning phase of the generator.

The facility will be used for low dose rate irradiation of engineered human tissues ("tissues on a chip").

APPENDIX E

Low dose rate γ-ray vivarium (MRB 06). This facility is used to irradiate small animals continuously with $_{137}$Cs γ-rays. A panoramic J.L. Shepherd Model 81-18 irradiator is positioned opposite an arc of cage racks that can house up to 250 mice. The section of the irradiator room containing the cages is enclosed by a bio-bubble that provides HEPA filtered air. This is a fully approved vivarium and mice can be housed in it for their entire life spans. The facility has also been used to irradiate Medaka fish.

MRB 06 was set up to provide a dose rate of 10 cGy per day. A day consists of 22 hours with the source exposed during which time the mice are irradiated and 2 hours with the source shielded so personnel can enter for animal husbandry. The dose rate can be adjusted by bringing the cages closer to the source and by adding or removing attenuators. A higher dose rate of 0.41 cGy/min was used in a radiation countermeasure study done by Cleveland BioLabs in the facility.

Low dose rate neutron vivarium. The neutron irradiator/vivarium is on the CSU Foothills Campus which is located in Fort Collins about 5 miles west of the Main campus. The facility is described in detail in Borak et al 2021 (see the reference section below). The irradiator building is a standalone structure built in 1964 consisting of an irradiator room, a control room, and two storage/equipment rooms. It was decommissioned as an irradiator facility in the 1970s. In 2016/2017, the building was renovated as a small animal vivarium housing a panoramic $_{252}$Cf neutron irradiator. Cage racks capable of housing 900 mice and 60 rats were positioned in a circle around the irradiator. Animal irradiation experiments were initiated there September 2017. The target dose rate is 1 mGy/day. Initially, a day was 16 hours with the source exposed and the animals being irradiated followed by 8 hours with the source shielded so personnel could enter the facility for animal care and maintenance. Because $_{252}$Cf decays (t$^{1/2}$ ~ 2.6 years), the daily exposure times must be steadily increased to deliver a 1 mGy dose. After about 2 years, a day becomes 22 hours of exposure followed by 2 hours with the source shielded. Two hours is the minimum needed for animal care, so at that point the source must be replaced or the dose rate reduced.

A scheduled replacement of the source was put on hold due to the COVID-19 pandemic. However, a new source has now been ordered and should be installed this calendar year (2021).

Availability

All of the described facilities are available to extramural investigators. We have previously provided access to CSU irradiators on a fee for service or collaborative basis. In the case of the NASA funded neutron irradiator/vivarium facility, five other extramural NASA funded research groups used the facility beginning on the first day it was operational. Some of these groups worked on site and we assisted them with finding accommodations, securing animal care and use protocols, and getting access to CSU computing networks and key cards.

None of the facilities is currently set up for inhalation work. However, we have considerable experience in this field. CSU used to conduct large inhalation studies, most notably on Beagles, in the past. The current Director of the Irradiation Services Laboratory has more than twenty years of experience in internal dosimetry. Recent work by his graduate students includes the measurement and modeling of the biokinetics of injected radionuclides utilizing murine and canine models at the CSU Veterinary Teaching Hospital.

There are no plans to decommission any of these facilities.

Additional infrastructure

Several other irradiators are available on the CSU campus, they are not listed here because they are used for treatment or for research involving acute exposures, including for large animals. Since acute exposure controls may be needed for some low dose rate experiments, note that a ^{137}Cs γ-ray panoramic irradiator is available in the MRB building. It is used to irradiate cells and mice. Using the standard distance to the source, the current dose rate is 0.77 Gy/min; this dose rate can be reduced by up to a factor of about 10. Also, using a tray immediately adjacent to the source allows small samples to be irradiated at 5.3 Gy/min.

Tissue culture and molecular biology laboratories are located on the 4$_{th}$ floor of the MRB building.

Small animal vivariums with procedure rooms are available on both the Main and Foothills campuses. CSU has a college of veterinary medicine. Large animals are housed on the Foothills and South campuses (South campus is 1 mile south of the Main campus). Veterinary residents have been recruited to assist in some experiments run by extramural investigators (e.g., slit lamp exams for cataracts in irradiated mice).

An additional irradiator building, the RSDF building, is located on the Foothills campus. It was constructed in 1967 for experiments requiring chronic low dose rate exposures of animals and is currently decommissioned. The RSDF contains two large irradiator rooms, both similar to the one in the low dose rate neutron irradiator/vivarium. This building may be available for renovation and recommissioning if additional facilities are needed.

Publications

MRB 08 Low dose rate tissue culture

Kato TA, Nagasawa H, Weil MM, Little JB, Bedford JS. Levels of gamma-H2AX Foci after low-dose-rate irradiation reveal a DNA DSB rejoining defect in cells from human ATM heterozygotes in two at families and in another apparently normal individual. Radiat Res. 2006 Sep;166(3):443-53. doi: 10.1667/RR3604.1. PMID: 16953663.

MRB 12 Low dose rate tissue culture

Amdur, R.J. and J.S. Bedford. Dose rate effects between 0.3 and 30 Gy/h in a normal and a malignant human cell line. Int. J. Radiat. Biol. 30:83-90, 1994.

Bedford, Joel S. The radiobiology of low dose-rate and fractionated irradiation. In: Principles and Practice of Brachytherapy (Joslin, Flynn, Hall, eds.), Arnold, London, 2001, pp. 161-179.

Huang, Q., Li, F., Liu, X., Li, W., Shi, W., Liu, F-F., O'Sullivan, B., He, Z., Peng, Y., Tan, A-C., Zhou, L., Chen, J., Han, G., Wang, X-J., Thorburn, J., Thorburn, A., Jimeno, A., Raben, D., Bedford, J.S., and Li, Chuan-Yuan, Caspase-mediated paracrine signaling from dying cells potently stimulates tumor cell repopulation during cancer radiotherapy. Nature Medicine 17, 860-866 (2011)

Kato, T. A., H. Nagasawa, M. M. Weil, J. B. Little and J. S. Bedford, Levels of gamma-H2AX Foci after low-dose-rate irradiation reveal a DNA DSB rejoining defect in cells from human ATM heterozygotes in two at families and in another apparently normal individual. Radiat. Res. 166, 443-453, 2006.

Kato TA, Nagasawa H, Weil MM, Genik PC, Little JB, Bedford JS. Gamma-H2AX foci after low-dose-rate irradiation reveal Atm haploinsufficiency in mice. Radiat Res. 2006 Jul;166(1 Pt 1):47-54. doi: 10.1667/RR3587.1.

Kato, T.A., P.F. Wilson, H. Nagasawa, M.M. Fitzek, M.M. Weil, J.B. Little, and J.S. Bedford, A defect in DNA double strand break processing in cells from unaffected parents of retinoblastoma patients and other apparently normal humans. DNA Repair (Amst.) 6, 818-829, 2007.

Lin, J.Y-D, M.C. Muhlmann-Diaz, M.A. Stackhouse, J.F. Robinson, G.E. Taccioli, D.J. Chen, and J.S. Bedford. An ionizing radiation-sensitive CHO mutant cell line: irs-20. IV. Genetic complementation, V(D)J recombination and the scid phenotype. Radiat. Res. 147:166-171, 1997.

Lin, J.Y-D. and J.S. Bedford. Regional gene mapping using mixed radiation hybrids and reverse chromosome painting. Radiat. Res. 148:405-412, 1997.

Ochola, D, Sharif R, Bedford JS, Keefe, T., Kato,T., Fallgren, C., Demant, P., Costes, S., and Weil, M., Persistence of Gamma-H2AX Foci in Bronchial Cells Correlates with Susceptibility to Radiation Associated Lung Cancer in Mice. Radiat Res 191.. 67-75 (2019).

Peng Y, Nagasawa H, Warner C, Bedford JS. Genetic susceptibility: radiation effects relevant to space travel. Health Phys. 103, 607-620 (2012).

Priestley, A., H.J. Beamish, D. Gell, A.G. Amatucci, M.C. Muhlmann-Diaz, B.K. Singleton, G.C. Smith, T. Blunt, L.C. Schalkwyk, J.S. Bedford, S.P. Jackson, P.A. Jeggo, and G.E. Taccioli. Molecular and biochemical characterization of DNA-dependent protein kinase-defective rodent mutant irs-20. Nucleic Acids Res. 26:1965-1973, 1998.

Stackhouse, M.A. and J.S. Bedford. IRS 20: An ionizing radiation sensitive mutant of CHO cells: irs cells. I. Isolation and Initial Characterization. Radiat. Res. 136: 241-249, 1993.

Stackhouse, M.A. and J.S. Bedford. IRS 20: An ionizing radiation sensitive mutant of CHO cells: irs cells. II. Dose-rate effects and cellular recovery process. Radiat. Res. 136: 250-254, 1993.

Stackhouse, M.A. and J.S. Bedford. An ionizing radiation sensitive mutant of CHO cells: irs-20. III. Chromosome aberrations DNA breaks and mitotic delay. Int. J. Radiat. Biol. 65(5):571-582, 1994.

Ulsh, B.A., F.W. Whicker, T.G. Hinton, J.D. Congdon and J.S. Bedford. Chromosome Translocations in T. scripta : The dose-rate effect and in vivo lymphocyte radiation response. Radiat. Res. 155: 63-73, 2001.

Ulsh, B.A., M.C. Mühlmann-Diaz, F.W. Whicker, T.G. Hinton, J.D. Congdon, and J.S. Bedford. Chromosome Translocations in Turtles: A biomarker in a sentinel animal for ecological dosimetry. Radiat. Res. 153:752-759, 2000.

Wilson, P.F., and Bedford, J.S., Radiobiological Principles. Chapter 1 (In Textbook of Radiation Oncology, 3rd Edition, S.A. Leibel, and T.L. Phillips, eds), Elsevier, Philadelphia. (In Press 2009).

Wilson PF, Nagasawa H, Warner CL, Fitzek MM, Little JB, Bedford JS. Radiation sensitivity of primary fibroblasts from hereditary retinoblastoma family members and some apparently normal controls: colony formation ability during continuous low-dose-rate gamma irradiation. Radiat Res. 2008 May;169(5):483-94. doi: 10.1667/RR1333.1.PMID: 18439048

MRB06 Low Dose Rate Gamma Ray Irradiator/Vivarium

Shakhov AN, Singh VK, Bone F, Cheney A, Kononov Y, Krasnov P, Bratanova-Toshkova TK, Shakhova VV, Young J, Weil MM, Panoskaltsis-Mortari A, Orschell CM, Baker PS, Gudkov A, Feinstein E. Prevention and mitigation of acute radiation syndrome in mice by synthetic lipopeptide agonists of Toll-like receptor 2 (TLR2). PLoS One. 2012;7(3):e33044. doi: 10.1371/journal.pone.0033044. Epub 2012 Mar 27. PMID: 22479357; PMCID: PMC3314012.

Ochola DO, Sharif R, Bedford JS, Keefe TJ, Kato TA, Fallgren CM, Demant P, Costes SV, Weil MM. Persistence of Gamma-H2AX Foci in Bronchial Cells Correlates with Susceptibility to Radiation Associated Lung Cancer in Mice. Radiat Res. 2019 Jan;191(1):67-75. doi: 10.1667/RR14979.1. Epub 2018 Nov 6. PMID: 30398394.

Foothills Campus Low Dose Rate Neutron Irradiator/Vivarium

Borak TB, Heilbronn LH, Krumland N, Weil MM. Design and dosimetry of a facility to study health effects following exposures to fission neutrons at low dose rates for long durations. Int J Radiat Biol. 2021;97(8):1063-1076. doi: 10.1080/09553002.2019.1688884. PMID: 31687872.

Perez RE, Younger S, Bertheau E, Fallgren CM, Weil MM, Raber J. Effects of chronic exposure to a mixed field of neutrons and photons on behavioral and cognitive performance in mice.

Behav Brain Res. 2020 Feb 3;379:112377. doi: 10.1016/j.bbr.2019.112377. Epub 2019 Nov 22. PMID: 31765722.

Acharya MM, Baulch JE, Klein PM, Baddour AAD, Apodaca LA, Kramár EA, Alikhani L, Garcia C Jr, Angulo MC, Batra RS, Fallgren CM, Borak TB, Stark CEL, Wood MA, Britten RA, Soltesz I, Limoli CL. New Concerns for Neurocognitive Function during Deep Space Exposures to Chronic, Low Dose-Rate, Neutron Radiation. eNeuro. 2019 Aug 22;6(4):ENEURO.0094-19.2019. doi: 10.1523/ENEURO.0094-19.2019. Erratum in: eNeuro. 2019 Oct 18;6(5): PMID: 31383727; PMCID: PMC6709229.

Loma Linda University
James M. Slater, M.D. Proton Treatment and Research Center
Radiation Biology Facilities and Logistic Support Report

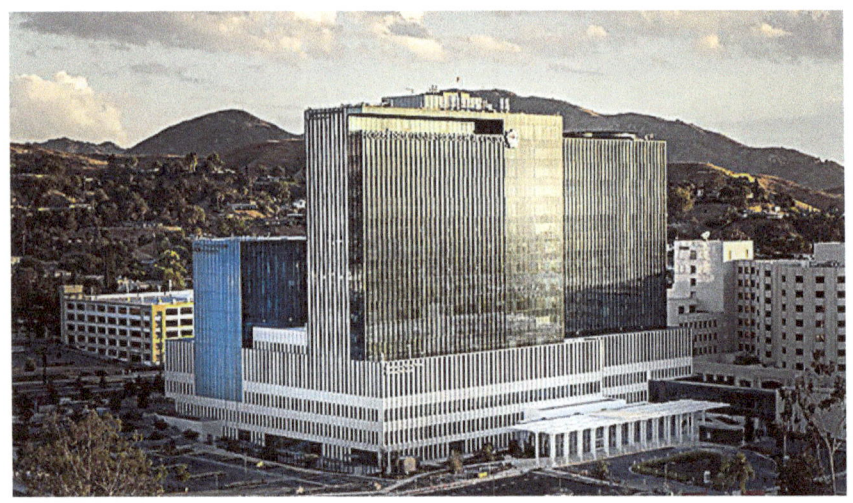

Marcelo E. Vazquez M.D., Ph.D.

October 25, 2021

LOCATION:

The James M. Slater, M.D. Proton Treatment and Research Center is located at Loma Linda University Medical Center (LLUMC) in the city of Loma Linda, located approximately 60 miles east of Los Angeles in San Bernardino County, California. Loma Linda is home to Loma Linda University (LLU). LLUMC and its Children's Hospital contain the largest neonatal intensive care unit in California, the Proton Accelerator Cancer Treatment Center, and the infant heart and multiple organ transplant center. Over 900 physicians are on the University and Medical Center staff.

The James M. Slater Proton Treatment and Research Center, operated and staffed by the Department of Radiation Medicine (LLURM), was the first proton facility in the world designed for patient treatment and related research in a hospital setting. Staff at the facility have treated more than 25,000 patients with protons since 1990. Protons have been used for patients with various tumors involving the prostate, brain, base of skull, eye, head and neck, spine, lung, liver, and various other sites. A significant number of patients are children. LLURM also provides other comprehensive radiation therapy services, including x-ray IMRT complementary to proton therapy. Patients treated with protons are followed for life and all events such as local or distal failure, side effects, and secondary cancers are recorded in computerized databases by dedicated LLURM clinical research staff.

FACILITIES

Proton Radiation Facilities

The LLURM synchrotron-based proton facility started operation in 1990. This facility supports patient treatments, clinical research, and radiobiological research. At present there are no plans/dates for the removal or decommissioning of this facility. The proton treatment center has three clinical gantry treatment rooms and two clinical horizontal fixed beamlines. In addition, the center has a research room equipped with three horizontal beam lines featuring semi-permanent experimental setups for physics and biological studies. Currently, biological experiments are conducted using one of the clinical gantries (G2) and one of the fixed horizontal beam lines (HBL). Research beam lines are dedicated to physics and technological development studies. However, these beam lines can be commissioned for biological studies as needed.

The clinical treatment rooms allow for image guidance and treatment planning support. The accelerator is available for research outside regular patient treatment hours and on weekends. Limited access during regular patient treatment hours is available. During the week, typically, short runs (30 minutes to 1 hour.) can be scheduled between patient treatments or at the end of the day after scheduled patient treatments are completed. Extended runs (of several hours) can be scheduled during weekends. Protons are delivered via a dedicated control system; accelerator and engineering personnel are available 24 hours/7 days per week. Engineering support staff are on site to maintain the facility and related proton research equipment.

The LLURM proton facility (maintained by Optivus Proton Therapy, Inc.) produces pulsed stream of proton radiation with variable energies (50 MeV – 250 MeV) and variable dose rates (standard setup: 100-200 cGy/min). The facility can provide very low dose rates settings if a non-clinical setup is arranged. Previous and current studies demonstrated that the facility could produce dose rates as low as **1 cGy/min** and even lower with a dedicated beam tuning. Therefore, lower dose rates can be produced as needed requiring special allocated time. Higher dose rates (up to about 300 cGy/min) can also be produced for small radiation fields.

Passive scattered beam delivery is accomplished in conventional ways: field size (**G2** max: 18 cm diameter circular field, **HBL** max: 14 cm diameter circular field) is achieved by means of scattering foils; spreading out the Bragg peak (SOBP) to irradiate different target volumes (from cells to animals) is done by a modulator wheel; absorber materials are used in addition to some electronic manipulations to control the depth of the Bragg peak; shaping the beam in the first two dimensions (height and width) is accomplished by Cerrobend or brass cut-outs; and beam shaping in the third dimension is achieved by compensators milled on a computer-controlled machine. Samples alignment is accomplished by a light field and multiple laser beams.

Conventional Radiation Facilities

One clinical **TrueBeam** linear accelerator (Varian Medical System, Palo Alto, CA) is available for clinical and research use at LLURM. This accelerator provides a range of X-ray energies, image guidance, lasers for alignment, and treatment planning support. The unit is used clinically for IMRT. For research purposes, the accelerator provides a vertical beam that can be used for *in vitro* and *in vivo* experiments as well as multidirectional beams for more complex animal studies. The maximum field size achievable is a square beam spot of 20 x 20 cm, while a light field and multiple laser beams can be used to aid in sample alignment. The linear accelerator provides an energy range from 6 to 22 MeV, with a dose rate range of 5 to 600 cGy/min. Access to this facility is limited, but short runs (30 minutes) can be scheduled between patient treatments during the week, or at the end of the day after scheduled patient treatment are completed.

Radiation Sources Characteristics Summary

	Protons		Photons
	G2	HBL	LINAC
Machine/Brand	synchrotron based (Optivus)	synchrotron based (Optivus)	LINAC (TrueBeam, Varian)
Energies (MeV)	50 to 250	50 to 250	2 to 22
Dose Rates (cGy/min)	<1 to 300	<1 to 300	5 to 600
Beam Spot	18 cm dia. (circular)	14 cm dia. (circular)	20 X 20 cm (square)
Beam direction	Vertical (any direction)	Horizontal (fixed)	Vertical (any direction)
Availability (hrs.): • Weekdays • Weekends	0.5 to 1 6 +	NA 6 +	0.5 to 1 NA
Experimental set up: • Biology • Physics	Yes No	Yes Yes	Yes No
Inhalation setup	Yes	Yes	Yes
Study type capability: • *In Vitro* • *In Vivo*	Yes TBD	Yes Yes	Yes TBD

LLURM Research and Development Team:

The LLURM's research and management activities are performed by the LLURM Research and Development Team. This team headed by Dr. Vazquez is a very active team focusing on studying mechanisms of biological effects of ionizing radiation on animals, tissues, and cells. Research projects currently underway at LLURM include: 1) proton radiobiology basic mechanisms; 2) combined therapies to improve clinical outcomes for aggressive cancers; 3) develop and validate new technologies in proton therapy; 4) CNS neurotoxicity induced by radiation; and 5) hypo- and hyper-fractionated studies. Laboratory space assigned to radiobiologic investigations is equipped to support tissue culture activities, cytogenetic research, and animal studies. The goal of this laboratory is development of technology and biological knowledge which can be rapidly translated into clinical practice. The LLURM research and development team coordinates the basic and translational research and proton beam planning activities for intra- and extra-mural scientists.

Core Research Laboratories:

The Department of Radiation Medicine at LLUMC has a well-equipped 6,700-square-feet core radiation research laboratory dedicated to physics, radiobiology, and translational research. In support of this mission the core laboratory facility is subdivided in modular areas with assigned benches and shared laboratory support rooms. Also available is a conference room equipped with a video conferencing system in addition to office space for researchers and administrative support personnel.

Collectively these facilities have their own Principal Investigators and staff and serve as resources for our investigators and external users. The laboratories' fundamental objective is to provide equipment and expertise that investigators may employ as needed to conduct research in photon/proton radiobiology and physics. Specifically, each component of the core laboratory research facility will provide the following resources:

Radiobiology Laboratories: These laboratories focus on providing a center for radiobiology translational research supporting cell and tissue culture activities and biochemistry for investigators conducting biological studies. The laboratories have specific equipment in support of this mission including:

> ***Biochemistry Laboratory:***
> - Image Capture and Analysis:
>   o Fluorescence microscopy (Olympus BX95 with Cell Sense imaging software).
> - Protein Determination (Western blot station, spectrophotometer)
> - Cytochemistry workstation
> - Cold storage capability: *4°, -20° and -80°C refrigerators and freezers.*
> - Bench top centrifuges
> - 3 chemical hoods.
> - *Waste disposal capability*

> ***Cell Culture Laboratory:***
> - Four CO_2 incubators for cell culture activities.
> - Two laminar flow hoods for sterile operations.
> - Inverted microscope (TCM4000 BIOMED) with image analysis system
> - Cell counter (Countess® II)
> - Liquid nitrogen storage
> - Ancillary Equipment: water baths, refrigerators/freezers, etc.

> ***Animal Studies:***

The LLURM radiation facilities are adjacent to the LLUMC Animal Care Facility, which provides assistance in acquiring, housing, feeding, preparing and treating vertebrate animals. Researchers have access to animals and can use equipment and surgical rooms to perform research within the facility. Research support services, such as CTs and MRIs, are available as well. In addition to animal husbandry areas, the LLUMC Animal Care Facility contains five surgical suites and an intensive care/recovery room for postoperative care. The facility also has fully equipped and staffed clinical pathology and microbiology laboratories and an animal necropsy laboratory. The diagnostic laboratories can perform hematology, clinical chemistry, urinalysis, cytology, coagulation profiles, parasitology examinations, blood gas examinations, and microbiologic and serological procedures.

LLURM's facilities and staff have extensive capabilities and experience in designing, planning, and running experiments using small (rodents, ferrets, flies, worms, and medium size animals (mini pigs)) for intra- and extra-mural investigators (NASA, NSBRI, etc.). Irradiation facilities can provide anesthesia and monitoring capabilities for *in vivo* studies.

Physics Laboratory:

This laboratory focusses on supporting medical physics research and additionally provides physics and dosimetry support for investigators conducting biological studies. The laboratory has specific equipment in support of this mission, including:
- Geant4 Monte Carlo Workstations
- A range of small-field dosimetry apparatuses, including ionization chambers, diodes and diamond detectors
- Gafchromic film imaging suite, including film scanner and dedicated software
- Treatment Planning workstations for proton and X-ray treatment planning

> **High-Powered Computing Center:**

This center supports Monte Carlo, treatment planning, and medical imaging development, while also providing data storage and handling for these activities. Specific facilities available include:
- 88 Tb Raid 6 storage server
- Fiver servers with 64 virtual nodes, each giving a total of 320 nodes for computer simulation support. Three of these servers have 512 Gb of RAM each to provide sufficient memory for intensive image-based research.
- A 19 quad core node cluster (providing 76 virtual processors) for computer simulation support.
- Battery backup power supplies to ensure uptime.

Utilization path

Proton and LINAC beam time are limited but free of charge for interested users. Scientists can access the LLURM radiation sources via collaborative agreement with the LLURM Research and Development team. Collaborative agreements and beam utilization are coordinated by Dr. Vazquez and review/approval are accomplished by an internal research committee (feasibility review), led by the Chair of the Department of Radiation Medicine.

Point of Contact:

Marcelo E. Vazquez, M.D., Ph.D.
Associate Professor
Director, Research and Development, Dept. of Radiation Medicine
James M. Slater, MD, Proton Treatment and Research Center
Department of Basic Sciences, School of Medicine
Loma Linda University Medical Center, B125
11234 Anderson Street
Loma Linda, CA 92354
Phone: 909 558 9490
Cell: 516 512 2032
E-mail: mvazquez@llu.edu

APPENDIX E

Other Resources:
LLU provides a unique environment for conducting scientific research. In addition to LLURM, LLU also houses the following core facilities available to intra- and extra-mural investigators:

- Center for Genomics (https://lluh.org/cancer-center/research/shared-resources/institute-genetics-translational-genomics)
- Mass Spectrometry Core Facility (https://medicine.llu.edu/research/core-facilities/mass-spectrometry-facility)
- Flow Cytometry Core (https://lluh.org/cancer-center/research/shared-resources/flow-cytometry-core)
- Advanced Imaging Microscopy (https://lluh.org/cancer-center/research/shared-resources/advanced-imaging-microscopy-core)
- Animal Care Facility (https://lluh.org/cancer-center/research/shared-resources/animal-care-facility-core)
- Imaging (https://lluh.org/cancer-center/research/shared-resources/center-imaging-research)
- PDX core (https://lluh.org/cancer-center/research/shared-resources/patient-derived-xenograft-core)

REFERENCES

a) M. Katerji, A. Bertucci, V. Filippov, M. Vazquez; P. Duerksen-Hughes; Ionizing radiation-induced DNA damage promotes integration of foreign plasmid DNA and HPV16 episome into human genome, (In preparation), 2021.

b) Unternaehrer-Hamm J, Chirshev E, Hojo N; Bertucci A, Sanderman L, Nguyen N, Wang H, Suzuki T, Brito E, Martinez S, Castañón C, Mirshahidi S, Vazquez ME, Oberg K and Ioffe Y; Epithelial/mesenchymal heterogeneity of high-grade serous ovarian carcinoma samples correlates with let-7 levels and predicts tumor growth and metastasis. Molecular Oncology, Vol. 14 (11): 2796-2813, November 2020.

c) E. Pariset; A. Bertucci; M.Petay; S. Malkani; A. Lopez Macha; I. G. Paulino Lima; V. Gomez Gonzalez; A. S. Tin; J. Tang; I. Plante; E. Cekanaviciute; M.Vazquez; S.V. Costes; DNA damage baseline predicts space radiation and radio-therapeutic resilience, Cell Report Cell Rep. 2020 Dec 8;33(10):108434, 2020.

d) Boyle KE, Boger DL, Wroe A, Vazquez M; Duocarmycin SA, a potent antitumor antibiotic, sensitizes glioblastoma to proton radiation. Bio. & Med. Chem. Letters Sep 1; 28(16):2688-2692, 2018.

e) Mao XW, Nishiyama NC, **Pecaut MJ**, Campbell-Beachler M, Gifford P, Haynes KE, Becronis C, Gridley DS. Simulated Microgravity and Low-Dose/Low-Dose-Rate Radiation Induces Oxidative Damage in the Mouse Brain. Radiat Res. 2016 Jun;185(6):647-57. doi: 10.1667/RR14267.1. Epub 2016 May 31.

f) Mao XW, Nishiyama NC, Campbell-Beachler M, Gifford P, Haynes KE, Gridley DS & **Pecaut MJ**. Role of NADPH oxidase as a mediator of oxidative damage in low-dose radiated and hindlimb unloaded mice. Radiat Rad. 2017 Aug 1. doi: 10.1667/RR14754.1.

g) **Slater JD**: Clinical applications of proton radiation treatment at Loma Linda University: review of a fifteen-year experience. Technology in Cancer Research and Treatment,5(2):81-89, 2006.

KNOWLEDGMENTS

I would like to thank Dr. Abiel Ghebremedhin, PhD, Baldev Patyal, PhD and Jerry D. Slater, MD for their support in preparing this report.

NASA Space Radiation Laboratory at Brookhaven National Laboratory

Date: October 25, 2021

Response to Letter dated Sept. 30, 2021: "National Academies' Study on Developing a Long-Term Strategy for Low-Dose Radiation Research: Request for Information on Radiation Sources and Facilities at the NASA Space Radiation Lab."

The committee would appreciate receiving responses/comments to the following questions:

1. Please provide a brief description of your radiation sources and facilities including location, type of source, first year of operation and expected date for removal/decommissioning, and types of activities these sources and facilities support (e.g., research, radiobiology experiments, radioisotope production, other).

NSRL Commissioning: first year of operations was 2003; expected decommissioning date >2040
Activities: Radiobiology research and electronics testing
Location: NSRL is located at DOE Brookhaven National Laboratory, Upton, New York on Long Island

Radiation sources: Accelerator-based ions and gamma;
  Protons: Linear Accelerator (LINAC) or Tandem Van de Graaff (> 40 yrs old)

  Ions of $Z \geq 2$: Electron Beam Ion Source (operational 2010) allows the creation of ion beams from almost any element.

  NASA investigators also use the **Gamma Radiation Facility** known as GRSF which houses a cesium-137 gamma ray source and can provide gamma rays at a variety of dose rates. These studies in conjunction with heavy ion and galactic cosmic ray simulations are used to determine RBE's. The gamma source is an industry standard J.L. Shepherd Mark I Model 68A $_{137}$Cs γ Irradiator. The photon energy from the source is 662 keV, with a Lineal Energy Transfer (LET) in water of approximately 0.8 keV/μm.

  Please see: https://www.bnl.gov/nsrl/grsf/

2. What are the dose ranges, radiation qualities, energy, and dose-rates delivered in your facilities? Is operation pulsed or steady-state? Are the facilities suitable for inhalation experiments?

Dose Rates: Typical dose rates of approximately 10 Gy/min and approximately 0.5 Gy/min are available for the 20 ˜ 20 cm$_2$ and the 60 ˜ 60 cm$_2$ configurations, respectively.

As demonstrated in our dose rate studies, individual beam fractions as low as 0.1 to 0.2 mGy can be reliably measured and delivered at the NSRL.

The spill structure during most radiobiology exposures has a 4 second repetition time. During the 4 second period, the ions are extracted more or less uniformly in time during a 0.3-0.4 second spill, followed by a ~3.6 second beam-off time. For protons, the maximum beam intensity is delivered when using the LINAC as the ion source. If using the Tandem as the ion source instead, the maximum proton beam intensity is 2.5 x 10$_{11}$ protons per spill.

APPENDIX E

The NSRL is not suitable for inhalation studies.

Ion Species [1]	Max Energy [2] (MeV/n)	LET in H_2O at Max Energy (keV/micron)	Peak LET (keV/micron)	Range in H_2O (mm)	Maximum Intensity [3] (ions per spill)
H^1	2500	0.206	84.3	10490	2.2×10^{11}
He^4	1500	0.84	237	5550	0.3×10^{10}
C^{12}	1500	7.55	922	1856	1.2×10^{10}
O^{16}	1500	13.4	1306	1391	0.4×10^{10}
Ne^{20}	1000	21.9	1637	657	0.10×10^{10}
Si^{28}	1000	43.4	2519	463	0.3×10^{10}
Ar^{40}	1000	74.2	3268	387	0.02×10^{10}
Ti^{48}	1000	105.6	3924	327	0.08×10^{10}
Fe^{56}	1000	147	4706	274	0.2×10^{10}
Kr^{84}	721	314	6221	132	2.0×10^7
Nb^{93}	520	594	6690	70	1×10^7
Ag^{107}	575	576	8470	70.7	3.5×10^6
Xe^{129}	589	761	9788	68.3	5.0×10^7
Ta^{181}	475	1449	12300	39.2	5.0×10^7
Au^{197}	400	1865	13140	27.7	1×10^8
Bi^{209}	359	21.8	138.7	22.6	7.0×10^7
Sequential Field	Various	Various	Various	Various	Various
Solar Particle Event [5]	Various	Various	Various	Various	Various
GCR Simulation	Various	Various	Various	Various	Various

https://www.bnl.gov/nsrl/userguide/beam-ion-species-and-energies.php

3. For radiobiology experiments, are your facilities mostly used for exposure of cells, tissues, or animals? Please describe and if possible provide publications that describe use of your radiation facilities to facilitate radiation research.

Facilities are used for all three - animal experiments accounts for over ~50% of work performed. Two relevant publications:

- Simonsen, L.C.; Slaba, T.C.; Guida, P., and Rusek, A. "NASA's first ground-based Galactic Cosmic Ray Simulator: Enabling a new era in space radiobiology research," PLOS Biology. Published May 19, 2020. https://doi.org/10.1371/journal.pbio.3000669

- La Tessa C, Sivertz M, Chiang IH, Lowenstein D, Rusek A. Overview of the NASA Space Radiation Laboratory. Life Sci Space Res (Amst), 11, 2016, pp. 18–23. https://doi.org/10.1016/j.lssr.2016.10.002

4. Are your facilities available for use to outside radiation researchers and other investigators?
   Yes, Brookhaven uses a Strategic Partnership Project (SPP) agreement when a partner seeks research and development to complete a project but does not intend to perform the work jointly. The partner fully covers the costs of the work to be performed. This is the mechanism typically used by non-NASA users at the NSRL. Please see:
   https://www.bnl.gov/techtransfer/partnerships.php

5. Is there available adjacent infrastructure that facilitates radiation research such as tissue culture and animal facilities?
   Yes, both tissue culture and animal facilities are available.

For more information please visit:

https://www.bnl.gov/nsrl/

The Columbia University Radiological Research Accelerator Facility
RARAF: www.raraf.org

The Radiological Research Accelerator Facility (RARAF) provides the radiation research community advanced irradiation techniques using charged particle and neutron beams. In particular, a number of the RARAF beams have been specifically designed to facilitate studies of radiobiological effects at very low doses. For example, the RARAF microbeam beamline is designed to allow delivery of the ultimate low dose of exactly one particle to targeted cells, and has been extensively used to facilitate studies of the effects of domestic radon exposures – the largest single source of background radiation exposure.

During the more than 50 years that RARAF has been in operation, experiments have been performed for over 50 different research groups from more than 40 institutions including universities, national laboratories, cancer centers, and private corporations. These experiments, performed with radiations such as protons, alpha particles, and neutrons, have resulted in more than 200 publications in refereed journals, proceedings, and books. Research has been conducted in the fields of radiation biology, radiological physics, radiation chemistry, health physics, and medicine.

All irradiations are supported by NIST-traceable doismetry where appropriate, and state-ofthe-art biology labs are available less than a 1-minute walk from the irradiation facilities.

Marino, S. A. (2017). *50 Years of the Radiological Research Accelerator Facility (RARAF)*. Radiation Research 187(4): 413-423.

1. Ion beams: Broad beams, Single-Particle Beams, and Microbeams

Our Singletron particle accelerator generates ion beams, including protons, helium ions (alpha particles), lithium ions, boron ions and carbon ions. These ions have ranges sufficient to irradiate cellular monolayers, if required targeting cellular or sub-cellular target (microbeams), or they can be used to irradiate thin tissues.

Specifically, these ion beams allow broad area irradiations or a focused sub-micron microbeam, with a range of dose rates spanning orders of magnitude from less than a single particle per cell (simulating low dose exposures from domestic radon) to hundreds of Gy.

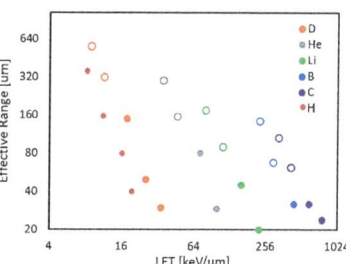

Ion beams available at RARAF

The recent installation of a linac booster allows irradiation of thicker samples beams enabling irradiation of thin tissue samples in addition to cell cultures.

Miller RC, Randers-Pehrson G, Geard CR, Hall EJ, Brenner DJ (1999). *The oncogenic transforming potential of the passage of single alpha particles through mammalian cell nuclei*. Proc Natl Acad Sci US A. **96**:19-22

Randers-Pehrson, G., et al. (2009). *The Columbia University sub-micron charged particle beam"*. Nuclear Instruments and Methods in Physics Research A: **609:** 294-9

2. Very Low Dose Rates

The **VA**riable **D**ose-rate **E**xternal $_{137}$Cs irradjato**R** (**VADER**) allows modeling of low dose rate $_{137}$Cs exposures in mice and other samples using $_{137}$Cs brachytherapy seeds to generate very low dose rates (0.1 to 1 Gy/day), mimicking fallout and ingestion exposures. Within the VADER, up to 15 mice can be housed in an IACUC approved "mouse hotel" for several weeks. A custom incubator is available for performing ex-vivo blood (or other tissue) irradiations.

Garty, G., et al. (2020). *VADER: a variable dose-rate external $_{137}$Cs irradiator for internal emitter and low dose rate studies*. Scientific Reports **10**(1): 19899.

3. Ultra High Dose Rates

The prompt exposure from nuclear device such as at Hiroshima or Nagasaki, or from an Improvised Nuclear Device (IND), will be delivered in less than 1 microsecond. Thus it is important to have facilities to investigate the effects of different doses of radiation delivered at ultra-high doses rates.

To mimic prompt exposures from an IND, we have adapted a clinical accelerator to deliver ultra high dose rates high dose rates. Using 9 MeV electrons, samples can be irradiated inside the Clinac head at average dose rates of up to 600 Gy/sec (3 Gy per 0.5 μsec pulse, 180 pulses per sec). In this mode multiple pulses are required for most irradiations. By modulating pulse repetition rate, dose rates of 1 Gy/sec to <1 Gy/min can be achieved at the isocenter, allowing comparison of very high dose rates vs. conventional irradiations with the same beam.

Using 6 MeV electrons, samples can be irradiated at instantaneous dose rates of up to 300 MGy/sec (0.2-150 Gy per 0.5 μsec pulse, 360 pulses per sec) and most irradiations can be performed with a single very high dose rate pulse.

In addition, an ultra-high dose rate (4 kGy/sec) 4.5 MeV proton beam is also available for irradiation of thin samples.

Grilj, V., et al. (2020), *"Proton Irradiation Platforms for Preclinical Studies of High-DoseRate (FLASH) Effects at RARAF"*. Radiat Res, **194**:646-55

4. Neutrons:

The **C**olumbia **IND** **N**eutron **F**acility (CINF), is a novel accelerator-based neutron source with an energy spectrum modeled on the Hiroshima atomic bomb spectrum at 1.5 km from the epicenter. Beams are generated by impinging a mixed proton/deuteron beam on a beryllium target generating a broad spectrum neutron beam peaked around 1 MeV. Mice and tissue samples can be irradiated at a dose rate of up to 3 Gy/h. The neutron energy spectrum obtained is also a good model for space radiations such as lunar albedo neutrons., as well as simulating the LET distribution from high-LET galactic cosmic rays.

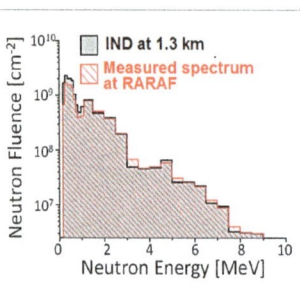

Xu, Y., et al. (2015). *Accelerator-Based Biological Irradiation Facility Simulating Neutron Exposure from an Improvised Nuclear Device*. Radiation Research **184**: 404-10.

APPENDIX E

Lab Facilities

All facilities are available for use by outside users. On-site fully equipped biology labs and a mouse housing facility are available to support experiments, less than 1-minute walk from the irradiation facilities.

Summary

	Neutrons	Ion beams	FLASH	VADER
Location	RARAF, Irvington, NY	RARAF, Irvington, NY	RARAF, Irvington, NY	CUIMC, New York, NY
Start year	2015	1980 <=150 keV/µm (H_+, D_+, He_{+2}) 2022 >150 keV/µm (Li_{+3}, B_{+5}, C_{+6})	2020	2017
Decommissioning	Not planned	Not planned	Not planned	Not planned
Activities	radiobiology experiments	radiobiology experiments	radiobiology experiments	radiobiology experiments
Dose range (max) (min)	Up to 10 Gy No lower limit	Up to 100 Gy Single particle	Up to 100 Gy .01 Gy	1 Gy/day 0.1 Gy/day
Radiation type	Neutrons	Ion beams (H_+, D_+, He_{+2}, C_{+6}, Li_{+3}, B_{+5}) LET=8-1000 keV/µm	6 or 9 MeV electrons	Cs137 gammas
Dose rate	Up to 3 Gy/h		Up to 150 Gy/usec	0.1-1 Gy/day
Spot size	10 cm	1 µm - 3cm	1-10 cm	35 cm
Pulsed	DC	DC or pulsed (10 Hz)	Pulsed (180-360 Hz)	DC
Inhalation experiments	No	No	No	No
Used for	Mice Tissue Cell culture	Cell culture Thin tissues	Mice Tissue Cell culture	Mice Cell culture

Contact:

Guy Garty, PhD
RARAF, Nevis Labs
136 S. Broadway,
Irvington NY 10533

gyg2101@cumc.columbia.edu
+1(914) 591 9244

List of recent publications using RARAF facilities:

Neutrons:

1. Klein, P.M., et al., Acute, Low-Dose Neutron Exposures Adversely Impact Central Nervous System Function. International Journal of Molecular Sciences, 2021. 22(16): p. 9020.
2. Oster, L., et al., Demonstration of the Potential and Difficulties of Combined TL and OSL Measurements of TLD-600 and TLD-700 for the Determination of the Dose Components in Complex Neutron-Gamma Radiation Fields. Radiat Prot Dosimetry, 2020. 188(3): p. 383-388.
3. Mukherjee, S., et al., Human Transcriptomic Response to Mixed Neutron-Photon Exposures Relevant to an Improvised Nuclear Device. Radiat Res, 2019. 192(2): p. 189-199.
4. Broustas, C.G., et al., Identification of differentially expressed genes and pathways in mice exposed to mixed field neutron/photon radiation. BMC Genomics, 2018. 19(1): p. 504.
5. Laiakis, E.C., et al., Metabolic Dysregulation after Neutron Exposures Expected from an Improvised Nuclear Device. Radiat Res, 2017. 188(1): p. 21-34.
6. Broustas, C.G., et al., Impact of Neutron Exposure on Global Gene Expression in a Human Peripheral Blood Model. Radiation Research, 2017. 187(4): p. 443-450.
7. Broustas, C.G., et al., Comparison of gene expression response to neutron and x-ray irradiation using mouse blood. BMC Genomics, 2017. 18: p. 2.

Low dose rate

1. Wang, Q., et al., DNA damage response in peripheral mouse blood leukocytes in vivo after variable, low-dose rate exposure. Radiation and Environmental Biophysics, 2020. 59(1): p. 89-98.
2. Pannkuk, E.L., et al., Biofluid Metabolomics of Mice Exposed to External Low-Dose Rate Radiation in a Novel Irradiation System, the Variable Dose-Rate External (137)Cs Irradiator. J Proteome Res, 2021.

High dose rate

1. Grilj, V., et al., Proton Irradiation Platforms for Preclinical Studies of High-Dose-Rate (FLASH) Effects at RARAF. Radiation Research, 2020. 194(6): p. 646-655.
2. Buonanno, M., V. Grilj, and D.J. Brenner, Biological effects in normal cells exposed to FLASH dose rate protons. Radiotherapy and Oncology, 2019. 139: p. 51-55.

Ion beams

1. Buonanno, M., et al., A Mouse Ear Model for Bystander Studies Induced by Microbeam Irradiation. Radiation Research, 2015. 184(2): p. 219-225.
2. Wu, J., et al., Cytoplasmic Irradiation Induces Metabolic Shift in Human Small Airway Epithelial Cells via Activation of Pim-1 Kinase. Radiation Research, 2017. 187(4): p. 451-463.
3. Wu, J., et al., Targeted cytoplasmic irradiation and autophagy. Mutat Res, 2017. 806: p. 88-97.
4. Miller RC, Randers-Pehrson G, Geard CR, Hall EJ, Brenner DJ. The oncogenic transforming potential of the passage of single alpha particles through mammalian cell nuclei. Proc Natl Acad Sci U S A. 1999 Jan 5;96(1):19-22.